Information Systems for Health Services Administration

* * *

5th Edition

Information
Systems
for
Health Services
Administration

*   *   *

5th Edition

Charles J. Austin
Stuart B. Boxerman

with collaboration and contributions by
Brian T. Malec

and with contributions by
Karen A. Wager

AUPHA

HAP

Health Administration Press
Chicago, Illinois

02 01 00 99   5 4 3

Library of Congress Cataloging-in-Publication Data

Information systems for health services administration / Charles J. Austin, Stuart B. Boxerman. — 5th ed.
  p.   cm.
Includes bibliographical references and index.
ISBN 1-56793-070-0
1. Hospitals—Administration—Data processing.   2. Information storage and retrieval systems—Hospitals.   I. Boxerman, Stuart B.   II. Title.
RA971.6.A928   1997
362.1'1'068—DC21   97-29106
                                                              CIP

The paper used in this publication meets the minimum requirements of American National Standard for Information Sciences—Permanence of Paper for Printed Library Materials, ANSI Z39.48-1984. ∞ ™

Health Administration Press
A division of the Foundation
  of the American College of
  Healthcare Executives
One North Franklin Street
Chicago, Illinois 60606-3491
(312) 424-2800

Association of University Programs
  in Health Administration
1911 North Fort Myer Drive, Suite 503
Arlington, VA 22209
(703) 524-5500

*To the students I have worked with throughout
a thirty-year career of teaching and research
in the field of health administration education*
—Charles J. Austin, Ph.D.

*To my wife and best friend, Susan,
who patiently relinquished her claim on my time
during this writing effort*
—Stuart B. Boxerman, D.Sc.

CONTENTS

List of Tables xii
List of Figures and Exhibit xiii
Preface xvii
Acknowledgments xix

Part I   Introduction and Essential Concepts

1   Information Technology Today 3
Categories of Information Systems   5
Historical Overview   6
The Changing Healthcare Environment   9
Information Technology in this Environment of Change   13
The Healthcare Information Professional   17
Summary   18

2   Essential Concepts 23
General Systems Theory   23
Management Control and Decision-Support Systems in
    Health Services Organizations   31
Information for Management Control   35
Principles of Information Resource Management   36
Management of Change   37
Concluding Comments   39
Summary   39

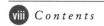

Part II   Information Technology

3   Computer Hardware **45**
An Overview of Computer Components   *46*
Classes of Computers   *68*
Summary   *73*

4   Computer Software **79**
An Introduction to Programming Languages   *80*
Language Translators   *89*
System Management Software   *91*
Application Software   *94*
Integrated vs. Interfaced Systems   *100*
A Final Note   *101*
Summary   *101*

5   Networking and Telecommunications **107**
A Rationale for Installing Computer Networks   *108*
Distributing the Processing Function   *109*
Network Components   *114*
Network Topologies   *119*
Electronic Data Interchange   *123*
Wireless Communication   *124*
Communicating via the Internet   *126*
Summary   *130*

6   Data Management **137**
Computer Files: A Brief Review   *138*
Databases: An Improvement over Files   *142*
An Overview of Database Models   *143*
Database Management Systems   *148*
Data Security   *152*
Developments in Database Technology   *154*
Data Warehouses   *157*
Summary   *161*

Part III   Information Systems Planning and Management

7   Strategic Information Systems Planning **169**
Purposes of Strategic IS Planning   *170*
Organizing the Planning Effort   *172*
Elements of an IS Master Plan   *174*

Goals and Objectives   *174*
Applications Priority List   *176*
System Architecture   *177*
Software Development Plan   *178*
Information Systems Management Plan   *179*
Statement of Resource Requirements   *179*
Review and Approval of the Plan   *180*
End-User Computing   *180*
Organizationwide Information System Standards
    and Policies   *181*
Strategic IS Planning for Integrated Delivery Systems   *187*
Summary   *189*

8 Systems Analysis **193**
The System Development Life Cycle   *194*
Project Organization   *195*
Systems Analysis   *197*
Systems Analysis Tools   *199*
CASE Tools   *207*
Process Reengineering   *207*
Benefits of Systems Analysis   *208*
Selection of a Design Approach   *209*
Conclusion: How Well Are We Doing?   *210*
Summary   *210*

9 System Design, Evaluation, and Selection **215**
Introduction   *215*
System Design Specifications   *216*
Evaluation of Application Software   *219*
Use of Contractual Services (Outsourcing)   *222*
The Selection Process   *222*
Alternatives to the RFP   *226*
Negotiation and Contracting   *227*
Role of Consultants   *228*
Summary   *229*

Appendix A: System Design Case Study 233
Appendix B: System Requirements Definition for Physician's
Practice Management Application 240

10 Managing Information Resources **245**
Managing System Implementation   *246*
System Operation and Maintenance   *249*
Continuous Quality Improvement   *250*

Organizing for Information Management: Role of the Chief
   Information Officer   *251*
Staffing Requirements   *252*
Outsourcing   *254*
Executive Management Responsibilities   *255*
Summary   *258*

Part IV   Information Systems Applications in Healthcare

11   Patient Care Applications 263
Introduction   *264*
Computer-Based Patient Records   *265*
Order Entry and Results Reporting   *268*
Clinical Services Applications   *269*
Ambulatory Care Information Systems   *273*
Nursing Information Systems   *275*
Clinical Decision-Support Systems   *278*
Computer-Assisted Medical Instrumentation   *280*
Other Clinical Applications   *281*
Summary   *284*

12   Administrative Applications
by Brian T. Malec 291
Introduction   *292*
Financial Information Systems   *293*
Human Resources Information Systems   *296*
Facility Utilization and Scheduling Systems   *298*
Materials Management Systems   *300*
Facilities Management Systems   *303*
Office Automation Systems   *304*
Summary   *305*

13   Strategic Decision-Support Applications 309
The Concept of Decision Support   *310*
An Overview of Decision-Support Systems   *312*
Information Needs for Decision Support   *317*
Approaches to Development of Decision-Support
   Systems   *323*
Applications of Decision-Support Systems   *326*
Expert Systems   *329*
Executive Information Systems   *331*
A Final Thought   *333*
Summary   *333*

14   Managed Care Applications
by Brian T. Malec **341**
Information Needs in the Managed Care Marketplace   *342*
Users of Managed Care Information   *345*
The Managed Care Software Market   *352*
Case Study: L.A. Care   *354*
Summary   *355*

15   Health Information Networks
by Karen A. Wager **359**
Definition and Evolution of Health Information Networks   *362*
Planning Activities in Establishing an HIN   *368*
Summary   *377*

16   Internet Applications
by Brian T. Malec **383**
History and Structure of the Internet   *384*
Internet Applications for Healthcare Organizations   *385*
Intranet Applications for Healthcare Organizations   *391*
Management of Internet Technologies in Healthcare
     Organizations   *393*
Summary   *396*

Case Study 1: Developing an Electronic Medical Record for an
Integrated Physician Office Practice
Andrea W. White and Gloria R. Wakefield 401

Case Study 2: Implementation of a Computer-Based Patient
Record in a Family Medicine Clinical Practice
Frances Wickham Lee, Steven M. Ornstein, and Ruth G. Jenkins 413

Case Study 3: Market Crisis in Metropolis: Opportunity for
Strategic Advantage Through Information Technology
Kathy S. Lassila and Karen A. Wager 419

Glossary of Technical Terms 429
Index 443
About the Authors 457

TABLES

4.1   Five Generations of Programming Languages 81

4.2   Representative Third-Generation Languages 83

4.3   Categories of Application-Specific Software in Healthcare 99

12.1   Estimated Number of Administrative Operations Software
Vendors as of December 1996 293

FIGURES AND EXHIBIT

Figures

1.1   Categories of Health Information Systems 6
1.2   Mainframe Computer.. 7
1.3   Personal Computer... 8
1.4   Objectives for Computer-Based Records 14

2.1   The Health Services Organization as a System 26
2.2   Health Services Organization Systems Network.................28
2.3   Diagram of a Simple System 28
2.4   Simple System with Feedback 29
2.5   Open System Diagram 29
2.6   Cybernetic System 31
2.7   Generalized Management Control System (Cybernetic) for a
       Health Services Organization 32
2.8   Clinical Laboratory as a Cybernetic System....................34
2.9   Characteristics of Useful Management Information 35

3.1   Major Components of a Computer System 47
3.2   A Typical Memory Chip....................................50
3.3   A Tape-Drive Autoloader...................................53
3.4   A Microcomputer Hard Drive and Floppy Drive 54
3.5   Typical Layout of a Disk 55
3.6   CD-ROM Drive 56
3.7   Optical Jukebox Storage System 57
3.8   Keyboard and Rollerball on a Portable Computer 60
3.9   Specimens with Bar-Code Labels in an Automated Laboratory
       System 62

3.10   Typical Pen-Based Computer 64

5.1   Central Mainframe Configuration 110
5.2   Client/Server Computing 111
5.3   File/Server Architecture 113
5.4   Distributed Data Processing 114
5.5   Communication Process 117
5.6   Function of a Multiplexer 118
5.7   Network Topologies 120

6.1   Hierarchy of a Field, Record, and File 139
6.2   Linkage between Application Programs and Associated Data
        Files 141
6.3   Hierarchical Data Model—Equipment Maintenance Database 144
6.4   Network Data Model—Equipment Maintenance Database 145
6.5   Relational Data Model—Equipment Maintenance Database 146
6.6   Illustration of Use of Query-by-Example .150

7.1   Purposes of Strategic Information Systems Planning 171
7.2   Organizing the Planning Effort 173
7.3   Elements of the Information Systems Strategic Plan 175
7.4   Information Security 182

8.1   Information Systems Development Life Cycle 194
8.2   Information Systems Project Organization 196
8.3   Information Systems Analysis 198
8.4   Tools of Systems Analysis 200
8.5   Interview Guide: Director of Clinical Laboratory 201
8.6   Guidelines for Questionnaire Development 202
8.7   System Flowchart—Ordering Tests, Obtaining Specimens,
        and Testing and Reporting 204

9.1   System Design Specifications 217
9.2   Sources of Information on Vendors and Software 220
9.3   Packaged Software Evaluation Criteria 221
9.4   Sample Output Screen—Emergency Service Note 237
9.5   Flowchart—Entry and Storage of Information in the Clinical
        Data Repository 238
9.6   Flowchart—Retrieval of Clinical Information in the Urgent
        Care/Trauma Department 239

10.1   Information System Implementation 246
10.2   Elements of a System Test 248
10.3   Information Systems Organization 253

11.1   Physician Office System 274
11.2   Point-of-Care Terminal 277
11.3   Ventricular Angiography Workstation 280

12.1   Financial Information System 295
12.2   Human Resources Information System 297
12.3   Materials Management Systems. 301

13.1   Summary of Steps for Deciding Whether to Sign Contract 312
13.2   Desirable Attributes of a Decision-Support System 313
13.3   Conceptual Model of a Decision-Support System. 314
13.4   DSS Systems Corresponding to Alter's Categorization of Uses . . .316
13.5   Some Sources of "External" Healthcare Data 319
13.6   Porter's Strategies for Competing in the Marketplace and
       Associated Information Needs. 320
13.7   Strategic Orientations to Marketing (Miles and Snow) and
       Associated Information Needs. 321
13.8   Categories of Outcomes Measurement Interests by
       Constituent Group 324
13.9   Number of Vendors Offering Decision-Support Systems by
       Category of System 325
13.10 Conceptual Model of an Expert System 330

14.1   Provider Functions and Associated Information Requirements. . . .347
14.2   Managed Care Organization Functions and Associated
       Information Requirements 350
14.3   Healthcare Software Vendors 353

15.1   Model of Integrated Service Delivery 361
15.2   The Community Health Care Management System 362
15.3   Defining the HIN Continuum 364
15.4   Three Levels of HIN 367

16.1   Business Strategies and Internet Applications 386
16.2   Health Care Financing Administration Web Page 388
16.3   PacifiCare Health Systems Web Page 389
16.4   Christ Hospital and Medical Center Web Page 390
16.5   Categories of Intranet Applications 391

Exhibit

4.1   The Structure and Syntax of Some Typical Programming
       Languages 85

PREFACE

T HIS BOOK is intended to assist health services administrators in understanding principles of analysis, design, evaluation, selection, and utilization of information systems in their organizations. The book reviews the state-of-the-art of information technology and describes how information systems can support high quality patient care and improve management decisions in healthcare organizations.

Sufficient technical detail on computer hardware, software, networks, and telecommunications is included to enable the manager to become conversant with modern information technology and its use in health services organizations. However, the material is written from a management perspective with emphasis on the intelligent use of information for strategic planning, decision support, program management, continuous quality improvement, and the provision of high-quality patient care.

The book is suitable as a textbook for a one-semester graduate or advanced undergraduate course on health information systems. It can also serve as a reference for health services administrators and others involved in the selection and utilization of health information systems. Extensive citations are included for those readers desiring additional information on the major topics covered.

Major changes have been made in this fifth edition. The new edition focuses on information management in the integrated delivery system and managed care environment. New chapters are included on health information networks, managed care applications, and the Internet. Three case studies are included for the first time. There is considerable emphasis

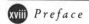

on evaluation and selection of commercial software for use in healthcare organizations. The chapters on information technology have been updated and expanded.

ACKNOWLEDGMENTS

WE ARE indebted to Brian Malec for significant collaboration and for contributing Chapters 12, 14, and 16 of this fifth edition. We appreciate also the work of Karen Wager who contributed Chapter 15 and was coauthor of one of the case studies. Important contributions to case studies and examples were made by Mark Daniels, Ruth Jenkins, Robert Johnson, Kathy Lassila, Frances Wickham Lee, Steven Ornstein, Gloria Wakefield, and Andrea White. Helen Coker provided invaluable library assistance. The responsibility for any errors or oversights lies entirely with the authors.

Introduction and Essential Concepts

INFORMATION TECHNOLOGY TODAY

THE DELIVERY of health services is an information-intensive process. High-quality patient care relies upon careful documentation of each patient's medical history, health status, current medical conditions, and treatment plans. Administrative and financial information is essential for efficient operational support of the patient care process. A strong argument can be made that the health services industry is

Concepts and Applications

To succeed in today's healthcare environment, executives must know what is happening with all facets of their organizations. Effective healthcare information systems can provide up-to-the-minute information on clinical and administrative matters, and they can process that information to allow a healthcare executive to make effective strategic decisions. In addition, a healthcare information system can provide computerized patient records, centralized patient data, and enhanced intra-organizational communication and data-sharing.

After completing this chapter, the reader will be able to discuss the many changes in healthcare that dictate the need for increased information, define the different types of information systems and their abilities and requirements, and list the different healthcare information management professional organizations.

one of the most information-intensive sectors of our economy. But health services organizations have been slow to adopt the use of modern information technology in the delivery of care and the management of services. This situation, however, is changing, given rapid advances in technology and the forces of change in the healthcare system itself.

This book is about management and how the management of health services organizations can be improved by the *intelligent* use of information. Some management theorists discount the value of information in the management process, stating that management is still more of an art than a science. They argue that experience, judgment, intuition, and a good sense of the political environment are the critical skills involved in making administrative decisions. On the other end of the spectrum are the technocrats, who argue that management and information are inseparable, that all management decisions need to be completely rational and based entirely on an analysis of comprehensive information. The focus of this book lies between these two extreme views of the managerial world. The use of information has both costs and benefits associated with it. These costs and benefits need to be assessed, and health administrators need to develop their skills in using information intelligently.

The health services industry is in the midst of a period of great change. Pressures for improved management information are growing as health services organizations face ever-increasing demands to lower costs, improve quality, and expand access to care. Market-driven healthcare reform has led to rapid expansion of managed care, development of integrated delivery systems through mergers and acquisitions, and radical changes in systems of payment for services. Health services organizations have grown larger and more complex, and information systems must keep pace with the dual effects of organizational complexity and continued advances in medical technology.

The intelligent use of information in health services management does not just happen. Rather, the administrator must ensure that it occurs in a systematic, formally planned way. This book, then, deals with two important matters: the management of information resources in health services organizations and the effective use of information in organizational management.

Careful distinction should be drawn between data and information. As used in this book, *data* are raw facts and figures collected by the organization. *Information*, on the other hand, is defined as data that have been processed and analyzed in a formal, intelligent way, so that the results are directly useful to clinicians and managers. All too often, computerized data banks are available, but are little used because of inadequate planning of information content and structure needed to support management planning and control.

An essential element for successful information systems implementation is carefully planned teamwork by clinicians, managers, and technical systems specialists. Information systems developed in isolation by technicians may be "technically pure and elegant in design," but rarely will they pass the test of reality in meeting organizational requirements. On the other hand, very few administrators and clinicians possess the equally important technical knowledge and skills of systems analysis and design, and the amateur analyst cannot hope to avoid the havoc that can result from a poorly designed system. A balanced effort is required: operational personnel contribute ideas on systems requirements and organizational realities, and technical personnel employ their skills in analysis and design.

Computer technology has advanced to a high level of sophistication in recent years. However, computers are only tools to aid in the accomplishment of a wider set of goals. Analysis of information requirements in the broader organizational context always should take precedence over a rush to computerize. Information technology by itself is not the answer to management problems; technology must be part of a broader restructuring of the organization, including reengineering of business processes. Alignment of information systems strategy with business goals of the health care organization is essential. (DeFauw and L'Heureux 1995)

Categories of Information Systems

Computerized information systems in healthcare fall into four categories: clinical, administrative, strategic decision-support, and electronic networking applications. (See Figure 1.1.)

Clinical information systems support patient care and provide information for use in strategic planning and management. Applications include computerized patient records systems, automated medical instrumentation, clinical decision-support systems (computer-aided diagnosis and treatment planning), and information systems that support clinical research and education.

Operational administrative systems support nonpatient care activities in the health services organization. Examples include financial information systems, payroll, purchasing and inventory control, outpatient clinic scheduling, office automation, and many others.

Strategic decision-support systems assist the executive management team in strategic planning, managerial control, performance monitoring, and outcomes assessment. Strategic information systems must draw on both internal data from clinical and administrative systems in the organization as well as external data on community health, market-area demography, and activities of competitors. Consequently, information

Figure 1.1   Categories of Health Information Systems

Clinical
  1. Computerized Patient Records
  2. Medical Decision Support
  3. Automated Instrumentation
  4. Clinical Research and Education
Administrative
  1. Financial
  2. Scheduling
  3. Human Resources
  4. Materials Management
  5. Office Automation
Strategic Decision Support
  1. Planning and Marketing
  2. Financial Forecasting
  3. Resource Allocation
  4. Performance Assessment
  5. Outcomes Measurement
Electronic Networking
  1. Insurance Billing and Claims Processing
  2. Regional/National Databases
  3. Online Purchasing
  4. Provider Networks

system integration—the ability of organizational information systems to communicate electronically with one another—becomes very important.

Most health services organizations also engage in electronic data interchange with external organizations for such activities as insurance billing and claims processing, accessing clinical information from regional and national databases, and communicating among providers in an integrated delivery system.

Computer applications in healthcare organizations are described in detail in Part IV of this book.

Historical Overview

The first computer systems in healthcare date to the early 1960s when a small number of hospitals began to automate selected administrative operations, usually beginning with payroll and patient accounting functions. These systems were developed by analysts and computer programmers hired by the hospital and were run on large and expensive centralized computers referred to as "mainframes." (See Figure 1.2.) Little attention was given to the development of clinical information systems to support

Figure 1.2 Mainframe Computer

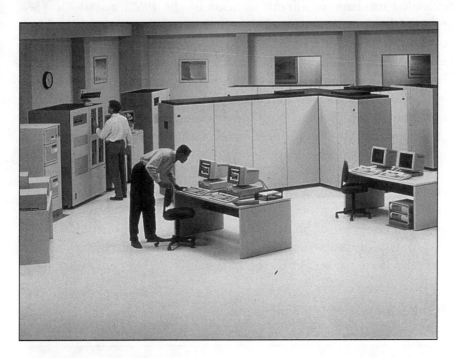

Courtesy of International Business Machines Corporation. Unauthorized use not permitted.

patient care. A few systems were developed for the electronic storage and retrieval of abstracts of inpatient medical records. But these systems contained limited information and were operated on a postdischarge, retrospective basis.

Advances in technology during the 1970s expanded the use of information systems in hospitals and marked the beginning of limited applications in other organizational settings, including clinics, physician practices, and long-term care facilities. Computers became smaller and less expensive, and some vendors began to develop "applications software packages," generalized computer programs that could be used by any hospital, clinic, or physician's office that purchased the system. Most of these early software packages supported administrative operations—patient accounting, general accounting, materials management, scheduling, and practice management. Some clinical systems were developed as well, particularly for hospital clinical laboratories, radiology departments, and pharmacies.

A revolution in computing occurred in the 1980s with the development of powerful and inexpensive personal computers (PCs), desktop devices with computing power and storage capacity that equaled or exceeded the large mainframe systems of the 1960s and 1970s. (See Figure 1.3.) A second major advance in this period was the development of electronic data networks in which personal computers and larger systems could be linked together to share information on a decentralized basis. An increasing number of vendors entered the healthcare software business, and a much larger array of products became available for both administrative and clinical support functions. The use of personal computers in physicians' offices, particularly for practice management, became commonplace.

The early 1990s were marked by dramatic changes in the healthcare environment with the advent of market-driven healthcare reform and rapid expansion of managed care. As a result, much greater attention began to be given to the development of clinical information systems and strategic decision-support systems to assist providers in achieving a critical balance between costs and quality in the delivery of care.

Figure 1.3 Personal Computer

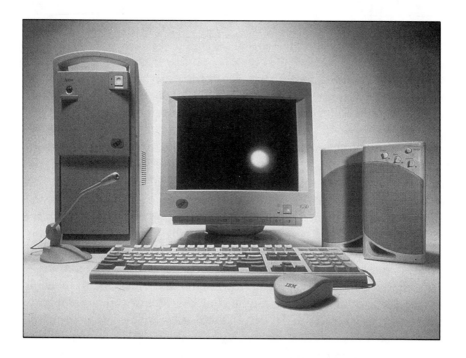

Courtesy of International Business Machines Corporation. Unauthorized use not permitted.

The Changing Healthcare Environment

The rapidly changing healthcare environment of the 1990s has made the employment of information technology more important than ever. Several factors are influencing this change. Most notable is the influence of market-driven healthcare reform, which has resulted in an expansion of managed care, the development of integrated delivery systems by providers of care, and major changes in insurance and payment mechanisms for the delivery of health services. Major forces of change in healthcare are discussed in the sections that follow.

Expansion of Managed Care

Managed care is a new paradigm for the delivery of health services, resulting from concern among large employers, insurance companies, and government agencies about rapid escalation in the costs of healthcare. There is no simple definition of *managed care* since it can assume many different forms. However, Wozmak (1995) provides the following functional definition:

> Managed care is a system of providing and paying for medical care that includes a panel of providers who agree to deliver services at an agreed upon fee. Financial incentives are included for patients to use the identified providers that make up the panel. (Wozmak 1995, 12)

Managed care can assume many different forms. Three of the more common arrangements are health maintenance organizations (HMOs); preferred provider organizations (PPOs); and exclusive provider arrangements (EPAs).

HMOs provide coverage of specified health services to plan members for a fixed premium, prepaid in advance (usually on a monthly basis). Physician services may be provided by employing a group of physicians on a salaried basis; contracting with physicians who have organized as a partnership, professional corporation, or association; contracting with multiple physician groups; or contracting with an individual practice association, which in turn contracts with individual physicians and medical groups.

PPOs are insurance programs in which plan members receive better benefits (usually through reduced deductible and copayment amounts) when they use services offered by preferred providers. Patients can use nonparticipating providers, but at a higher cost. Providers are usually paid on a fee-for-service basis, but agree to discounts in order to receive the preferred provider designation.

EPAs have been initiated "by major self-insured employers who decided to cut out the middlemen—health insurers and third party

administrators—and make their own deals in the medical marketplace."
(Coile 1990, 135) Pricing is established using the company's actual
experience with its own employees' utilization of health services. Strong
financial incentives are employed to limit or exclude services by providers
who are not part of the company's EPA plan.

Membership in managed care plans has increased rapidly. Enrollment
in HMOs grew to 59 million covered individuals in 1995. (Kertesz 1996)

Health services organizations operating in this environment must
have vastly improved financial and clinical information about their operation in order to monitor the costs and quality of services and negotiate
successfully with managed care plans.

Development of Integrated Delivery Systems (IDS)

In responding to the imperatives of managed care, many hospitals, medical group practices, and other health services organizations have come
together to form integrated delivery systems. An IDS can be defined as
"an organization that is accountable for the costs and clinical outcomes
associated with delivery of a continuum of health services to a defined
population." An IDS is composed of a network of hospitals, physicians,
and other healthcare providers who furnish all needed services to a patient
population, in some cases for a fixed annual payment.

Integrated delivery systems build on the HMO concept but are more
flexible in the organizational relationships that are established among
providers. Most networks will either own or be closely aligned with an
insurance product.

Physicians are actively engaged in IDS development activities. Medical group practices may enter directly as partners in a system. Hospitals
and physicians are joining together to form physician-hospital organizations (PHOs) in order to compete for managed care business. In some
cases, hospitals are buying physician practices in order to be able to
employ their own cadre of physicians, particularly those in primary care
(family practice, internal medicine, pediatrics, and obstetrics).

Integrated delivery systems are tied together by information about
the patients being served. Success will be heavily dependent upon the ability to provide good clinical, financial, and customer service information
to those who purchase health services from the IDS.

Changes in Reimbursement

Managed care will result in significant changes in methods of payment
for health services. Traditional systems of fee-for-service payment are
increasingly being replaced by *contractual discounts* and *capitation*. These

systems of reimbursement are designed to reduce costs. Providers are being asked to share in the financial risks traditionally assumed by insurers and purchasers of care.

All managed care plans require that physicians, hospitals, and other healthcare providers accept discounts from their regular prices or fee schedules in order to be included in the plan as participating or preferred providers.

An increasing number of plans are moving toward capitated payment in which a provider agrees to accept a fixed fee (monthly or annual) for all patient care provided to a defined population (the enrollees in the managed care health plan). Results from a recent survey of 19 HMOs revealed that 17 employ capitation in contracting for specialty medical services. (Wong 1994)

Capitation requires that providers assume some of the financial risk in providing patient care. Capitated payment systems offer incentives for reducing unnecessary utilization of services, and place a premium on prevention and strategies for keeping people healthy.

Capitated contracting makes it essential that health services organizations have good information about their own service patterns as well as information on the health needs of the population to be covered by the contract. Without such information, it is impossible to determine an acceptable capitation rate for the practice.

Outcomes Assessment

Balancing the costs and quality of patient care is an important requirement in today's healthcare delivery system. Purchasers of care, insurance companies, and managed care plans are placing emphasis on *outcomes assessment* as a method for striking this delicate balance between costs and quality.

Outcomes assessment involves measuring the effectiveness of alternative treatment modalities on clinical outcomes for specific groups of patients and specific medical conditions. Outcomes assessment can be used to compare the quality of care delivered by individual providers. Managed care plans are using outcomes information in seeking out the *lowest cost* treatment protocols that have been shown to have *at least equal medical effectiveness* to other available treatment modalities. Much of the impetus behind outcomes research stems from a desire to use the results of the research for cost-control purposes.

The federal government's Agency for Health Care Policy and Research has established a grant program to support outcomes research. The results of these research studies will likely be used in the following ways:

1. Effectiveness results will be used in determining what types of treatments will be eligible for reimbursement under public and private health insurance plans.
2. Large purchasers of care will use effectiveness results in making selections among HMOs and individual providers.
3. Healthcare providers will use effectiveness results in measuring their own performance and implementing programs of continuous quality improvement.
4. Individual physicians will use effectiveness information to explain treatment options to patients and involve them in decision making.
5. At the national level, outcomes information will be use to establish practice guidelines for common and high-cost medical conditions, such as treatment of prostate cancer and hip replacement. (Unger 1992)

Health services organizations will need to develop good clinical information systems to monitor their operations and develop their own clinical effectiveness measures. Computerization of patient records will take on increasing importance as we move into the 21st century.

Report Cards

The concept of outcomes measurement is being extended to formal systems of quality reporting. These "report cards" are used by consumers and purchasers to assist in selection of a health plan. Report cards have been developed by individual employers, industry coalitions, some of the larger HMOs, accrediting organizations, and professional associations.

The Cleveland Health Quality Choice Coalition is a voluntary collaborative effort involving hospitals, the medical society, corporate CEOs, human resource and benefits managers, and small businesses in the Cleveland, Ohio, metropolitan area. The purpose of the Coalition is to assess the quality and efficiency of healthcare in the community and distribute the results to Coalition members. Outcomes information has been reported for 31 hospitals, including the following measures:

1. Patient satisfaction
2. In-hospital mortality
3. Length of stay for different procedures
4. Hospital acquired complications
5. Severity adjusted outcomes for medical, surgical, and obstetrical patients. (Rosenthal and Harper 1994)

Some of the nation's largest HMOs are developing their own quality report cards as well. Efforts are under way to develop reporting standards in order to minimize variations and facilitate comparisons among plans. The National Committee for Quality Assurance has developed the Health Plan Employer Data and Information Set (HEDIS) to facilitate standardized reporting on a national basis.

Information Technology in this Environment of Change

Healthcare organizations operating in this environment of change must develop sophisticated information systems to support clinical operations and strategic management. The major priorities for system development include:

1. development of repositories of computerized patient records;
2. a shift in emphasis from inpatient systems to ambulatory care systems;
3. development of enterprisewide computer networks to support integrated delivery systems;
4. development of strategic decision-support systems for risk analysis, financial forecasting, outcomes assessment, and quality improvement; and
5. development of new applications as some integrated delivery systems take on the dual roles of provider and insurer.

Computerized Patient Records

In 1991, a distinguished committee of the Institute of Medicine, National Academy of Science, issued a report calling for the development of a national system of computer-based patient records (CPRs). (Dick and Steen 1991) Such a system would serve multiple objectives. (See Figure 1.4.) The ready availability of complete medical records should improve the quality of patient care to an aging and highly mobile population. The productivity of healthcare workers would be enhanced since essential demographic and medical information would need to be captured and entered into the system only once, avoiding unnecessary duplication of effort. Information on insurance coverage and eligibility would be available electronically to physicians, hospitals, and other providers of health services. Data captured in such a system would be very useful in health services research and policy formulation.

The Institute of Medicine (IOM) Committee envisioned a standardized patient record format that would be available on a national basis through electronic data interchange (EDI) technology. This massive undertaking would ultimately require computerization of all records, from those maintained in large medical centers to those in solo physician practices. Many problems would need to be addressed to bring such a system to reality, including funds for developmental costs and systems

Figure 1.4 Objectives for Computer-Based Records

Institute of Medicine Report
1. Support patient care and improve its quality.
2. Enhance productivity of healthcare professionals.
3. Reduce administrative costs associated with healthcare delivery and financing.
4. Support clinical and health services research.
5. Accommodate future developments in healthcare technology, policy, management, and finance.
6. Protect patient data confidentiality.

to protect the confidentiality of patient information. The Committee recommended that a developmental effort be undertaken by a follow-up organization, the Computer-Based Patient Record Institute (CPRI) which would "promote and facilitate development, implementation, and dissemination of the CPR."

Market-based healthcare reform is providing additional impetus to the development of computerized patient records and clinical information systems. As integrated delivery systems are formed, clinical and financial information must be readily available and shared electronically with all providers in the system—hospitals, physician offices, long-term care facilities, home health agencies, etc. Emphasis seems to be shifting from a single, national system of electronic patient records to systems developed at the local or regional level.

In discussing the major barriers to effective integration of healthcare delivery systems, Shortell, Gillies, and Anderson (1994, 56) state that " . . . systems must expand their information capabilities to link patients and providers across all settings involved in the continuum of care, from acute inpatient care to care provided in the physician's office to care provided in the patient's home."

Barea (1993) describes the development of a clinical information system at Egleston Children's Hospital at Emory University in Atlanta:

> Having measurable outcomes and tracking this information in a clinical database will save the institution money as physicians improve utilization. . . . Proven success will be critical as contracts are negotiated with employers, HMOs and other entities. (Barea 1993, 44)

Many healthcare organizations are planning to build "data warehouses" containing complete clinical, financial, and administrative data on every patient. These repositories of patient records can be centralized in one large computer file or they may be "virtual" systems in which the data are distributed across a number of departmental systems. These data warehouses require solid computer architecture in their design and must employ industrywide standards for data definition and coding. Security is essential to protect privacy and confidentiality of patient information. (Talbott 1994)

Ambulatory Care Systems

Managed care and market-based reform have caused a major shift in emphasis from acute inpatient care to services delivered on an outpatient basis (including surgery). As a result, health services organizations are placing increased emphasis on the development of ambulatory care information systems.

Park Nicollet Medical Center in Minneapolis, Minnesota, has developed an advanced ambulatory care information system to support patient care and strategic management in the multiple clinics operated by the Center. All clinic sites are linked electronically to a centralized patient database and accounting system. The system enables physicians and staff members at any clinic to access patient records from other sites, schedule appointments with other physicians, and schedule laboratory and radiology procedures at the central facility.

Data from the information system are used to generate a number of performance reports, including patient satisfaction, ratios of patients to staff, and other key indicators of cost and quality. Outcome reports are generated on the cost-effectiveness of alternative treatment modalities, with data from these assessments used to create practice guidelines for the clinics. The system also generates strategic management reports. Population-based data are used to monitor health status, illness patterns, prevention and wellness practices, and service utilization rates. (Kralewski et. al. 1994, 22–23)

Enterprisewide Systems

As healthcare organizations band together to form integrated delivery systems, development of enterprisewide information and communications networks becomes a high priority. Often this involves the need to integrate diverse information systems developed by individual provider organizations who have come together through mergers, acquisitions, or joint ventures.

An enterprisewide system must include an electronic network infrastructure to facilitate sharing of clinical and financial information among members of the integrated delivery system: physicians, hospitals, ambulatory care centers, home health service agencies, long-term care facilities, and other components of the system.

One approach to establishing an information infrastructure that can support the goals of an integrated delivery system is to participate in or promote the development of a community health information network (CHIN). (Weaver 1993) A CHIN expands the communications network to include employers, insurers, government agencies, and other providers in the community. CHINs provide authorized users access to relevant patient and financial information from multiple sources. There is some skepticism about CHIN development among healthcare executives:

> Executives are coming to realize that they are often ill-positioned—technologically, operationally, and strategically—to move toward a true community information network. Instead, many hospital-based integrated delivery systems are going back a few steps and regrouping, putting in place plans that span the entire system before making the leap to community-wide information management. (Appleby 1995, 43)

The Internet provides one option for development of intrasystem communications among components of an integrated delivery system. Applications include intercompany messaging, e-mail, Web browsing, and access to knowledge-based resources for physicians.

Strategic Decision-Support Systems

Historically, information systems in hospitals and other health services organizations have focused on day-to-day operations: admitting and discharging patients, ordering lab tests, reporting results from radiology, processing the payroll, preparing bills for insurance payments, and the like. Until recently, very little priority was assigned to the use of information for strategic planning and management in healthcare facilities. Managed care and market-driven reform have quickly changed this situation. Organizations that wish to survive in the current environment must be able to:

1. assess the health risks of the populations they serve or plan to serve in the future;
2. forecast the costs and revenues anticipated from contracts with HMOs and exclusive provider arrangements; and
3. measure the clinical outcomes of services provided and continuously improve service quality in order to compete successfully for business in the medical marketplace.

Meeting these strategic objectives requires development of databases of clinical and financial information plus decision-analysis programs to support executive management.

Some vendors are developing software products for decision-support purposes. Dilts, Kappeler, Durham & Co. established a data repository for health networks used to develop computer models of treatment costs. The software will search the database and build a profile of resource consumption for a typical patient for a given procedure. The profiles are used to forecast the profitability of capitation proposals. (Morrissey 1994, 82)

New Types of Applications

With the expansion of managed care and concurrent development of integrated delivery systems, many healthcare organizations are now playing dual roles as providers of care and insurers of populations served by the network. For example, Intermountain Health Care System of Salt Lake City, Utah, includes multiple hospitals, clinics, and other facilities providing health services to patients in its region. In 1992, Intermountain also operated three managed care plans with enrollment of more than 200,000 individuals. (Hard 1992)

Systems such as Intermountain must develop a full range of information systems to support patient care (clinical, administrative, and decision support). In addition, integrated delivery systems involved in direct contracting and offering insurance products such as HMOs or PPOs must develop a complete range of insurance products to support sales and marketing; actuarial and underwriting activities; service contracting; eligibility; billing; utilization review; and claims processing (among others). (Austin and Sobczak 1993)

Recent surveys of leaders in healthcare confirm these trends. Executives responding to the fifth annual survey of information systems trends sponsored by *Modern Healthcare* indicated that redesigning their computer systems for managed care was their highest information technology priority. (Morrissey 1995) These findings are supported by results from the 1996 Leadership Survey conducted by the Healthcare Information and Management Systems Society and Hewlett-Packard Corporation. Respondents indicated that the most significant force driving information technology investments was the need to control costs due to pressures of managed care. The survey also indicated movement of computer technology to outpatient settings, including ambulatory clinics, physicians' offices, and group practices—far out pacing development of applications in traditional inpatient settings. (HIMSS/HP 1996)

The Healthcare Information Professional

A number of trade and professional organizations support the work of information professionals in the healthcare field.

1. American College of Healthcare Information Administrators (ACHIA). A subunit of the American Academy of Medical Administrators, ACHIA is a personal membership organization for information

administrators with special focus on continuing education and research in healthcare information administration.

2. American Health Information Management Association (AHIMA). Formerly the American Medical Record Association, AHIMA is comprised of information professionals who specialize in the utilization and management of clinical data.

3. American Medical Informatics Association (AMIA). "Medical informatics" is a term used to describe the science of storage, retrieval, and optimal use of biomedical information for problem solving and medical decision making. AMIA is a personal membership organization of professionals interested in computer applications in biomedicine.

4. Center for Healthcare Information Management (CHIM). CHIM is a trade association of corporate members representing the leading firms (hardware, software, and consulting) in the healthcare information technology industry.

5. College of Healthcare Information Management Executives (CHIME). CHIME is a personal membership organization of chief information officers (CIOs) in the healthcare field. CHIME provides professional development and networking opportunities for its members.

6. Healthcare Information and Management Systems Society (HIMSS). HIMSS is a personal membership organization representing professionals in four areas: clinical systems, information systems, management engineering, and telecommunications. HIMSS provides professional development opportunities to its members through publications and educational programs.

For more information on these and other related professional organizations, the reader is directed to the Annual Market Directory issue of *Health Management Technology*. The 1996 Directory lists 41 associations and includes addresses and contact information for each organization in the listing.

Summary

Healthcare is an information-intensive process. The management of health services organizations can be improved through intelligent use of information. This requires systematic planning and management of information resources in order to develop information systems that support patient care, administrative operations, and strategic management.

Health information systems fall into four categories: clinical, administrative, strategic decision-support, and electronic network applications. Clinical information systems support patient care and provide information for strategic planning and management. Administrative systems support nonpatient care activities such as financial management, human resource management, materials management, scheduling, and office automation. Strategic decision-support systems assist executives in planning, marketing, management control of operations, performance evaluation, and outcomes assessment. Electronic network applications are used for insurance billing and claims processing, ordering medical supplies, and exchanging information across provider networks.

Change is occurring rapidly in healthcare. Major forces of change include:

1. expansion of managed care;
2. development of integrated delivery systems;
3. changes in reimbursement, including contractual discounts and capitation;
4. outcomes assessment to improve quality and reduce costs; and
5. demand for "report cards" on the performance of health plans and providers of care.

These environmental forces have resulted in reordering of the information system priorities of health services organizations. These new priorities include:

1. development of computerized patient records systems;
2. shift in emphasis from inpatient to ambulatory care systems;
3. development of enterprisewide electronic networks within integrated delivery systems;
4. development of strategic decision-support systems for risk analysis, financial forecasting, outcomes assessment, and quality improvement; and
5. development of new insurance-type applications within integrated delivery systems.

Discussion Questions

1.1 Why is healthcare one of the most information-intensive sectors of the U.S. economy?

1.2 Describe the following categories of information systems in health services organizations: clinical, administrative, and strategic decision support. How important is integration of information among these three categories of systems?

1.3 In what ways has managed care affected the use of information technology in health services organizations?

1.4 As integrated delivery systems develop in response to managed care, what are some of the major information system priorities for these organizations?

1.5 Define *outcomes assessment*. Are information systems important in assessing outcomes? in what ways?

1.6 How do changes in reimbursement (i.e., capitation and contractual discounts) affect information systems in health services organizations?

1.7 Develop a profile (mission, membership, programs, etc.) of one of the major professional organizations in the healthcare information management field.

References

Appleby, C. 1995. "The Trouble with CHINs." *Hospitals & Health Networks* 69 (9): 42–44.

Austin, C. J., and P. M. Sobczak. 1993. "Information Technology and Managed Care." *Hospital Topics* 71 (3): 33–37.

Barea, A. 1993. "Links to Physicians as Requirements of Reform?" *Healthcare Informatics* (September): 42–44.

Coile, R. C. 1990. *The New Medicine: Reshaping Medical Practice and Health Care Management*. Rockville, MD: Aspen Publishers.

DeFauw, T. D., and D. L'Heureux. 1995. "How to Strategically Align Information Resources with the Goals of an Integrated Delivery System." *Healthcare Information Management* 9 (4): 3–10.

Dick, R. S., and E. B. Steen, eds. 1991. *The Computer-Based Patient Record: An Essential Technology for Health Care*. Washington, DC: National Academy Press.

Hard, R. 1992. "Well-managed Information Vital to Effective Managed Care Contracting." *Hospitals* 66 (11): 50.

Healthcare Information and Management Systems Society and Hewlett-Packard Company (HIMSS/HP). 1996. *Seventh Annual Leadership Survey: Trends in Health Care Computing*. Chicago: Healthcare Information and Management Systems Society.

Kertesz, L. 1996. "HMO Enrollment Soars." *Modern Healthcare* October 28: 10.

Kralewski, J. E., A. deVries, B. Dowd, and S. Potthoff. 1994. *The Development of Integrated Service Networks (ISNs)*. A Report for the MinnesotaCare Legislative Oversight Committee. University of Minnesota, School of Public Health, February 21.

Morrissey, J. 1994. "Hunting for Data to Limit Risks of Managed Care." *Modern Healthcare* 24 (46): 80–82.

———. 1995. "Information Systems Refocus Priorities." *Modern Healthcare* (February 13): 65–66.

Rosenthal, G. E., and D. L. Harper. 1994. "Cleveland Health Quality Choice: A Model for Collaborative Community-Based Outcomes Assessment." *Journal on Quality Improvement* 20 (8): 425–42.

Shortell, S. M., R. R. Gillies, and D. A. Anderson. 1994. "The New World of Managed Care: Creating Organized Delivery Systems." *Health Affairs* (Winter): 46–64.

Talbott, N. 1994. "Managing Information: Today's Integrated Healthcare Enterprises." *Healthcare Informatics* (June): 24–28.

Unger, W. J. 1992. "The Interdependence of Outcomes Management." *Decisions in Imaging Economics*. 5 (4): 4–7.

Weaver, C. 1993. "CHINs: Infrastructure for the Future." *Trustee* 46 (12): 12.

Wong, L. K. 1994. "Specialty Services Capitation Contracting by HMOs." *Medical Group Management Journal* (September–October): 96–100.

Wozmak, M. S. 1995. "Managed Care: A Primer." *American Academy of Medical Administrators Executive* (January–February): 12–14.

Additional Readings

American Hospital Association. 1993. *Transforming Health Care Delivery: Toward Community Care Networks*. Chicago: The Association.

Catholic Health Association. 1993. *A Handbook for Planning and Developing Integrated Delivery* St. Louis, MO: The Association.

Coile, R. C. 1995. "Assessing Healthcare Market Trends and Capital Needs: 1996–2000." *Healthcare Financial Management* 49 (8): 60–2, 64–5.

Health Care Advisory Board. 1994. *Report on Capitation*. Washington, DC: The Board.

Health Management Technology. 1996. *Annual Market Directory* Atlanta, GA: Argus, Inc.

Norman, K. C., and J. J. Moynihan. 1994. "Electronic Data Interchange: An Electronic Network Strategy for Managed Care." *Managed Care* 2 (1): 54–61.

Rontal, R. 1993. "Information and Decision Support in Managed Care." *Managed Care* 1 (3): 3–14.

Shortell, S. M., R. R. Gillies, D. A. Anderson, J. B. Mitchell, and K. L. Morgan. 1993. "Creating Organized Delivery Systems: The Barriers and Facilitators." *Hospital & Health Services Administration* (Winter): 447–66.

2

ESSENTIAL CONCEPTS

ERTAIN BACKGROUND concepts are important to an understanding of the effective application of information technology in health services organizations. These concepts, the subjects of this chapter, include a review of general systems theory, key principles of management related to the development and operation of information systems, and the need for change management in adapting systems to the organizational culture.

General Systems Theory

Systems theory provides the conceptual foundation upon which the development of information systems is based. Healthcare administrators

Concepts and Applications

A **system** is a term used to describe the relationships among a group of components that function together to achieve a common purpose. Cybernetic systems use continuous feedback of information to monitor and control the functioning of the system.

At the conclusion of this chapter, the reader will be able to define and discuss general systems theory, list the different types of systems and how they work, and discuss the role of information in a healthcare system.

should have a general understanding of this theory in order to understand how information systems function in their organizations, particularly in using information for management control. The systems approach is important because it concentrates on examining a process in its entirety rather than focusing on the parts, and it relates the parts to each other in order to achieve total system goals. Management control requires that performance be compared against expectations and that feedback be used to adjust the system when performance goals are not being met.

As discussed in detail in Chapter 8, systems analysis is a fundamental tool for the design and development of information systems. It is the process of studying organizational operations and determining information system requirements for a given application. Systems analysis employs concepts from *general systems theory* in analyzing inputs, processes, outputs, and feedback in defining requirements for an information system.

The remainder of this section presents a general overview of systems theory and its application in healthcare organizations.

A variety of systems comprise the functioning of health services organizations. These can be categorized into three groups: mechanical systems, human systems, and man-machine systems. *Mechanical systems* are an integral part of the physical plant, serving such purposes as heating and cooling; monitoring temperature, pressure, and humidity; and supplying chilled and heated water.

Most of the essential functions of the health services organizations are carried out through *human systems*—organized relationships among patients, physicians, employees, family members of patients, and others. Many of these systems are formally defined. For example, nursing care is provided in accordance with a scheduled set of predetermined protocols and procedures, and nursing service personnel are trained and supervised in the proper execution of this "system of care." Many things also happen through informal relationships, which through time often become well-defined and known to those in the organization. Thus certain activities get accomplished by "knowing the right person" or sending informal signals to key individuals about actions that need to be taken.

With the development of modern information technology, many systems fall into the third category, *man-machine systems*. These are formally defined systems in which human effort is assisted by various kinds of automated equipment. For example, computer systems have been developed to monitor continuously the vital signs of critically ill patients in intensive care units of medical centers.

Information systems in health services organizations fall into the second and third categories of this simple taxonomy; that is, information systems will either be human systems or man-machine systems designed to support operations. Information systems that operate without any type of machine processing of data are referred to as *manual* systems. Although much of this book deals with computer-aided information processing, most of the principles that are set forth, particularly those dealing with systems analysis and design, apply equally to the development of manual systems for processing of information.

Health services organizations also can be described in a broader context. Figure 2.1 is a systems diagram for a health services organization, showing the relationships among various inputs and environmental factors as these factors influence the provision of services to the community. In this context, mechanical, human, and man-machine systems would constitute elements, or subsystems, of the conversion process. The theoretical concepts on which this diagram is based are described in the section on general systems theory which follows.

Considerable research has been carried out by scientists on systems and how they function in all phases of our society. Interest in general systems theory developed in the post–World War II period. Initial research efforts were focused primarily on the physical sciences, with the study of strategic military weapons systems, systems for space exploration, and automated systems of all kinds to reduce manual labor and improve the overall quality of life.

In the 1960s, attention shifted to the application of systems theory to the social sciences, including organizational theory and management. Although much of this work is highly theoretical and of primary interest to those involved in basic research, some general discussion of systems theory is useful as background for understanding management control systems in health service delivery and for setting forth principles of information systems analysis and design.

Social scientists have defined systems in various ways. Simply defined, a system is "a set of objects and the relationships between the objects and their attributes." (Hall and Fagen 1968, 81–92) *Objects* in this definition constitute the component parts of the system. *Attributes* are the properties of these objects, abstract descriptors that characterize and define the component parts of the system. Essential to the concept of a system are defined relations, which tie the component parts together, thus enabling the parts to equal some greater unity rather than simply constituting an uncoordinated assemblage of objects or people. Relationships can be planned or unplanned, formal or informal, but they must exist if the collection of components is to constitute a system.

Certain basic concepts are central to a general understanding of systems and how they function. First, a system must have *unity*, or *integrity*. That is, the system must be something that can be viewed as an

Figure 2.1 The Health Services Organization as a System

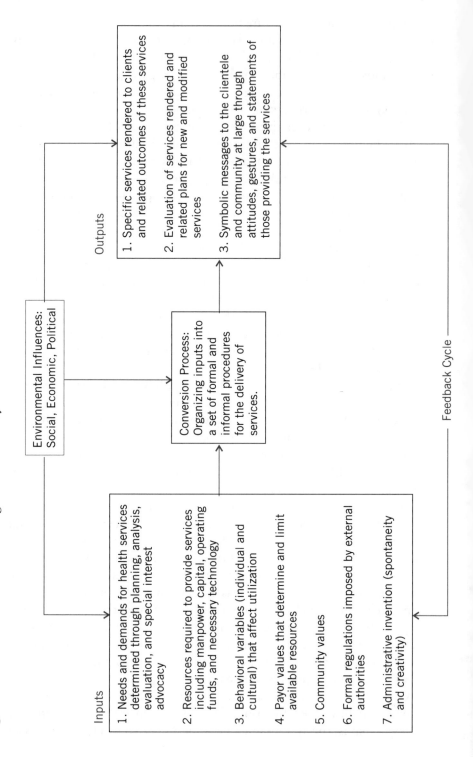

entity in its own right, with unity of purpose in the accomplishment of some goal or function. A system must have an identity and must have describable boundaries that allow it to be defined without reference to external events or objects.

Systems in health services organizations are for the most part very *complex*. The intricate web of complex relationships that constitutes most social systems often makes it difficult to describe simple cause-and-effect relationships among individual components of the system. The phenomenon of system complexity is often described by stating that a system is more than the sum of its parts.

Complex systems are further defined by their *hierarchical structure*. That is, large systems in health services organizations can be divided into several subsystems, and these subsystems in turn are subject to further subdivision in a nested format. For example, the patient care component of an integrated delivery system is composed of several subsystems: a diagnostic subsystem, a therapeutic subsystem, a rehabilitative subsystem, and so forth. Each of these subsystems in turn can be further described by a series of smaller systems. The entire network of systems and subsystems nests together in a structured way to describe the patient care system of the organization. (See Figure 2.2.)

Although most organizational systems are dynamic and subject to frequent change, they nonetheless must possess some *stability* and *equilibrium*. That is, the system must continue to function in the face of changing requirements and changes in the external environment in which it operates. To accomplish this, procedures must be sufficiently generalized to accommodate a variety of situations that can be expected to develop. Complex systems must be self-adapting and must include control functions that are continuous and automatic. At that time when the system can no longer adapt to changing requirements or major changes in the external environment, it no longer functions as a system and breakdown has occurred.

Systems can be further categorized as either *deterministic* or *probabilistic*. In a deterministic system, the component parts function according to completely predictable or definable relationships. Most mechanical systems are deterministic. On the other hand, human systems or man-machine systems (including information systems) are probabilistic, since all relationships cannot be perfectly predicted. In health services organizations, for example, most clinical systems are subject to fairly extreme fluctuations in the quantity and nature of the demand for patient services.

Systems theory, then, provides a perspective, a way of viewing not just the parts, not just the whole, but rather the spectrum of relationships

Figure 2.2 Health Services Organization Systems Network

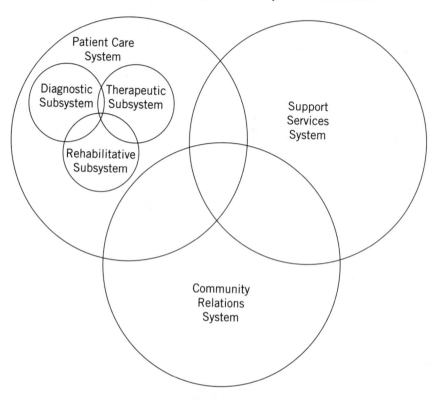

of the parts viewed in the context of the unitary purposes of the system as a whole.

The simplest of all systems will consist of three essential components: one or more inputs, a conversion process, and one or more outputs. (See Figure 2.3.)

Consider for example the appointment scheduling process of an ambulatory care center as a simple system. Inputs to the system consist of appointment requests from patients; physician schedules; and clinic resources, including personnel, treatment rooms, and supporting materials. The conversion process includes a set of actions in which the scheduling

Figure 2.3 Diagram of a Simple System

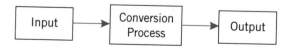

clerks collect information from patients, match patient requirements to available time slots, and make appointments. Output of this simple system consists of patients scheduled for service in the clinic. Note that the output of this system becomes the input for several other functional systems of the clinic—medical records, patient accounting, and others.

Most systems also involve *feedback*, a process by which one or more items of output information "feeds back" and influences future inputs. (See Figure 2.4.)

In the example just cited, feedback would occur in the form of adjusted information on the number of time slots available as patients are scheduled for the clinic. Each time an appointment is made, input data on times available would be revised and updated.

Systems are either *open* or *closed*. A closed system is completely self-contained and is not influenced by external events. In an open system, the components of the system exchange materials, energies, or information with their environment. (See Figure 2.5.) That is, they are influenced by, and themselves influence, the environment in which they operate. All closed systems eventually die (cease to function as a system). Only open systems that adjust to the environment can survive as systems over time.

Health services systems, with the exception of certain purely mechanical systems in the physical plant, fall into the category of open systems.

Figure 2.4 Simple System with Feedback

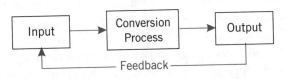

Figure 2.5 Open System Diagram

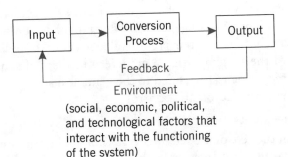

Human or man-machine systems in health services organizations are influenced by a variety of environmental factors (sometimes referred to as exogenous factors, or variables), and these are important to consider in understanding how a system functions. These environmental factors fall into four broad categories.

Health systems are influenced by *social factors*, characteristics of individuals and groups of people involved in the transactions that organizations undertake. Social factors affect patient behavior and patterns of utilization of services. Informal patterns of behavior develop among employees, and these have definite effects on the way operating systems function. Role-playing by physicians and other health professionals interacts with the formal functioning of systems. Social factors are important determinants of system functioning, and systems analysts need to be well versed in the art of human-factors engineering when designing systems.

A second major category of environmental factors is *economic* in nature. Systems are directly dependent on the availability of resources, and fluctuations in the local and national economy will influence both demand and resources. It is well-known, for example, that elective procedures are often deferred by patients during times of economic recession.

Health services systems are also affected by *political factors*. There are competing demands placed upon health services organizations by a variety of special interest groups, and systems are influenced both by community politics and by organizational politics. These political realities must be considered in the analysis and design of systems for the institution.

The *physical environment* constitutes the final category of environmental factors affecting organizational systems. The amount of space available and the way in which system components relate physically to each other will influence the effectiveness of a system.

To summarize briefly, health services systems are open systems influenced by a variety of social, economic, and political factors and by the physical environment in which they function.

The final concept to be introduced in this brief review of general systems theory is the concept of a cybernetic, or self-regulating, system. (Weiner 1954) Figure 2.6 is a generalized diagram of a cybernetic system. Feedback in a cybernetic system is controlled in order to adjust the future functioning of the system within a predetermined set of standards. The following three elements are added to the general system components in order to provide this automatic control:

1. a *sensor* element continuously gathers data on system outputs;
2. data from the sensor are fed into a *monitor* for continuous matching of the quantity or quality, or both, of performance against *standards*, predetermined expectations of system performance; and

Figure 2.6 Cybernetic System

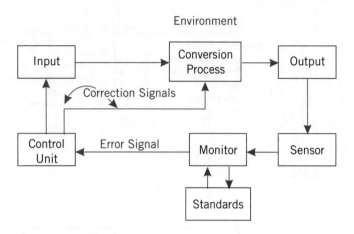

3. error signals from the monitor are sent to a *control unit* whose purpose is to generate correctional signals that automatically modify inputs and conversion processes to bring the functioning of the system back into control.

The most often cited example of a cybernetic system is a thermostatic control system for the automatic heating and cooling of a building. The sensor unit continuously measures ambient temperature and sends signals to the monitor, which compares the current temperature to preset standards. Through the control process, automatic correction signals are sent back to the heating/cooling units of the system to keep the temperature within control limits.

Management Control and Decision-Support Systems in Health Services Organizations

Organized systems in health services organizations should be designed as cybernetic systems with formal management controls built in as an integral part of the design. Figure 2.7 is a conceptual diagram of a generalized cybernetic system for a health services organization.

The inputs to this generalized system include demand for services by patients and those who represent them and also the resources required to provide services—labor, materials, capital, and technology. The conversion process consists of actions taken by employees of the health services organization aided by formalized procedures, informal patterns of functioning, and supporting equipment. System outputs include services

Figure 2.7 Generalized Management Control System (Cybernetic) for a Health Services Organization

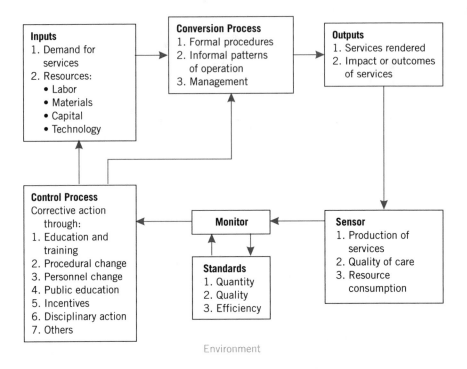

rendered to patients and the specific patient and community outcomes related to these services.

Management control is introduced in cybernetic components of the system. The sensor component continuously gathers data on the quantity of services rendered, the quality and other characteristics of these services, and the resources consumed in their provision. Data from the sensor (management reports) are monitored against preestablished standards of quantity (production and service goals), quality of care, efficiency of the service process, and patient outcomes. When standards are not met, a control process is activated to initiate necessary changes and improvements. The control process contains several elements, including education and training of personnel, community education programs, reengineering of the process of care, personnel changes in order to improve service, utilization of employee incentives, initiation of disciplinary action, and many others.

A key element in the establishment of management control systems is the establishment of standards for performance and quality control. The task of developing standards is not an easy one and requires considerable effort and thoughtful planning among administrators and professional personnel practicing in or employed by the health services organization. Standards can be developed in a number of ways. They can be established by administrative or medical authority in the institution. In some cases they may be developed through negotiation and subsequent agreement between employees and supervisors. Empirical studies of previous performance, using industrial engineering techniques, offer another approach to standards setting. In certain areas of operation, standards are mandated by external regulations, legal requirements, or accrediting agencies.

Whatever the approach to their development, standards are essential if management control is to operate on other than an ad hoc basis. Standards require careful management planning, continual review and revision, and frequent reinforcement through incorporation into the formal reward system. They are essential to effective management control.

As an example of these concepts, the operation of a centralized clinical laboratory in an integrated delivery system (IDS) can be described as a cybernetic system with planned controls built into the system for quality assurance and performance control purposes. Figure 2.8 is a schematic diagram describing the functioning of the laboratory in system terms.

System inputs include scheduled demand (laboratory tests planned, ordered, and scheduled in advance) and also unscheduled demand (tests required to be processed on an emergency, or stat, basis). Resource inputs include technical personnel in the laboratory, materials and equipment used in the testing process, and related technology. The conversion process consists of those formal and informal organizational actions related to collecting of specimens, conducting the lab tests, and reporting results to appropriate points in the hospitals, outpatient clinics, and other service units of the IDS. System outputs include the test reports sent back to clinicians ordering the tests, charges for services transmitted to the patient accounting department for billing purposes, and various statistical reports.

Cybernetic components for management control are also included in Figure 2.8. The sensor component is the management reporting system of the laboratory by which data on the number of tests conducted by various categories, quality control data, and records of resources consumed (including personnel time of laboratory technicians) are collected and recorded. These data are used by laboratory managers who monitor actual performance against predetermined standards, including those established by the Joint Commission on Accreditation of Healthcare Organizations (JCAHO), professional standards of quality established by the chief pathologist and medical staff, and cost and efficiency (productivity) goals established jointly by administrative and medical personnel

Figure 2.8 Clinical Laboratory as a Cybernetic System

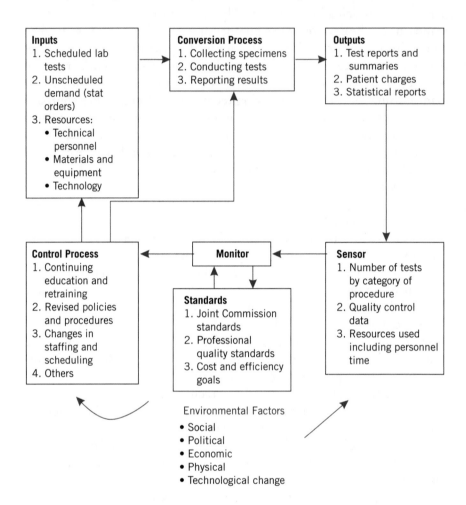

in the organization. When standards are not met, corrective actions are initiated, including activation of continuing education and retraining; revision of operating policies and procedures including recalibration of test equipment if necessary; change in staffing patterns and scheduling; and the like. The laboratory operates overall as an open system influenced by several contextual or environmental factors including the physical environment of the laboratory facility, current economic conditions of the IDS, social and political factors related to interaction of personnel in the laboratory, and the advancement of technology.

Information for Management Control

Any management control system is information-dependent. Information requirements permeate the system diagrams presented in the preceding parts of this chapter. In order for health programs to be properly managed, information is needed about each of the major system components previously described.

Input information must be collected to monitor demand continuously, both scheduled and unscheduled, as well as the resources consumed in the provision of services. Operational procedures must be constantly observed through information on exceptions, error rates, system malfunctions, and similar performance measures on a management-by-exception basis. Output information on the quantity and quality of services rendered must be matched with information on related outcomes of the provision of specific services.

In addition, the effective manager must keep in close contact with the environment in which his department or institution functions. Environmental information is essential to this task—data such as demographic characteristics of the service population, previous utilization patterns, services offered by other organizations, and recent changes in community values. An effective information system will be designed with these kinds of management information needs in mind.

What, then, are the attributes of information useful for management control in the delivery of health services? Some of the more important characteristics of effective management information are discussed below. (See Figure 2.9.)

The first, and perhaps most essential, characteristic is that information, to be useful, must be *information, not just raw data*. That is, data must

Figure 2.9 Characteristics of Useful Management Information

- Information—not data
- Relevant
- Sensitive
- Unbiased
- Comprehensive
- Timely
- Action-oriented
- Uniform (for comparative purposes)
- Performance-targeted
- Cost-effective

be intelligently processed in accordance with predesigned plans before they become information useful to management or operating personnel.

Health information must be *relevant* to the purposes for which it is to be used. It must be sufficiently *sensitive* to provide discrimination and meaningful comparisons for operating managers. Many information systems provide data that are so aggregated as to provide no meaningful indicators for management planning or control purposes. Overall hospital cost per patient day is a good example. By contrast, separating costs into fixed and variable components and allocating variable costs by diagnostic groupings and level of care would provide more useful information to management.

Useful information must be *unbiased* and not collected or analyzed in such a way as to meet self-fulfilling prophecies. Information should be *comprehensive*, so that all elements or components of a system are visible to those responsible for administering that system.

Information must be *timely*, presented to users in advance of the time when decisions or actions are required. Many information systems produce beautiful reports that are completely useless because of failure to meet operational time requirements. Information should be *action-oriented*, designed to aid the manager directly in the decision process rather than just presenting passive facts about current operations. For example, information from an inventory control and materials management system should include direct indicators of when specific items need to be reordered rather than just presenting data on current numbers in stock.

Information systems should have as their goal the production of *uniform* reports so that performance indicators can be compared over time both internally against previous performance and externally against the experience of other comparable organizations. Good information will also be *performance-targeted*, that is, designed and collected in reference to predetermined goals and objectives of the institution.

Finally, information should be *cost-effective*. The anticipated benefits to be obtained from having the information available should be worth the costs of collecting and processing that same information.

Principles of Information Resource Management

Listed below are three key management principles that are very important for successful application of information technology in health services organizations. Many other principles could have been included, some of which are discussed in later chapters of this book. However, the items presented here are overarching principles critical to successful information resource management. (Austin and Howe 1994, 230)

1. Treat information as an essential organizational resource. Managers in health services organizations should treat information as a fourth major type of resource required to do business, on a par with human resources, financial resources, and capital facilities and equipment. As such, information resource management should receive the same care and attention that is given to human resources management, financial management, and materials management in the organization.

2. Obtain top executive support for information systems planning and management. Given the importance of information resources and the costs and complexities involved in information systems development, top level support is essential to success. The chief executive officer and key members of the executive management team should be knowledgeable and involved in information systems planning and establishment of priorities for system development. Information resource management should be the responsibility of a corporate-level executive, the chief information officer (CIO) in larger organizations and health systems. (See Chapter 10 for more details on the role and responsibility of the CIO.)

3. Develop a strategic vision and plan. Health services organizations need an enterprisewide vision of how information technology will be used to support patient care and strategic management. An information systems plan must be strategically aligned with the vision, mission, goals, and objectives of the organization. Alignment with organizational strategy

> " . . . involves the review of the organization's 'formal' strategic plan (if it has one), as well as interviews with key executives and stakeholders. . . . Regional alliances, new care-delivery locations, product-line changes, marketing plans and other projects must be thoroughly, creatively and cost effectively addressed as part of the I/S planning process." (Spitzer 1993, 30)

In summary, strategic information systems planning must be driven by the business plans of the health services organization. (See Chapter 7 for more details.)

Management of Change

The application of information technology in health services organizations inevitably involves change, often major change, in the way business is done. Change is threatening to organizational stakeholders, particularly employees. Careful attention must be paid to human factors and the organizational culture within which information systems must function.

Fear of change, with resultant anxiety and tension, is a common problem encountered in many system development efforts. Employees may have concerns about possible effects of the new system on their own jobs and possible changes in the work environment that may be required. Managers may have concerns about changes that could result in the redistribution of power, greater centralization of authority, or increased demand for accountability as by-products of the new system. Some may have concerns that the information system will result in more rigid and less flexible patterns of operation, with resultant lack of discretion in carrying out the task. Often these concerns are unfounded and based upon misunderstanding of the technology. Nevertheless, they are concerns that are very real to the individuals involved.

Mann (1988) conducted a study of personnel affected by changes resulting from installation of a new information system at a large health science center. Interviews were conducted with clerical personnel, professional staff, and administrators affected by the system. Major findings included the following:

- the beliefs, attitudes, and behavioral intentions of individuals toward the change tended to be influenced by their groups in in the workplace;
- individuals who were motivated by the needs for self-esteem and self-fulfillment had beliefs and attitudes more supportive of the information system; and
- persons with considerate managers—managers who were concerned with the comfort, well-being, and status of their subordinates—were more likely to have behavioral intentions supportive of the change.

Effective change management requires an understanding of these behavioral and cultural factors in information system development. Open communications are essential. Avoid being secretive and provide a comprehensive program of staff orientation and training prior to initiation of a major project. Structure the project in such a way that users will be active participants and will "buy in" from the beginning. Make top level support visible and reinforce that support regularly.

Active management of change should be planned and implemented in advance of the implementation of an information system:

> A lot of money is spent on consultants brought in to put out the fires caused by technical implementations that did not consider the people and organizational issues. . . . The use of change management strategies at an early stage might have saved a great deal of money and organizational pain, i.e., the pain experienced by everyone connected with the information system regardless of his or her organizational position or attitude about the technology, the process, or the circumstances. (Lorenzi et. al. 1995, 152)

The best technology in the world will be ineffective if system planning is not accompanied by careful attention to change management.

Concluding Comments

In concluding this brief review of essential concepts, two final points are offered.

First, as noted above, information has both costs and benefits associated with its use. Before initiating major system development projects, managers should consider whether the benefits to be obtained from information (tangible and intangible) will be worth the investment required to install the system.

Second, it is important to recognize the difference between the ability to use a personal computer (PC) and the ability to understand the management of information in complex organizations. Sophistication in PC use does little to enhance knowledge of information systems development and the application of computer systems to problems of patient care, administration, and strategic management in health services organizations. For this reason, the emphasis throughout this book is on the management of information resources with personal computers being only one component of a complex information architecture found in most organizations.

Summary

An understanding of general systems theory is useful for health administrators in designing and developing management control systems and in obtaining the kinds of information required to enable such systems to function effectively.

A system is a set of objects together with the relationships between the objects and their attributes. Systems are characterized by unity of purpose, complexity, hierarchical relationships with other systems, and a need for stability in the face of a dynamic environment. Most health systems are probabilistic, in that relationships cannot be perfectly predicted or described in the design of the systems.

A simple system consists of one or more elements of input, a conversion process, and one or more outputs that flow from that process. Most systems also include feedback, by which system outputs influence future inputs and processes. Open systems are influenced by the environment in which they function, and they exchange information and energy with that environment. Environmental factors include political, social, and economic variables that influence system performance, as well as the physical environment in which the system functions.

Cybernetic systems include formally planned components that introduce automatic control into the systems. Cybernetic components include sensors to gather data on current system functioning, monitors to compare these data against predetermined standards, and control elements to change inputs or processes, or both, when system functioning is out of control. Management control systems in health services organizations can be designed according to principles of cybernetic system theory.

Health services delivery viewed in a systems context is information-dependent. Effective information for management control purposes has several important characteristics, including relevance, timeliness, sensitivity, comprehensiveness, objectivity, action-orientation, uniformity, performance-targeting, and cost-effectiveness. Good information systems will be developed with these characteristics constantly in view of those charged with design and implementation.

Key management principles essential to success in application of information technology in healthcare include:

1. Information should be treated as an essential organizational resource.
2. It is important to obtain top executive support for information systems planning and management.
3. Health services organizations need an enterprisewide strategic vision and plan for the application of information systems to patient care and strategic management.

Information systems operate within an organizational culture. Key stakeholders are affected by the changes associated with installation of information systems in the organization. Effective change management is an important component of an information systems development project.

Discussion Questions

2.1 Define the term *system*. What are the three general kinds of systems that will be found in health services organizations?

2.2 What is the difference between an open and a closed system?

2.3 What are some of the environmental factors that will influence open systems in integrated delivery systems? How important are these factors in systems design?

2.4 What is a cybernetic system? Explain how cybernetic theory can be utilized in the development of management systems in health services organizations.

2.5 Why is stability an important characteristic of a system? How can system stability be achieved in the dynamic environment of a modern health services organization?

2.6 Why are most systems in health services organizations described as probabilistic rather than deterministic?

2.7 What are some of the attributes of information that make it useful for management control purposes?

2.8 What is change management? Why is it important in information system development projects?

Problems

2.1 For the functions listed below, use cybernetic theory to describe the operation and management control of each in systems terms:
a. the emergency room of an acute care general hospital
b. the medical records department of an ambulatory care center
c. the enrollment management section of an HMO
d. the patient billing function in a long-term care institution
e. the nurse scheduling function of a home health agency
f. an outpatient rehabilitation and physical therapy program
g. the patient registration process of a medical group practice

2.2 For each of the systems listed in Problem 2.1, develop a list of information elements that would be needed for each system to operate effectively.

2.3 Prepare a brief report to the board of directors of an integrated delivery system commenting on the general characteristics of useful information for assisting in strategic planning and management of the system.

References

Austin, C. J., and R. C. Howe. 1994. "Information Systems Management." In *The AUPHA Manual of Health Services Management*, edited by R. J. Taylor and S. B. Taylor. Gaithersburg, MD: Aspen Publishers.

Hall, A. D., and R. E. Fagen. 1968. "Definition of System." In *Modern Systems Research for the Behavioral Scientist*, edited by W. Buckley. Chicago: Aldine Publishing Co.

Lorenzi, N. M., M. J. Ball, R. T. Riley, and J. V. Douglas. 1995. *Transforming Health Care Through Information*. New York: Springer-Verlag, Inc.

Mann, G. J. 1988. "Managers, Groups, and People: Some Considerations in Information System Change." *Health Care Management Review* (Fall): 47.

Spitzer, P. G. 1993. "A Comprehensive Framework for I/S Planning." *Computers in Healthcare* (May): 28–33.

Weiner, N. 1954. *The Human Use of Human Beings: Cybernetics and Society*. Garden City, NY: Doubleday Anchor. (Dr. Weiner is the father of cybernetic systems theory.)

Additional Readings

Baker, F., ed. 1973. *Organizational Systems: General Systems Approaches to Complex Organization*. Homewood, IL: Richard D. Irwin.

Bertalanffy, L. V. 1968. *General Systems Theory*. New York: Braziller.

Cummings, T. G., ed. 1980. *Systems Theory for Organization Development*. New York: John Wiley and Sons.

Griffith, J. R. 1995. *The Well-Managed Community Health Care Organization*, 3rd Ed. Chicago: AUPHA Press/Health Administration Press.

Reynolds, G. W. 1995. *Information Systems for Managers*, 3rd Ed. St. Paul, MN: West Publishing Company.

Schmitz, H. H. 1987. *Managing Health Care Information Resources*. Rockville, MD: Aspen Publishers. (Note particularly Chapter 1, "The Theory of Systems.")

Starkweather, D. B., and D. G. Shropshire. 1994. "Management Effectiveness." In *The AUPHA Manual of Health Services Management*, edited by R. J. Taylor and S. B. Taylor. Gaithersburg, MD: Aspen Publishers.

Studnicki, J., C. E. Stevens, and L. Knisely. 1985. "Impact of a Cybernetic System of Feedback to Physicians on Inappropriate Hospital Use." *Journal of Medical Education* 60 (June): 454–60.

Warner, D. M., D. C. Holloway, and K. L. Grazier. 1984. *Decision Making and Control for Health Administration*. Chicago: Health Administration Press.

Information Technology

CHAPTER

3

COMPUTER HARDWARE

T
HE MANAGEMENT of information resources and the effective
use of information typically do not require that the healthcare executive have an in-depth knowledge of computer technology. However,
as the leader of an information intensive organization, the healthcare
executive must have at least a basic understanding of computers and their
components. Such an understanding is of particular importance when the
executive is part of a multidisciplinary team, along with physicians, other
clinicians, financial experts, and computer system specialists, charged

Concepts and Applications

Hardware refers to the physical devices that make up a computer
system. Basically, a system must possess the means to store and
retrieve data, as well as manipulate and display them.

A healthcare executive must understand the components that allow
the computer system to work, how those components function,
and the different classes of computers, such as mainframes, personal
computers, etc.

This chapter will enable readers to define and explain how and where
data are stored, the different ways that the data can be retrieved and
displayed, and how data can be manipulated. Further, readers will be
able to determine which hardware technology can be used in, and
which is most appropriate for, their healthcare organizations.

with the responsibility of defining system needs, acquiring new systems, or implementing new applications. In order to be effective, the executive must not be intimidated by technical computer concepts or "buzzwords."

This chapter discusses the physical components that comprise a computer and the physical devices that combine to form a computer system. These components and devices are known collectively as hardware. The personal computer, or PC, used by a large segment of the population, is an example of computer hardware. No attempt is made here to present an exhaustive treatment comparable to what is found in computer science texts. Readers interested in such coverage of the topic are referred to the Additional Readings listed at the end of the chapter.

Rather, an overview is offered that provides the healthcare executive with an appropriate background to understand the important role that hardware plays in making possible the implementation of the information system applications discussed in later chapters of this book.

An Overview of Computer Components

The Electronic Numerical Integrator and Calculator (ENIAC) was the first electronic digital computer built in the United States. (Rosen 1969) Completed in 1946 at the University of Pennsylvania, this computer launched what has since become known as the first generation of computer hardware. Today, a half century later, the computer world has evolved to the fourth generation of hardware and is at the threshold of the fifth generation. A small desktop can now hold the computing power that once required a large room with special air-conditioning equipment.

Although this hardware evolution has been quite impressive, the basic schematic of a computer remains the same. Figure 3.1 depicts the major components of a computer system. Five categories of components comprise this system: the Central Processing Unit (CPU); primary storage; secondary storage; input units; and output units. Each of these categories will be discussed and illustrated in this chapter. In addition, today's computer systems typically have hardware to allow the computer to communicate with other computers, either within the organization or external to the organization. Such communication gives rise to the concepts of networking and telecommunications. Discussion of the hardware necessary to support this communication can be found in Chapter 5.

Central Processing Unit

The CPU might be called the "brains" of the computer. It is here that the actual "computing" takes place. The CPU consists of three major

Figure 3.1 Major Components of a Computer System

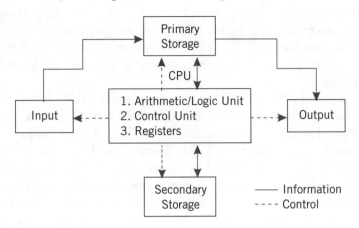

subcomponents: the Arithmetic/Logic Unit; the Control Unit; and Registers.

Arithmetic/Logic Unit (ALU). The basic computational and comparison capability of the computer lies in the ALU. The ALU has the ability to perform addition and subtraction, and thus, by extension, multiplication and division. Of course, it is capable of performing these operations quite rapidly. In addition, the ALU can perform the logical operation of comparison—that is, determining if two quantities are equal or if one is greater than the second. This logical comparison can be performed on both numeric as well as character (non-numeric) data. The speed of the ALU is an important performance characteristic of a computer, and faster processing speeds can improve the performance of applications that involve a large number of arithmetic operations. Examples of such applications—sometimes known as computation-bound applications—include image processing, interpretation of EKG data, and statistical analysis of very large sets of data.

Control Unit. No matter what "language" is used to communicate a problem to the computer, the problem description is ultimately converted to a series of machine instructions that the computer is able to "understand." The instructions are stored in primary storage. (How this conversion takes place is described in the chapter on software; the notion of primary storage is described below.) The sequential processing of these machine instructions is orchestrated by the control unit.

In order to process one machine instruction, the control unit must coordinate two distinct operations. First, the instruction must be retrieved from primary storage and interpreted. This operation is known as an instruction cycle. Then, the control unit must locate any required data (also stored in primary storage), instruct the ALU to perform the necessary operation, and ensure that the result gets put into the proper primary storage location. These operations constitute the execution cycle. The instruction cycle and execution cycle together are known as a machine cycle.

Frankenfeld (1993, 718) describes two measures of the speed with which the control unit can orchestrate the processing of a machine instruction. The first measure indicates how long it takes for the system to execute a simple instruction. This measure can be stated in terms of elapsed time, usually expressed in nanoseconds (a nanosecond is 10^{-9} seconds), or in terms of CPU speed, typically expressed in units of hertz (abbreviated Hz and equivalent to cycles per second). For example, computers with clock speeds of 200 MHz (1 MHz = 10^6 Hz) require only 5 nanoseconds to execute one simple instruction. The second measure provides the number of simple instructions that can be executed in a second. It is typically expressed in units of millions of instructions per second (MIPS).

The computer world has become so complex today that these simple measures of the control unit's performance have become essentially meaningless. A variety of benchmarks have been created to provide indices of performance for comparing alternative computer systems. (Yager 1996; Slater 1996) These indices attempt to account for the variety of configurations that are incorporated into today's CPUs in order to optimize the computer's performance for specific applications. However, as Yager (1996, 145) so appropriately indicates, for many users "the only worthwhile benchmarks are the ones that they create and run themselves using real applications."

Registers. When program instructions or data are transferred from primary storage to the CPU for processing, they are held in a high-speed memory area within the CPU known as registers. The instruction to be processed is held in the *instruction register* and the address of the data to be operated on is held in the *address register*. When the data value is retrieved from primary memory, it is put into a *storage register*. When the desired operation is performed on this data value, the result is placed into the *accumulator* from which it is transferred back to primary memory. Once this cycle is completed, the process begins all over again. The computer's performance can be enhanced by increasing the number of operations performed within the CPU (using the CPU's registers) and minimizing the number of accesses to data stored in memory.

Three additional CPU characteristics that affect the computer's performance bear mention. The first is the CPU *word length*, or the number of bits that the CPU can process at one time. Larger word lengths will increase the speed of the computer. Secondly, the speed of the computer is affected by the *data bus width*. The *data bus* refers to the pipeline through which data flow into and out of the CPU. Larger bus widths allow for the simultaneous transfer of larger amounts of information, thus increasing the processing speed of the computer. Finally, the introduction of reduced instruction-set computing (RISC) technology is being touted by many as a great improvement over the conventional complex instruction-set computing (CISC) technology. Computers employing RISC technology execute most of their instructions in one machine cycle, as opposed to CISC machines, which might require multiple cycles to execute an instruction. Prosise (1995) presents an interesting tutorial comparing the two technologies.

Primary Storage

The primary storage in early computers consisted of a large number of small toroidal pieces of magnetic material called *magnetic cores* with a wire looped several times around the core. Current passing through the wire could affect the direction of the magnetism in the core, and depending on this direction the core could be said to be storing a "0" or a "1." Because of the use of these core elements, early computer users often referred to primary storage as "core memory." Today, small silicon chips, known as semiconductors, have replaced the magnetic cores as the basis for primary storage. (See Figure 3.2.) Each chip contains a large number of transistors printed on it, which allows millions of pieces of information to be stored.

Information is stored within the computer using the binary number system because it is straightforward to equate a 0 or 1 with the absence or presence of an electrical signal. Numeric data are stored simply as their binary equivalent. Non-numeric, or character, data are represented by unique binary values that are distinguishable from numerical data. Each "digit" in the binary system is known as a *bit*. Depending upon the particular computer design, 8, 16, 32, or more bits are clustered together to form a "word." For convenience, the bits of a word are separated into groups of eight and each group of eight bits is called a *byte*.

A group of 1,000 bytes is called a *kilobyte* (kb). Because computers operate in the binary system, a kilobyte actually equals the power of two which is closest to 1,000, or 1,024 bytes (1,024 is equal to 2^{10}). Similarly, a group of one million bytes is known as a *megabyte* (mb). Again, consistent with the binary system, a megabyte actually is equal to 1,048,576 bytes (1,048,576 is equal to 2^{20}). The size of a computer's primary storage is typically stated in units of megabytes.

Figure 3.2   A Typical Memory Chip

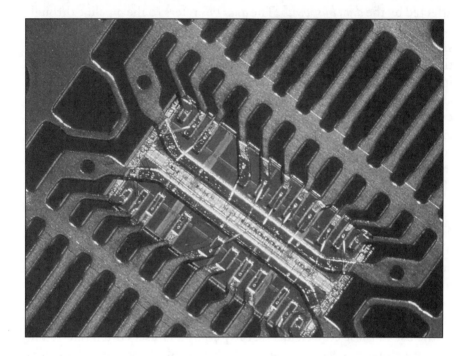

Courtesy of International Business Machines Corporation. Unauthorized use not permitted.

Whereas the "core" memory in early computers was quite expensive, memory "chips" found in today's computers are relatively inexpensive. As a result, the amount of primary storage contained in today's computer systems continues to increase, thus enabling these systems to run increasingly complex and sophisticated applications.

Several types of primary storage can be found in the computer. Specifications for a computer system will typically indicate the amount of each type that the computer contains. Therefore, a brief definition of each type will help the executive to understand better the meaning of these specifications.

Read-Only Memory (ROM). The first type of primary storage is known as read-only memory, or ROM. The contents of this type of memory can be read, but nothing can be written into these storage locations. ROM is typically used to store small sets of instructions used by a computer to perform special tasks, such as the sequence to be followed when the computer is first turned on. These instructions remain in ROM even when the computer is turned off. Memory that retains its contents in this way is said to be *nonvolatile*.

Random-Access Memory (RAM). Random access memory (RAM), the second type of storage, constitutes the majority of primary storage. It is in RAM that data and program instructions are held until needed for processing. Recall that the control unit is responsible for retrieving the data and instructions as they are needed for program execution. Each location in memory has an *address* associated with it. The control unit is able to locate the needed data or instructions by knowing the address at which they are stored.

The notion of "random access" refers to the fact that the control unit is able to proceed directly to a given address. By contrast, a "sequential access" device would require that the control unit proceed through the memory contents sequentially from the beginning, until the desired address is reached. Tape devices (described below) are examples of sequential devices. Even though the control unit can go directly to the desired address, a finite time is required to read the contents of a memory location or to write a value into such a location. This time (typically of the order of magnitude of nanoseconds, or 10^{-9} seconds) is important since it affects the overall speed of operation of a given computer.

In general, RAM is *volatile* memory so that its contents are lost when the computer's power is turned off. On some computers a portion of RAM can be designated to be nonvolatile memory. Its contents are preserved by means of a battery. This is of particular value in a portable computer (described later in the chapter).

Cache Memory. Finally, the third type of primary storage is known as cache memory. The speed of this type of memory is generally higher than that of conventional RAM, but its cost is typically higher as well. Cache memory is often used in conjunction with other components in the computer, including the CPU itself as well as disk drives. In all cases, the goal is to achieve higher processing speed by keeping important data or instructions available where it can be read more quickly. While the amount of RAM in today's computers might be in the hundreds of megabytes, the amount of cache memory is more typically in the hundreds of kilobytes.

Secondary Storage

Despite the decreasing cost of primary storage, it is not practical for a computer system to have sufficient primary storage to accommodate all of the information that must be maintained to support the many healthcare information system applications in use today. And, of course, it would be quite inconvenient if this information were to "disappear" when the computers were turned off. What is needed is large capacity, nonvolatile storage media from which desired information can be obtained as necessary. Secondary storage media are designed to meet this need. Several such storage media are available today, and each will be described below.

Magnetic Tape. Magnetic tape is one of the older secondary storage media. Like the tape used in the "reel-to-reel" audio tape recorders, magnetic tape travels from one reel to a second on a *tape drive*, passing over a transducer capable of detecting the sequence of magnetized and nonmagnetized spots on the tape. These spots, typically arranged in nine "tracks" running the length of the tape, correspond to 0's and 1's and can thus store a series of nine-bit binary values representing either data or program instructions. Large amounts of data or programs can be stored on a single reel of tape.

Advantages of magnetic tape include its low cost, relative stability, and large storage capacity. Disadvantages are its relatively slow speed and the fact that tape drives are sequential devices. In order to find a particular piece of information on a tape, one must start reading the tape at the beginning and proceed until the desired information is found. As a result, the use of tape is decreasing, often limited to the archiving of inactive data in "tape libraries." In addition, on small computer systems, tape cassettes are frequently used as a medium for "backing up" (making copies of) other secondary media to protect against the loss of data from these media. These tape backup units have capacities of 800 megabytes or more. A cartridge-based disk drive used on a microcomputer system is shown in Figure 3.3.

Magnetic Disks. The secondary storage medium most widely used today is the magnetic disk. This disk can either be rigid, in which case it is called a *hard disk*, or flexible, in which case it is called a *floppy disk*. In either case, the disk stores data or program information as magnetized spots. The storage capacity of a popular 3.5" floppy disk is 1.44 mb, while hard disk capacities can be in the order of magnitude of gigabytes. (A gigabyte (gb) is equal to 2^{30}, or 1,073,741,820 bytes.) Developments within the field suggest that the capacity of floppy disks could also increase into the gigabyte range.

The disk rotates at a fairly high rate of speed on a *disk drive*. (See Figure 3.4.) By sliding along the diameter of the disk, a transducer can position itself over one of a number of concentric rings called *tracks*. If the surface of the disk is equated to a pie that has been cut into a large number of equal pieces, then each piece of the pie is analogous to a *sector* of the disk. The segment of a particular track that lies within a given sector is known as a *block*. The transducer, called the *read/write head*, can

Figure 3.3   A Tape-Drive Autoloader

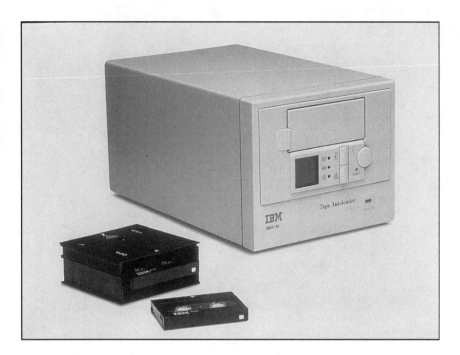

Courtesy of International Business Machines Corporation. Unauthorized use not permitted.

be directed to read data from, or write data to, any desired block. For this reason, disk drives are known as *direct-access storage devices* (DASDs). Figure 3.5 illustrates the typical layout of a disk.

Typically hard disk drives are an integral part of the computer and cannot be removed. Floppy disk drives, on the other hand, are built so that the floppy disk can be removed. There are some hard disk drives that are designed to allow removal of part of the drive from the computer. In this way, the data on these disks can be stored away from the computer and carried from one machine to another. These removable disks are mounted in a cartridge into which the arm holding the read/write head can slide, or, in more expensive removable disk configurations, which contains its own arm and read/write head assembly.

Even though disk drives are direct-access devices, a finite time is required to read or write data. This required time is known as disk access time and typically measures in the millisecond range. Many healthcare information system applications involve frequent interactions with the disk drive so that disk access time becomes an important specification of any hardware system under consideration.

Figure 3.4 A Microcomputer Hard Drive and Floppy Disk

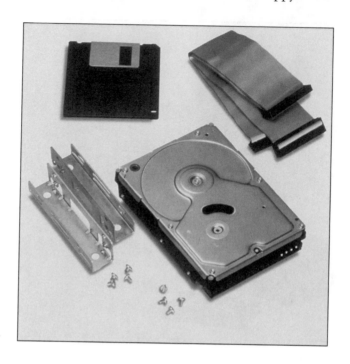

Courtesy of International Business Machines Corporation. Unauthorized use not permitted.

Optical Disks. Optical storage offers the advantage of being able to store a large amount of information on a relatively small disk. An optical disk is a rigid disk of plastic on which crevices have been burned by a special laser. Just as the presence or absence of magnetism can be used to represent 1's or 0's on magnetic disks, so can the presence or absence of a crevice represent a 0 or 1 on an optical disk. Three forms of optical disks are in general use: compact-disk read-only memory (CD-ROM); write-once, read-many (WORM) optical disks; and magneto-optical (MO) disks.

Most personal computers sold today are equipped with a *CD-ROM* drive, capable of reading a CD-ROM disk. (See Figure 3.6.) Millman and Lee (1995) present an easy-to-read overview of CD-ROMs. They indicate that a single CD-ROM disk has a capacity of over 600 megabytes, which is equivalent to more than 400 floppy disks. Since a CD-ROM disk can store up to 300,000 pages of text, it is ideal for storing bibliographic material, journal articles, meeting abstracts, and government reports. In addition to text, color photographs, video clips, animations, stereo

Figure 3.5 Typical Layout of a Disk

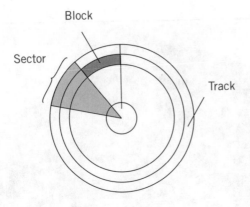

sound, and software are being released in this medium. Schwartz and Lossef (1995) describe an interesting application of these disks in storing radiology images.

Data are stored on CDs differently from magnetic disks. Rather than being arranged in concentric circles, the data form a single track that winds in spiral-fashion from the inside of the disk to its outside. This design results from the fact that CD-ROMs originally were used in audio applications where the "data" on the disk were typically accessed sequentially. In fact, the CD-ROM drives used in computers are capable of "reading" audio-compact disks as well.

Since, as their name indicates, CD-ROMs are read-only devices, data cannot be written to them. Therefore, they are not appropriate for use as a medium for files that are continuously updated to reflect transactions being processed.

One variation of the CD-ROM to which data can be written (only once, however) is the *WORM* disk. Once data have been written to this disk, they cannot be changed, but the data can be read as often as desired. The data are stored in concentric tracks and arranged in sectors like magnetic disks.

WORM disks serve as a cost-effective medium for archiving data, or for providing a backup for a magnetic disk. They have been used along with a variety of other storage media as part of a picture archiving and communication system (PACS), a system used by radiology departments to support the capture, storage, retrieval, distribution, and display of digital images at multiple sites. (Wong et al. 1994) This system archives 1.5 Gbytes (1 Gbyte = 10^9 bytes) of radiologic images daily. The goal was to optimize access time for both current and historical images. Their

Figure 3.6 CD-Rom Drive

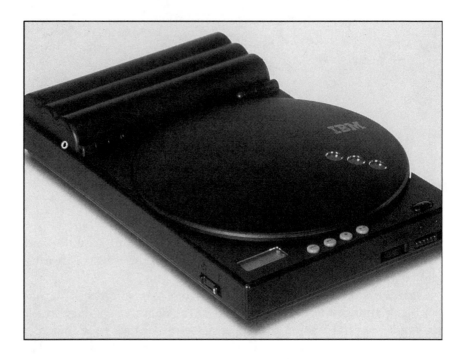

Courtesy of International Business Machines Corporation. Unauthorized use not permitted.

design indicates how the appropriate arrangement of secondary storage devices can be an important design consideration in a PACS system.

Magneto-optical (MO) disks are the third type of optical disks in use today. Sometimes known as erasable optical disks, these devices enjoy the cost and capacity advantages of an optical device while having the ability to have data written to them like magnetic disks. Their capacity can range up to the gigabyte range and, like the WORM disks, data are arranged on them in concentric rings divided into sectors.

The name magneto-optical reflects the fact that a laser is used to heat the alloy coating of the disk to a sufficiently high temperature at which the material responds to magnetism. The data are written by magnetically altering the alloy in one direction or the other. A laser beam can then "read" this direction and determine the presence of a "0" or "1."

Large numbers of MO disks can be aggregated in what is known as an optical jukebox storage system, or simply a jukebox. (See Figure 3.7.) These systems can make large amounts of data available for immediate online access. One system, for example, described by Stanczak (1996)

Figure 3.7 Optical Jukebox Storage System

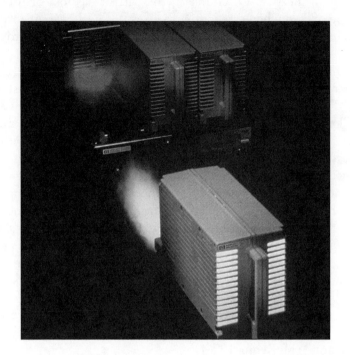

Courtesy of Hewlett-Packard Company.

is capable of providing up to 100 Gbytes of storage, using dual-sided 5.25-inch cartridges.

Optical or *Laser Cards.* Resembling a small plastic credit card, an optical or laser card uses a laser to permanently store data. The data are nonerasable, but new data can be added as appropriate. Optical cards can hold from 4–6 Mbytes of data. They are touted as being capable of storing a variety of inputs including signatures, photographs, x-ray films, and voice. Chatfield (1996) indicates that demand for these cards has been 100,000 in the United States and 75,000 in western Europe. The Defense Logistics Agency successfully used them in the Persian Gulf and in Somalia.

Smart Cards. Like a laser card, a smart card also resembles a plastic credit card. However, in addition to memory, the smart card "contains a central processing unit that has the ability to store and secure information, and 'make decisions,' as required by the card issuer's specific applications needs." (Smart Card Forum 1996) These cards can potentially store an individual's medical record, determine eligibility for specific procedures, and even maintain a cash balance to cover insurance copayments as needed. Of course, if the patient has lost or forgotten either type of card when care is sought, previous healthcare records will be unavailable, and it will not be possible to update the records with new data.

It is interesting to compare the advantages of smart cards relative to optical cards. Chatfield (1996, 613) presents a very interesting summary, stating, "The Smart Card is soon to be the state of the art. The Optical Card will store more computer data for a complete, unalterable medical record . . . and cost/benefit advantage favor the Smart Card now; in time the Optical Card with complete history will demonstrate more advantage."

On the other hand, a number of authors have touted the important role that smart cards can play in improving healthcare delivery, including its role in the emergency department (Quick 1994), its ability to assist in routine communication (Branger and Duisterhout 1995), and its role in protecting medical information in hospitals (Allaert and Dusserre 1994). In fact, interest in this technology is so widespread that a users' group was established in 1993 "to accelerate the widespread acceptance of smart cards that support multiple applications by bringing together in an open environment leading users and technologists from both the public and private sector." (McKenna 1996)

Input Units

The power of an information system can only be realized when data (and programs) have been entered into its storage. The process of entering data into the computer can often be a very time-consuming and costly operation. Fortunately, the field has progressed from the era in which keypunched cards served as the exclusive input medium. The variety of techniques used to input data today are reviewed below.

Keyboards. A common device for entering data into a computer is a keyboard. It resembles a typewriter but has a number of extra keys with special characters or commands. In addition to keys containing the 26 letters of the alphabet, there are ten keys arranged like a calculator for entering the digits zero through nine; several keys for controlling the position of a pointer, or *cursor*, on the display screen (described below); and a set of keys called *function keys* that perform specific operations depending upon the particular software being implemented.

It is interesting to note that many people who spend extended periods of time using a keyboard are experiencing symptoms of physical stress, like carpal tunnel syndrome. As a result ergonomically designed keyboards are available, which divide the keys into two sections and allow each of the user's hands to be held in a more comfortable and natural position.

Comfort aside, the need to use a keyboard is often viewed as a deterrent to potential computer users, especially physicians. As Wyatt (1994, 1610) points out, "Many clinicians resent having to type in their data: although an experienced operator can enter 200 characters a minute with a 4% error rate, most clinicians will reach only 80 (with more errors)." As a result, healthcare executives wanting clinician support for information systems must be sensitive to the type of input media that the system utilizes.

Pointing Devices. The use of pointing devices provides an alternative to typing text into a keyboard. However, these devices can be used for data entry only if the software makes available on the screen a list of data choices known as a *menu*. By pointing to a given choice, the user is able to select that data value for entry into the computer. The several ways of implementing this process are described briefly below.

A common way of pointing to a menu item is to use a handheld device known as a *mouse*. This device has a "ball" on its bottom that rolls along the desk surface as the user moves it. This rolling motion causes the cursor on the screen to move. A special kind of mouse, known as a *rollerball*, is typically integrated into the keyboard of a portable computer. (See Figure 3.8.) When the cursor is pointing to the desired menu item (or in some applications when the selection is "highlighted"), the user can depress a button on the mouse to complete the selection process. The combination of moving the cursor so it points to a menu item and pressing a button to enter the selection is known as "point-and-click" data entry.

A simple application is the selection of a patient whose vital signs are to be entered. By pointing to the correct patient's name and "clicking" on that choice, the nurse can ensure that vital signs will be associated with the correct patient. Of course it might be necessary to use the keyboard in order to enter the actual value of the vital sign. To avoid the need for typing, some software designers create a menu consisting of the digits from 0 to 9 along with a decimal point. Thus, a temperature of 99.3 would be entered by "clicking" on the 9, followed by the 9 again, followed by a decimal point, followed by a 3. It remains for a prospective purchaser to decide the comparative advantage of this approach relative to simply typing the value "99.3" directly into a keyboard.

Rather than using a mouse to move a cursor to a desired menu item, two alternative methods can be employed. The first method requires that the video display monitor be sensitive to the presence of a finger or other

Figure 3.8 Keyboard and Rollerball on a Portable Computer

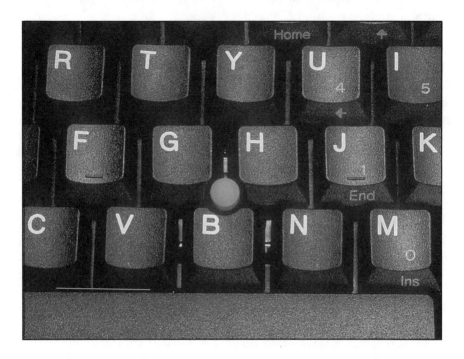

Courtesy of International Business Machines Corporation. Unauthorized use not permitted.

pointer on the surface of the screen. Called a *touch screen*, this monitor allows data to be entered into the computer by simply pointing to the desired choice. The computer actually detects the location being chosen by using infrared light beams that "shine" across the screen surface in a checkerboard fashion. The user's finger interrupts the beams in both the "horizontal" as well as the "vertical" direction, allowing the computer to pinpoint where the user is pointing.

Touch screens are found in a wide range of applications, from locating the aisle where a given item can be found in a supermarket to choosing descriptions of items of interest to a visitor in a museum. One interesting application is a community-based touch-screen public-access health information system in Scotland. (Jones, Navin, and Murray 1993) The touch screen units, located at various community and health service sites, make accessing the information quite easy. Hawley, Cudd, and Cherry (1994) describe a computer-based control system to assist children with severe physical disabilities. A variety of input devices is included in the system including a touch screen. The system can be tailored to the user's requirements and helps the child carry out fundamental everyday tasks.

Some users might experience difficulty in pointing to the exact spot on the screen that they wish to select. A second alternative pointing method, the *light pen*, overcomes this difficulty. The user points the light pen at the spot on the screen containing the desired data selection. The position of the pen is determined by the photodetector built into the pen, which responds to the light being emitted by the screen. Again, the capability to support the use of a light pen must be built into the software system that the user wants to run. Light pens have been part of clinical information systems, (see Figure 11.2), and are also being found in some of the office-based electronic medical record systems being released. These systems are discussed later in this book.

Scanning Devices. Healthcare information systems utilize a variety of scanning devices to input data. These devices are designed to scan the assortment of source documents generated within healthcare organizations: documents containing specially designed characters or codes; special forms such as questionnaires or evaluation sheets; and documents containing text and/or graphics. Each is discussed below.

Printed labels containing sets of vertical black/white bars can be "read" by a *bar-code scanner*. Each bar-code pattern denotes a different character. (See Figure 3.9.) Many types of bar-code printers may be used to print bar codes for pharmacy prescription dispensing and inventory, laboratory tests, equipment inventory, medical records, and other areas. The scanning itself may be performed using a bar-code wand connected to a computer with an interface cable or a wireless handheld unit, containing a wand or built-in gun-type scanner, which transmits data to a central computer.

Willard and Shanholtzer (1995) describe an implementation of bar-code scanning in their microbiology laboratory. They indicate three key roles that bar codes can play in such a setting: labeling of specimens; labeling of internal worksheets to link subspecimens back to the primary specimen; and the use of bar-code "scripts" to reduce keyboard data entry. Their article provides an excellent overview of bar-code scanning.

In a desire to assess customer satisfaction and the quality of the care being provided, healthcare organizations are utilizing increasing numbers of questionnaires and evaluation instruments. Inputting the data from these documents can be time-consuming. *Optical mark readers* can be used if the documents have been designed as "multiple-choice" questions on which the respondent shades a box adjacent to his or her response.

Figure 3.9 Specimens with Bar-Code Labels in an Automated Laboratory System

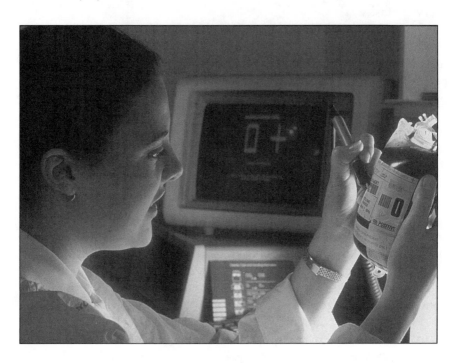

Courtesy of International Business Machines Corporation. Unauthorized use not permitted.

Finally, *optical scanners* can be used to enter a variety of source documents containing both text and graphics. Their role is to "turn documents, illustrations, and photographs into patterns of tiny dots that can be stored, edited, or transmitted electronically." (Himowitz 1996, 183) Several types of scanners are available. The flatbed scanner looks and functions like a desktop personal photocopier. Page-feed models are about the size of a rolled-up newspaper. The source document is slid through the unit. They carry a relatively low price and are generally available only in black and white. Even smaller are handheld scanners, which are passed over the page to be entered.

Himowitz (1996) explains the scanner characteristics that are important to the prospective purchaser. "Optical" resolution, measured in dots per inch, indicates how detailed an image the scanner can produce. "Gray scale levels" denotes the number of levels of gray that a black-and-white scanner can distinguish. Similarly, "bit depth" is related to the number of colors distinguishable by a color scanner. The bit-depth value is the exponent to which two must be raised to obtain the actual number of colors that the scanner can handle. Thus, a 24-bit scanner can distinguish 2^{24}, or more than 16 million colors.

It is important to remember that scanners are hardware devices that convert source documents into "tiny dots" (called pixels). Even text characters are converted into pixels, so the computer cannot recognize individual letters or words. This picture of the original page can be viewed and stored, but, because it lacks structure, it cannot be manipulated. What is needed is software that converts text into a structured form that can be processed or graphics into a form that can be altered. The subject of software is discussed in the next chapter.

Areas where optical scanners may be useful in healthcare settings are varied. Text material like a radiology report or consultant's evaluation can be added to the patient record without the time-consuming process of keypunching. Graphical material like EKG traces can also be incorporated into the computerized record and thus be conveniently accessible to a clinician. In the administrative areas, scanning documents that are only available as "hard copy" can potentially avoid large amounts of word processing. Xakellis, Gjerde, and Emerson (1994) describe the use of optical scanning in a family medicine teaching program. Optically scannable forms replace the 1,000 manually processed evaluation forms as the input to the process of generating a series of administrative reports. Reports are generated in a more timely fashion and at a lower cost.

Handwriting Recognition Devices. A *pen-based computer* allows a user to input data by touching or writing on its pressure sensitive screen. (See Figure 3.10.) Known also as a tablet, notebook, notepad, or palm-top computer, the popularity of this device "has 'taken off' in the field of health-care. The pen strokes, in some cases, can be converted to text or retained as original handwriting, . . . Typical yes/no statements and vital signs can be easily recorded and then transferred into either digital or paper medical records." (Guiannulli 1996, 369)

Retention of the original handwriting is appropriate, for example, if the desire is to maintain a record of the physician's signature on an order. However, frequently the objective is to translate handwritten entries into recognizable text. "Many experts say handwriting recognition still has a way to go before it is reliable. In fact, some doubt whether it will ever approach the reliability needed in medicine, where mistaking a '1' for a '7' could be disastrous." (Bunschoten and Deming 1995, 54) On the positive side, however, is the fact that in many cases the software provides a list of menu choices. In this case, the pen is not used for writing but rather as a pointing device to touch the screen to indicate the desired selection from the menu.

Figure 3.10 Typical Pen-Based Computer

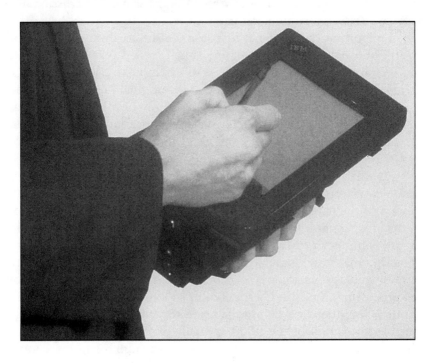

Courtesy of International Business Machines Corporation. Unauthorized use not permitted.

Despite the fact that refinements still need to be made in handwriting recognition devices, "compared to keyboard-based systems, pen-based systems are easier to use and more intuitive in their form and function. If designed properly, many older physicians feel that they are significantly less intimidating." (Guiannulli 1996, 372)

Voice Input. Many people would define voice input as the ultimate computer input medium. For what could be easier than simply "telling" the computer what operations you wish it to perform and then "dictating" the input data you want the instructions to operate on. Certainly practitioners who have refused to use "conventional" input media would have difficulty finding a basis for criticism of voice input techniques. "As a matter of fact, speech technology has some of the greatest potential for success in the health care market. However, it also has some of the greatest obstacles to overcome in order to become a standard application means." (Clark 1996, 460)

Like handwriting recognition, voice input has several levels of implementation. Devices capable of voice input are designed to change sound waves into digitized data that can simply be stored and later replayed. While the data can be modified in order to change its sound, no interpretation or translation of the data is possible. By contrast, *voice recognition* is the "machine processing of speech to extract its content." (Clark 1996, 461) Other levels that Clark (1996) defines are speech-to-text transcription; voice control, which permits voice commands to control action or function of a device; and speaker recognition, which allows identification of the speaker based upon previous examples of speech.

In summary then, "The technology of voice recognition is finally overcoming some early limitations that required users to speak haltingly and to use a tightly restricted vocabulary. However it still has a long way to go, experts say. Eventually, it may be possible for clinicians to enter and receive information without touching a computer." (Bunschoten and Deming 1995, 54)

Output Units

An important objective of information systems is to produce output of value to the user. Types of output that are of particular value to healthcare executives include visual displays, printed output, and voice output.

Visual Displays. The oldest and still most widely used form of displaying output from an information system is a *video display terminal* (VDT). Typically called a "monitor," the VDT has evolved from the small monochrome screens commonly used just a few short years ago. Although it resembles a television screen, a VDT is generally designed to display a much sharper, detailed image. Its text display is typically 80 columns by 24 rows.

Two important characteristics associated with a VDT are screen size and resolution. The screen size is usually measured in inches diagonally across the screen. Resolution indicates the quality or clarity of the display. It is measured in units of *pixels*, individual dots that can be illuminated to help form a particular character or graphical pattern. Higher resolution monitors present images that have greater detail and accuracy and are important in applications such as radiology systems. "Once you've experienced a big screen, it's really hard to return to a 15-inch box. Becoming less of a luxury, a 21-inch monitor can support 1600- by 1200-pixel resolutions, . . . Power users will appreciate running multiple applications on the desktop . . . and heavy-duty spreadsheet junkies absolutely require a large, high-resolution tube for mission-critical work." (Mysore 1996, 116)

A second visual display is the *liquid crystal display* (LCD). Using what is known as flat-panel technology, this display consists of a "sandwich" of fluorescent light, filters, liquid crystal cells, and a glass plate.

Monochrome displays have a single liquid crystal cell for each pixel while color displays have three cells for each pixel. Signals from the computer are applied to cells, which in turn affect the polarization of the fluorescent light. One of the filters then affects the brightness of the light reaching the glass plate. Howard (1992) presents more details on this technology.

Two types of color LCD screens are available—active matrix display and passive matrix display. The difference lies in the number of transistors used to apply a charge to the cells. Active matrix displays utilize many more transistors, thus charging each cell repetitively and achieving a brighter picture. Of course, active matrix displays are more expensive than passive matrix displays.

The flat-panel technology can also be implemented in a device that can be placed on the glass of an overhead projector. In this way, computer output can be projected on a screen and incorporated into presentations. Projectors that combine the features of an overhead projector and LCD panel are also available.

Printed Output. Printers, too, have developed extensively from the early devices used to create "hard" output. These devices were quite similar to typewriters, using raised characters that impacted the paper through an inked ribbon. Because they were capable of only printing those raised characters that comprised their "character set," they were unable to print graphics. Today, healthcare executives will generally encounter one of three printing technologies: dot matrix, inkjet, or laser printers. In addition, when shopping for a printer to be used with a portable computer, the executive may encounter thermal printers.

Dot matrix printers are also known as impact printers because they contain a print head that impacts the paper in order to produce the printed output. Early print heads contained nine pins, but today's dot matrix printers generally contain 24 pins. The print head is capable of sliding horizontally across the page. As it slides, electromagnets control whether a given pin strikes the paper through an inked ribbon. Electronics within the computer control the movement of the print head and the individual pins.

After a row has been printed, the paper is advanced vertically and printing continues onto the next row. In this way the contents of an entire page can be printed. The paper used with dot matrix printers consists of a continuous roll of pages joined together with "perforations." After a given document has been printed, these pages can be separated into a completed stack of output. The sophistication of the computer's electronics greatly influences the quality of the output, including the high-quality graphics that can now be achieved with dot matrix printers. Although several inked ribbons can theoretically be combined to print color output, dot matrix printers are generally not used for color applications.

In the past, dot matrix printers were a popular choice because they had a lower purchase price and generally lower maintenance costs. Today, however, the cost of competing technology is comparable, maintenance is less of a problem, and the noise associated with dot matrix printers can be a problem in many healthcare settings. As a result, other types of printers are being increasingly used.

Inkjet printers are similar mechanically to dot matrix printers. Instead of a print head, however, an inkjet printer contains a print cartridge. As the cartridge slides across the page, ink is sprayed from a reservoir through very small nozzles, which produces dots on the page. Once a row has been printed, the paper moves vertically so the next row can be printed. Single-sheet plain paper is used in these printers. When a page has been completed, it is mechanically moved "out of the way" and allowed to dry, and a new blank page is positioned for printing.

Black-and-white printers have a single reservoir of black ink, whereas color printers have three ink reservoirs. The quality of color printing that can be achieved with an inkjet printer is quite good, particularly in view of their very reasonable cost.

Laser printers are becoming the most popular type of printers in use today. The quality of laser printer output is quite high, and color laser printers are available that can produce copies of sufficient quality to be used in reproducing artwork.

Purchasers of laser printers should be aware of several of their characteristics. First is the size of the printer's memory, where pixel information is stored in preparation for pages to be printed. Graphical images can quickly exhaust the memory capacity and result in a "Memory Overflow" error message. Memory capacities can range from a standard of 2 Mbytes to 80 Mbytes or more. Second is resolution, which is a measure of the print quality. Higher resolution requires more memory and slows down the printing. Standard resolution is now 600 dots per inch, but can range up to 1,200 dots per inch or more. Finally, print speed is also of importance. This can range from 4 to 12 pages per minute for printers typically used with microcomputers. In large volume, mainframe settings, one can find laser printers capable of printing more than 100 pages per minute. Poor (1996) reviews 11 laser printers that are designed for use in a computer network.

The technology of laser printers is quite similar to that of photocopying, except that the image source is information in the computer controlling a laser rather than an original hard copy, bright light, and mirrors. In both systems, however, a photosensitive drum becomes electrically charged wherever a dot is to be printed, and a black powder, known as toner, sticks to those electrically charged locations. A sheet of paper, given the opposite charge, is fed over the drum and picks up the toner from the drum. A heating process, known as fusing, causes the toner to stick permanently to the paper and produces a finished copy.

Portable printers, used in conjunction with portable computers allow the traveling executive to produce printed copies of computer work performed "on the road." Three technologies are typically employed in portable printers: inkjet, which works like the desk-model version; thermal transfer printers, which use heat and pressure to transfer images from a ribbon to paper; and thermal printers, which operate like the old-style fax machine by heating images on special heat-sensitive paper. (Lee 1996, 21a)

Voice Output. A potentially useful form of computer output for healthcare applications is voice output. Here the digital text of the computer's memory is converted to understandable speech by means of a process known as voice synthesis. The sounds that comprise the words and phrases of speech are assembled electronically using basic sound components. A major objective is to create an output that sounds natural and pleasant rather than synthetic and robot-like. Available hardware works moderately well at very reasonable prices.

A potential application for voice output in a healthcare setting would involve situations where clinicians want to use an ordinary telephone to obtain information stored within the information system. For example, laboratory systems typically create output records within the computer containing the results of a particular test. A physician needing those results could use a telephone to "call" the laboratory system and hear the results "read" by a voice synthesizer. The financial community uses similar technology to supply account balances to its customers at any time that they might call into the system.

Poole and Millman (1995) describe an electronic reading machine that converts printed text to electronic speech. This machine utilizes text scanning as an input modality along with voice synthesis as an output. A comprehensive overview of text-to-speech techniques is presented in a two-part publication by Edgington et al. (1996a, 1996b). The authors focus on linguistic analysis as the basis for identifying important features of text that need to be incorporated into speech synthesis to make the result sound natural and intelligible.

Classes of Computers

Until recently it was not very difficult to construct a classification of computers based upon their capabilities. Large, expensive, mainframe systems were clearly more powerful than small, less expensive PCs. The categories of computers were relatively easy to define. Today, however, the picture is somewhat blurred. Most healthcare executives have laptop computers that have more capabilities than the computers that ran their organization's financial systems just a few years ago. Nevertheless, the classification paradigm persists, and the industry continues to use the terms "supercomputers," "mainframes," "minicomputers," "workstations," and "personal computers." The meaning of these terms is reviewed next.

Supercomputers

By definition, the class of computers known as supercomputers have more processing power than other computers available. Typically these machines are used in military and scientific applications. Their strength lies in their ability to perform a large number of complex calculations with considerable speed. This performance is achieved in two ways. First, the processors themselves are quite fast. But in addition, many processors are linked together into a *parallel processing* configuration. This means that the problem being solved is broken down into a number of smaller parts, and each part is solved by a different processor. Special consideration must be given to the software design in order to take full advantage of the power of these parallel processors.

The rapid pace of development in the supercomputer area is demonstrated by a front-page newspaper article that announced IBM's plans to build a computer designed to work 300 times faster than any existing machine. (Anonymous 1996) This new computer is able to perform 3 trillion operations per second and has a memory of 2.5 trillion bytes. The computer manufacturer indicates that the most advanced existing machines have only 10 billion bytes. An understanding of the speed of this supercomputer can be gained from an analogy presented in the article. If one equates home computers to the current world record of nine seconds for the 100-meter dash, then the newly announced computer could run from New York to Philadelphia in the same nine seconds.

Mainframe Computers

Healthcare information processing has historically been performed on large mainframe computer processors, centrally located and under the tight control of the Data Processing Department. These machines are characterized by their large size, fast processing speed, primary storage of several hundred megabytes, online secondary storage in the order of magnitude of billions of bytes, and large magnetic tapes used for off-line secondary storage.

Originally, mainframe computers typically were stand-alone processors, usually with only dumb terminals connected. (A dumb terminal has a keyboard and screen but no processing capability.) However, stand-alone systems have frequently not been able to keep up with the large volume of data processing needed by more and more data end-users and by more sophisticated software systems. Many mainframe systems, therefore, now use shared processing techniques to increase computing power and data transfer.

Shared configurations include processor clusters, front-end processors, and networks with microcomputers and workstations. *Processor clusters* can greatly increase processing power without a great increase in cost. Clusters consist of several CPUs that share the processing load. The Information Services (IS) manager can use operating system software to perform load balancing so that no one processor is slowed down too much.

Front-end processors typically are small minicomputer processors or powerful microcomputers that can perform selected processing tasks or share general computing with the mainframe processor, thus taking a large part of the processing load off the main CPU. Often these specialized computers manage all of the routine communications with peripheral devices.

Mainframes are also being configured in *networks* with minicomputers and microcomputers. The configuration of these networks and the role that mainframe computers play in their operation is discussed in Chapter 5.

The long-term future of mainframe computers is an interesting topic of speculation and discussion. Many people have predicted the demise of this hardware and are frankly surprised at its persistence. Alsop (1996, 114) shares three interesting observations that help to explain the continued interest in mainframe computers. First, "personal computers aren't interesting anymore." People are focusing "on how to make their information systems work," and not "whether their PC runs at 150 or 160 MHz." Second, "centralization has some benefits." Thus, people are beginning to realize that the corporation needs to be a "mixture of central resources and highly developed systems." And finally, "IS departments are still at war with users." The shift to heavy PC usage did not make the relationships between the user and the IS department any smoother.

In addition, it is always important to bear in mind that the value of a piece of hardware is ultimately its ability to allow some application to be processed. Many software packages today are still only available on mainframes. Thus, so long as a program is available and supported by its vendor for processing on a mainframe computer, one can build a strong case for continuing its use.

What, then, should be the healthcare executive's position on the organization's mainframe computer? As Grochow (1996, E12) so appropriately indicates, "It is getting less and less likely that anyone wants to develop a brand new 'from scratch' system on a mainframe. . . . On the other hand, there are lots of mainframe applications that are going to be upgraded over the next several years, and keeping parts of them on that box will still be a viable option."

Minicomputers

Minicomputers have a physical size and computing capability between the mainframe and the microcomputer (although the continuum of computing power is increasingly blurred). In addition to their role as front-end processors to mainframe computers or as part of a network with mainframes, minicomputers are often used as stand-alone systems. Several integrated software systems (discussed in more detail in the next chapter) have been designed to run on a minicomputer and are targeted specifically for small to medium-size healthcare institutions.

Even in large health services organizations, minicomputer systems are used for specific processing tasks that can be performed separately from the main processor, thus alleviating the main data processing load. The minicomputer system may still be networked to the mainframe if needed.

Minicomputers have been used in a variety of applications within healthcare settings. Wagener and Pridlides (1993) describe a tool that assists radiology managers to obtain the necessary data to plan equipment replacement and facility project renovation. Hohnloser et al. (1994) have built a cytology report database. From terminals connected to the central minicomputer pathological findings can be entered and subsequently made available to all of the wards within the hospital. Claxton et al. (1995) have used both a personal computer as well as a minicomputer to support the collection, organization, and analysis of microbial mutagenicity data generated in the laboratory while also supporting a quality assurance program. Tabular and graphical summaries of the data are available and specialized statistical analyses can be performed.

Workstations

The term "workstation" is generally used to refer to a high-end microcomputer with a large amount of primary storage, a fast processor, high-resolution graphics capability, and in many cases a CD-ROM drive and sound card. Initially, these machines were targeted at the engineering, design, and technical communities. Today, however, workstations are used in a variety of application settings, including the healthcare environment.

Radiology Imaging Units. High-resolution workstations connected to imaging equipment support the recording, storage, and retrieval of patient x-rays by radiologists and technicians. These systems generally have very large amounts of disk storage so x-ray images can be kept for a certain period of time, and they may be connected to a mainframe computer to allow incorporation of the images into electronic patient files for permanent storage. Interestingly, Steckel et al. (1995) demonstrated that in some cases no significant clinical information is lost with the use of lower resolution equipment.

Patient Monitoring Units. These mobile or stationary bedside workstations are typically found in intensive care units (ICUs) of hospitals. They have very high resolution graphics capabilities for display of heart rate, blood pressure, respiration, and other patient data collected at each bedside unit. Friesdorf et al. (1994) describe a research workstation in an ICU that they designed and built. They were able to evaluate data/information processing and presentation concepts as well as a variety of new devices and functions.

Simulation. The computing power of workstations enables them to be an important component of a simulation tool. For example, a surgical workstation is part of a virtual reality simulator designed to re-create the human abdomen with several essential organs. (Satava 1995) The system includes a helmet-mounted display and DataGlove and allows the user to practice surgical procedures with a scalpel and clamps. Sinclair et al. (1995) describe an eye surgery simulator that uses a high-speed graphics workstation, a stereo operating system, a wrist rest, and a position-tracking stylus connected to force feedback motors. The object is to allow ophthalmic surgeons of all experience levels to enhance their surgical skills. The advantage, of course, is that the surgeons can achieve a satisfactory level of proficiency before performing a procedure on an actual patient.

Personal Computers

Technological advances in PCs have caused the distinction between them and workstations to become quite blurred. As a result, many healthcare applications are currently being performed on PCs, either in a "stand-alone" mode or in a distributed processing configuration. (See Chapter 5 for details.) The processor in a personal computer typically consists of a single electronic chip known as a microchip. Therefore, PCs are also called microcomputers and are characterized by relatively low-cost, small-size, and easy-to-maintain hardware components.

From its initial function of helping managers perform analyses of the raw data contained in printed reports, the microcomputer has evolved into a powerful platform for significant information processing in health-care settings. Microcomputers support the analysis of clinical data in research studies, help managers make strategic decisions, support major clinical systems, provide the computing power for medical office finan-cial systems, and provide word-processing capability for manager and secretary alike. The list of applications seems almost endless. In fact, in some cases microcomputers can provide the computing power for the entire healthcare organization. (Glaser et al. 1991)

Smaller versions of microcomputers are gaining popularity in the healthcare setting. These include laptop computers (about the size of a small briefcase), notebook computers (about the size of a small three-ring binder), and palmtop computers (able to be held and operated in a single hand). Runion (1995) describes the use of a laptop computer in the examining room to capture computer-generated notes. Yamamoto (1995) has studied the feasibility of using a pocket cellular phone and a notebook computer to obtain immediate access to consultants at any location. Benefits cited were the expediting of therapy decisions in questionable cases and reduction of operating room preparation times in severe head trauma. Palmtop computers are described as an ideal platform to main-tain communication between busy physicians and medical information systems. (Ram and Block 1993) The authors indicate that physicians can access information in the hospital information system as well as the Family Health Center's ambulatory medical record system.

Summary

Computer hardware spans a broad spectrum, from small palmtop com-puters that can be held in one hand to extremely large and powerful supercomputers. No matter where on the spectrum a given system lies, it is comprised of five basic components: a CPU; primary storage; sec-ondary storage; input units; and output units. The CPU is the "brains" of the computer and its speed and power greatly influence the computer's capabilities. The capacity and speed of the primary storage also impact the computer system's performance, and fortunately the cost of this component is generally falling.

Secondary storage devices include a variety of disk and tape units and are designed to maintain the large quantities of data common to healthcare applications. Optical storage is becoming more prevalent and will likely become increasingly important. The speed with which data are entered into and retrieved from secondary storage devices is also an important specification within the overall system.

A number of peripheral devices are available to facilitate the process of entering data into the computer in a variety of formats, including keyboard entry, scanning, and voice input. Similarly, data can be obtained from the computer on a display screen, in printed form, magnetically for future processing, or in spoken form. The goal of the industry is to make data entry and retrieval as simple as possible.

Computer hardware technology changes at such a rapid pace that it is difficult for even the information systems specialist to keep up, let alone the healthcare executive. Like any other investment decision, consideration must be given to the size and power of the computer that is appropriate for a given application. Nevertheless, the hardware fundamentals discussed in this chapter are designed to make the executive feel comfortable participating in the planning, implementation, and evaluation of new hardware systems.

Discussion Questions

3.1 Name each of the five components of a computer system and indicate the function of each.

3.2 Give a brief description of three secondary storage media.

3.3 Discuss the relative advantage of using a pointing device to enter a patient's vital signs compared to simply typing in the values using a keyboard.

3.4 Suggest how the use of a patient ID bracelet containing a bar-code representation of the patient's ID and a bar-code scanner can lead to improved quality of care in a hospital.

3.5 Explain the difference between devices capable of voice input and voice recognition.

3.6 Explain what is meant by the resolution of a video display terminal, and indicate applications where high resolution is quite important.

3.7 Name three types of printers and briefly explain the major characteristics of each.

3.8 Give a brief description of three applications of workstations.

Problems

3.1 Interview the chief information officer in a medical center of your choice to obtain a list of their currently installed computer hardware and the applications running on each hardware platform. Determine the rationale for their allocation of applications to each hardware platform.

3.2 Design and administer a survey to a group of physicians in order to identify their attitudes toward the various types of input devices. In particular, determine the extent to which the need to type data serves as an impediment to their use of information systems.

3.3 Assume that a large multispecialty physician group is considering scanning reports and letters from consultants into their patients' electronic medical record. Obtain vendor data on document scanners including performance, price, and staffing information. Make a recommendation as to whether they should indeed scan these documents or maintain a separate paper chart.

3.4 Using the literature as well as vendors as sources of information, determine the feasibility of using optical storage devices as a backup medium for an electronic medical record system.

3.5 Choose a sample of patients utilizing a clinic in an institution to which you have access. Conduct a survey of these patients to determine their attitude toward the use of a palmtop computer to enter data during a patient visit.

References

Allaert, F. A., and L. Dusserre. 1994. "Security of Health Information System in France: What We Do Will No Longer Be Different from What We Tell." *International Journal of Bio-Medical Computing* 35 (Supplement): 201–4.

Alsop, S. 1996. "Five Years Later, We're Still Waiting for the Unplugging of the Last Mainframe." *InfoWorld* 18 (11): 114.

Anonymous, 1996, "New Computer to Be Fastest in World," *St. Louis Post Dispatch* 118 (209): 1a, 5a.

Branger, P. J., and J. S. Duisterhout. 1995. "Communication in Health Care." *Methods of Information in Medicine* 34 (3): 244–52.

Bunschoten, B., and B. Deming. 1995. "Hardware Issues in the Movement to Computer-Based Patient Records." *Health Data Management* 3 (2): 45–8, 50, 54.

Chatfield, J. N. 1996. "Marketing an HMO by 'Smart' ID Cards with Patient History on an Electronic Medical Record." In *Proceedings: Toward an Electronic Patient Record '96*. 12th International Symposium on the Creation of Electronic Health Record System and Global Conference on Patient Cards. May 11–18: 608–20.

Clark, M. 1996. "Fully Integrated Hybrid Speech and Dictation Technology and Its Effect on Provider Use." In *Proceedings: Toward an Electronic Patient Record '96*. 12th International Symposium on the Creation of Electronic Health Record System and Global Conference on Patient Cards. May 11–18: 460–66.

Claxton, L. D., J. Creason, J. A. Nader, W. Poteat, and J. D. Orr. 1995. "GeneTox Manager for Bacterial Mutagenicity Assays: A Personal Computer and Minicomputer System." *Mutation Research* 342 (1–2): 87–94.

Edgington, M., A. Lowry, P. Jackson, A. P. Breen, and S. Minnis. 1996a. "Overview of Current Text-to-Speech Techniques: Part I—Text and Linguistic Analysis." *BT Technology Journal* 14 (1): 68–83.

————. 1996b. "Overview of Current Text-to-Speech Techniques: Part II—Prosody and Speech Generation." *BT Technology Journal* 14 (1): 84–99.

Frankenfeld, F. M. 1993. "Basics of Computer Hardware and Software." *American Journal of Hospital Pharmacy* 50 (4): 717–24.

Friesdorf, W., F. Gross-Alltag, S. Konichezky, B. Schwilk, A. Fattroth, and P. Fett. 1994. "Lessons Learned While Building an Integrated ICU Workstation." *International Journal of Clinical Monitoring and Computing* 11 (2): 89–97.

Glaser, J. P., R. F. Beckley 3d., P. Roberts, J. K. Marra, F. L. Hiltz, and J. Hurley. 1991. "A Very Large PC LAN As the Basis for a Hospital Information System." *Journal of Medical Systems* 15 (2): 133–37.

Grochow, J. M. 1996. "The Reincarnation of the Mainframe." *PC Week* 13 (14): E12.

Guiannulli, T. 1996. "Mobile Point of Care Computing." In *Proceedings: Toward an Electronic Patient Record '96*. 12th International Symposium on the Creation of Electronic Health Record System and Global Conference on Patient Cards. May 11–18: 368–73.

Hawley, M. S., P. A. Cudd, and A. D. Cherry. 1994. "Implementation of a PC-Based Integrated Control System for Children." *Medical Engineering and Physics* 16 (3): 237–42.

Himowitz, M. J. 1996. "A Cure for Too Much Paper." *Fortune* 133 (9): 183–84.

Hohnloser, J. H., A. Konig, M. R. Fischer, B. Hertenstein, and B. Emmerich. 1994. "Building a Cytology Report Database: A Computer-Assisted System for Documentation, Evaluation and Hospital-Wide Recall of Haematological Biopsy Reports." *Medical Informatics* 19 (3): 199–208.

Howard, W. E. 1992. "Thin-Film-Transistor/Liquid Crystal Display Technology—An Introduction." *IBM Journal of Research and Development* 36 (January): 3–10.

Jones, R. B., L. M. Navin, and K. J. Murray. 1993. "Use of a Community-Based Touch-Screen Public-Access Health Information System." *Health Bulletin* 51 (1): 34–42.

Lee, M. Y. 1996. "Portable Printers Necessary for Traveling Businesspeople." *St. Louis Business Journal* 16 (39): 21a.

McKenna, J. 1996. Letter from the President. Internet Homepage—http://www.smart crd.com/info/more/letter.html.

Millman, A., and N. Lee. 1995. "ABC of Medical Computing: CD ROMS, MULTI-MEDIA, and OPTICAL STORAGE SYSTEMS." *British Medical Journal* 311 (7006): 675–78.

Mysore, C. 1996. "Lab Report: 20 Big-Picture Monitors." *Byte* 21 (1): 116–18, 125–26, 128, 128a.

Poole, C. J. M., and A. Millman. 1995. "ABC of Medical Computing: Adaptive Computer Technology." *British Medical Journal* 311 (7013): 1149–51.

Poor, A. 1996. "Share and Share A Lot." *PC Magazine* 15 (11): 185–87, 191–94, 196, 198–200, 204, 208–10, 212, 215, 219.

Prosise, J. 1995. "RISC vs. CISC: The Real Story." *PC Magazine* 14 (18): 247–48, 50.

Quick, G. 1994. "Introduction to Smart Card Technology and Initial Medical Application." *Journal—Oklahoma State Medical Association* 87 (10): 454–57.

Ram, R., and B. Block. 1993. "Development of a Portable Information System: Connecting Palmtop Computers with Medical Records Systems and Clinical Reference Resources." *Proceedings of the Annual Symposium on Computer Applications in Medical Care:*125–28.

Rosen, S. 1969. "Electronic Computers: A Historical Survey." *Computing Surveys* 1 (1): 7–36.

Runion, H. J. 1995. "Using a Laptop Computer to Improve Clinical Performance." *Physician Assistant* 19 (1): 79–84.

Satava, R. M. 1995. "Medical Applications of Virtual Reality." *Journal of Medical Systems* 19 (3): 275–80.

Schwartz, L. H., and S. V. Lossef. 1995. "A Low-Cost CD-ROM–Based Image Archival System." *Radiographics* 15 (1): 151–54.

Sinclair, M. J., J. W. Peifer, R. Haleblian, M. N. Luxenberg, K. Green, and D. S. Hull. 1995. "Computer-Simulated Eye Surgery. A Novel Teaching Method for Residents and Practitioners." *Ophthalmology* 102 (3): 517–21.

Slater, M. 1996. "Beyond the Pentium." *PC Magazine* 15 (10): 100–2, 106–7, 110–13.

Smart Card Forum. 1996. "What Is a Smartcard?" Internet Homepage—http://www. smartcrd.com/info/what is/whatis.html.

Stanczak, M. 1996. "HP Eases Storage Indigestion—SureStore Archive Server Offers Plug-and-Play Archiving." *PC Week* 13 (5): N7, N11, N23.

Steckel, R. J., P. Batra, S. Johnson, J. Sayre, K. Brown, K. Haker, D. Young, and M. Zucker. 1995. "Comparison of Hard- and Soft-Copy Digital Chest Images With Different Matrix Sizes for Managing Coronary Care Unit Patients." *AJR. American Journal of Roentgenology* 164 (4): 837–41.

Wagener, G. N., and A. J. Pridlides. 1993. "Radiology Capital Asset Management." *Journal of Clinical Engineering* 18 (5): 419–23.

Willard, K. E., and C. J. Shanholtzer. 1995. "User Interface Reengineering: Innovative Applications of Bar Coding in a Clinical Microbiology Laboratory." *Archives of Pathology and Laboratory Medicine* 119 (8): 706–12.

Wong, A. W., H. K. Huang, R. L. Arenson, and J. K. Lee. 1994. "Digital Archive System For Radiologic Images." *Radiographics* 14 (5): 1119–26.

Wyatt, J. C. 1994. "Clinical Data Systems, Part 2: Components and Techniques." *Lancet* 344 (8937): 1609–14.

Xakellis, G. C., C. L. Gjerde, and M. Emerson. 1994. "Using an Optical Scanner and Data Base Program to Manage a Family Medicine Teaching Program." *Family Medicine* 26 (7): 421–24.

Yager, T. 1996. "Bringing Benchmarks up to SPEC." *Byte* 21 (3): 145–46.

Yamamoto, L. G. 1995. "Wireless Teleradiology and Fax Using Cellular Phones and Notebook PCs for Instant Access to Consultants." *American Journal of Emergency Medicine* 13 (2): 184–87.

Additional Readings

Adebonojo, L. G. 1994. "Clinical Department Use of Three CD-ROM Databases: A Case Study." *Bulletin of the Medical Library Association* 82 (3): 318–20.

Englander, I. 1996. *The Architecture of Computer Hardware and Systems Software*. New York: John Wiley and Sons.

Grasso, M. A. 1995. "Automated Speech Recognition in Medical Applications." *M.D. Computing* 12 (1): 16–23.

Haber, S. L. 1995. "CD-ROM: An On-Ramp to the Information Superhighway." *MLO: Medical Laboratory Observer* 27 (1): 20–22.

Hammer, J. S., J. J. Strain, A. Friedberg, and G. Fulop. 1995. "Operationalizing a Bedside Pen Entry Notebook Clinical Database System in Consultation-Liaison Psychiatry." *General Hospital Psychiatry* 17 (3): 165–72.

Kühnel, E., G. Klepser, and R. Engelbrecht. 1994. "Smart Cards and Their Opportunities for Controlling Health Information Systems." *International Journal of Bio-Medical Computing* 35 (Supplement 1): 153–57.

Liberman, M. 1995. "Computer Speech Synthesis: Its Status and Prospects." *Proceedings of the National Academy of Sciences of the United States of America* 92 (22): 9928–31.

Poss, R., M. Koris, R. Santore, and H. Mevis. 1995. Computer Applications for Orthopaedic Surgeons: CD-ROM and Beyond." *Instructional Course Lectures* 44: 519–26.

Saunders, R. R., M. D. Saunders, and J. L. Saunders. 1994. "Data Collection With Bar Code Technology." In *Destructive Behavior in Developmental Disabilities: Diagnosis and Treatment*, Sage Focus Editions, Vol. 170, edited by T. Thompson and D. B. Gray, 102–16. Thousands Oaks, CA: Sage Publications, Inc.

Stair, R. 1996. *Principles of Information Systems: A Managerial Approach*, 2nd Ed. Danvers, MA: Boyd and Fraser Publishing Company.

4

COMPUTER SOFTWARE

T HE HARDWARE components of even the most powerful super-computer cannot by themselves produce output of value to the healthcare executive. These components need a detailed set of instructions that describe, step-by-step, the tasks they should perform in order to achieve a desired objective. This detailed set of instructions is known collectively as a *program*.

Concepts and Applications

Without software, hardware is useless. Simply, software provides the instructions that tell the hardware what to do. Like hardware, software has evolved: From arcane scientific and academic origins, today's software packages are easily used and versatile, able to perform many general and specific functions.

Healthcare executives must understand the capabilities and limitations of software programs, and how those programs affect clinical and management decisions. This chapter provides an overview of programming languages, reviews applications software, and lists various packages that healthcare executives should be familiar with.

After reading this chapter, readers will be able to discuss the role of operating systems, understand the difference between interfaced and integrated systems, and list the different software applications available that could be used in a healthcare environment.

It is possible for a program to be permanently stored within the computer's read-only memory (ROM). In fact, as was mentioned in Chapter 3, small special-purpose sets of instructions are maintained within ROM, such as the sequence followed by the computer when it is first turned on. However, it is much more practical for a program to be stored on secondary storage devices—a disk for example—and read into the computer's primary storage when the user wishes to run it. In the early days of computing, programs were stored on tape or even on punched cards. Perhaps these "soft" storage media gave rise to the use of the term *software* as a synonym for computer programs.

The tasks of selecting, implementing, and testing software are at least as complex as the corresponding hardware tasks, and are often more important for the success of the overall computer implementation. Healthcare executives must therefore have an understanding of basic software concepts, including an introduction to programming languages, the functions of language translators, system management software, application software, and the distinction between integrated and interfaced systems. This chapter presents these basic concepts.

An Introduction to Programming Languages

As mentioned, the hardware components of a computer are capable of performing useful functions only when directed to do so with carefully written step-by-step instructions. Just as two people communicate in a specific language, so does a problem solver tell a computer what to do in a specific *programming language*.

The format of a particular programming language is known as the *syntax* of that language. It is interesting to note that humans are much more forgiving with regard to language errors than are computers. If, for example, the programming language syntax calls for a comma at a particular point in the "conversation," omission of that comma can lead to unpredictable, if not disastrous, results.

A discussion of computer programming languages can be organized along a time continuum. Each decade between the 1940s and the 1980s roughly marked the beginning of a new "generation" of programming languages. These five generations of programming languages, summarized in Table 4.1, are described in the following paragraphs.

First-Generation Programming Languages

When computers were first developed, it was necessary for users to provide instructions in *machine language*, which consisted of strings of zeros and ones. The collection of strings understood by the computer

Table 4.1   Five Generations of Programming Languages

Generation	General Characteristics
1	Machine Language; Strings of Zeros and Ones
2	Assembly Language; Uses Mnemonics
3	Procedural Language; Focuses on Solution to Problem
4	Variety of Application and Program-Generating Languages; Focuses on Description of Problem Itself
5	Natural Languages; Easy Communication with Computer

is known as that computer's instruction set and allows the user to perform a variety of arithmetic operations, data comparisons, and data movement within the computer's central processor and memory. Each instruction provides a numeric code for the desired operation and, where applicable, the location in memory of the data on which the operation is to be performed. In general, the machine language is unique to a given computer make (and perhaps model). Machine languages represent the first generation of computer programming languages.

Although machine language is the only language that the computer is capable of "understanding," the average prospective computer user did not find learning the complex sequences of zeros and ones particularly appealing. It was obvious to computer developers that widespread use of these machines would occur only if communication with them were made easier. This recognition led to the development of assembly languages and ushered in the second generation of programming languages.

Second-Generation Programming Languages

An *assembly language* essentially replaces a string of zeros and ones with an alphabetic symbol known as a *mnemonic*. Thus, the "code" for addition might be AD, for subtraction SUB, etc. In addition, memory address locations can also be replaced with mnemonics so that the user does not need to keep track of these locations. Although these mnemonics were somewhat easier for the user to learn, the computer can only deal with binary strings of zeros and ones. Thus, it is necessary for the set of instructions written by the user in an assembly language to be converted or translated to the binary codes recognized by the computer. This translation is accomplished by special software described later in this chapter.

Even the use of mnemonics, which bore some resemblance to the corresponding computer operation, was considered intimidating to the average computer user. These users were accustomed to thinking of their problems in a language associated with their particular problem area. Thus, engineers and scientists typically model their problems as equations, while business analysts frequently describe their business processes verbally. Problem solvers still considered the tedious process of constructing a sequence of mnemonics to describe their problem to be a burden.

Third-Generation Programming Languages

The desire to enable a user to focus more on the structure of the solution to a problem and less on the computer's internal processes led to the development of *procedural, high-level languages*, the third generation of programming languages (3GL).

The term *procedural* signifies that these languages still require the user to describe to the computer, in a structured format, the detailed solution steps that are to be followed. However, the term *high-level* indicates that the format of the user's description resembles the language of the problem more closely than do the zeros and ones of machine language or the mnemonics used in an assembly language. In fact, one high-level language statement might generate several machine language instructions. The details of how this occurs will be covered later in the chapter.

Key milestones in the development of programming languages are highlighted in a special twentieth anniversary report in *Byte* magazine (Anonymous 1995). Table 4.2 presents a summary of representative third-generation languages, and a brief description of each is presented below.

FORTRAN. The first higher level language, which appeared in 1957, is known as FORTRAN (an acronym for FORmula TRANslation). This language was quickly embraced by scientists and mathematicians because of its use of mathematical notation. The language has undergone many revisions, and despite the introduction of other scientific and engineering languages, FORTRAN maintains its popularity for numerical analysis.

COBOL. Shortly after the release of FORTRAN, a committee of representatives from business, manufacturing, government, and academia was formed to create a computer language. Programs written in that language were to be capable of running on a variety of computers and were

Table 4.2 Representative Third-Generation Languages

Language	Major Characteristic
FORTRAN	Early Scientific Language
COBOL	Early Business-Oriented Language
ALGOL	Influenced the Development of Several Contemporary Languages
PL/1	Intended to Combine Best Features of FORTRAN, COBOL, and ALGOL
BASIC	Important Language in Early Days of Personal Computing
MUMPS (renamed M)	Specifically Developed for Use in Healthcare Environments
Pascal	Replacement for BASIC that is Suitable for Business and Scientific Applications
C (newer version is C++)	Suitable for Business and Scientific Applications; Allows Operations Close to Machine Language

to use a syntax closely resembling simple English sentences. The result of the committee's efforts was the COBOL programming language, which quickly gained a popularity among the business community comparable to that afforded FORTRAN by scientific users.

COBOL has also been revised several times since its introduction. Nevertheless, because a large portion of computer applications have been in the business area, many computer systems have been developed in COBOL. For example, as Collen (1994, 97) indicates, "From the 1960s through the 1980s, COBOL was used almost universally for the business and accounting functions in hospitals." In fact, many healthcare executives are now trying to decide whether to keep these COBOL-based systems, typically running on mainframe hardware, or replace them with alternative technology.

ALGOL. Although never widely used, ALGOL (Algorithmic Language) "was the precursor of several more widely used languages." (Collen 1994, 98) Its instructions were "English-like" and its statements employed conventional algebraic terms. ALGOL greatly influenced the development of other third-generation languages—PL/1, PASCAL, and C.

PL/1. Initially called NPL (New Programming Language), PL/1 was intended to combine the best features of FORTRAN, COBOL, and ALGOL into a single language attractive to both the scientific and business communities. The language finds less frequent use today, although it has been used in healthcare settings. "Since the 1970s, PL/1 has been used to develop several hospital information systems." (Collen 1994, 98)

BASIC. A relatively easy high-level language to learn, BASIC was developed in the mid-1960s at Dartmouth College in New Hampshire. BASIC (Beginner's All-Purpose Symbolic Instruction Code) was intended for use in introductory computer programming courses. Early personal computer manufacturers typically included the BASIC language with their hardware. While the language has had widespread use among personal computer (PC) users, it has found little use among serious business users.

MUMPS. The MUMPS programming language was developed in the 1960s at Massachusetts General Hospital for healthcare environments. Subsequently renamed M, MUMPS (Massachusetts General Hospital Utility Multi-Programming System) is expressly set up for a multiuser environment with data stored in a tree structure rather than the traditional file structure of most other languages.

MUMPS works well in many healthcare applications that need multiuser access to many central files and report generation capabilities, such as patient admitting and records, patient bed scheduling, and nurse personnel staffing and scheduling, among others. As Collen (1994, 98) indicates, "MUMPS was probably the most commonly used programming language in the United States for clinically oriented medical applications during the 1970s and 1980s." Successful applications include COSTAR, an outpatient record system; DXplain, a diagnostic decision-support system; and a variety of systems developed by the Department of Defense and the Veterans Administration.

Pascal. Developed in the late 1960s, Pascal was meant to be a good medium for teaching computer programming. In fact, Pascal replaced BASIC as the language taught in many introductory university computing courses. It is well-suited for both business and scientific applications. For example, Grouven, Bergel, and Schultz (1996) have used the Pascal language to develop a PC program which, unlike widely available statistical software, incorporates unequal misclassification costs as part of a discriminant analysis with more than two groups. Kingma et al. (1994) describe a program, written in Pascal, that converts ICD-9CM coded diagnoses into one of two severity of injury scores. The program, which eliminates the need for manual coding or translation, can be used in a "stand-alone" mode or as a procedure in a database management system

C. The C programming language was developed at Bell Laboratories in 1972. C is a high-level language that is appropriate for both business and scientific applications. It incorporates some features that allow its users to perform operations typically possible only with an assembly or machine language (Donovan 1993). For this reason, the C language was used to program the UNIX operating system (discussed later in this chapter).

This language is popular because programs written in C can be run on most computers, a property known as machine portability. In fact, a number of healthcare applications described in the literature have been developed in the C language or its enhanced successor, C++. Examples include a teleradiology system designed for image transfer between two hospitals (Heinila et al. 1994), a graphical portrayal system to assess spinal deformities (Vandegriend et al. 1995), and a discrete-event simulation designed to determine the optimal base location for a trauma system helicopter in Maine (Clark et al. 1994). Exhibit 4.1 illustrates a simple program written in each of four third-generation programming languages. Using an annual interest rate and time period provided by the user, each program computes the amount to which $1,000 will grow if compounded daily at the specified interest rate for the specified time period. Although the illustration is relatively straightforward, these sets of programming code allow the reader to compare the syntax of four commonly used languages—FORTRAN, BASIC, C++, and Pascal.

Exhibit 4.1 The Structure and Syntax of Some Typical Programming Languages

FORTRAN Programming Language

```
    integer n
    real*16 r,di,nd,a
    write(*,*) "Enter the number of years the investment is held "
    read(5,*) n
    write(*,*) "Enter the annual interest rate (as a percent) "
    read(5,*) r
    di=r/36500
    nd=n*365
    a=1000*(1+di)**nd
    write(*,*)
    write(*,*)
    write(*,*) "An investment of $1000 held for ", n, " years"
    write(*,10) a
10  format(" will grow to ",f10.2, " at an interest rate")
    write(*,20) r
20  format(" of ",f6.1, "% compounded daily")
    end
```

Output
Enter the number of years the investment is held   8
Enter the annual interest rate (as a percent)   10.2

An investment of $1000 held for 8 years
will grow to 2261.18 at an interest rate
of 10.2% compounded daily

continued

Exhibit 4.1 Continued

BASIC Programming Language

```
CLS
INPUT "Enter the Number of Years the Investment is Held ", n
INPUT "Enter the Annual Interest Rate (as a Percent) ", i#
di# = i# / 36500
nd# = n * 365
a# = 1000 * (1 + di#) ^ nd#
PRINT
PRINT
PRINT USING "An Investment of $1,000 held for ###.### years"; n
PRINT USING "will grow to $$###,###,###.## "; a#;
PRINT "at an interest rate"
PRINT USING "of ###.#% compounded daily"; i#
```

Output

Enter the Number of Years the Investment is Held 8
Enter the Annual Interest Rate (as a Percent) 10.2

An Investment of $1,000 held for 8.000 years
will grow to $2,261.18 at an interest rate
of 10.2% compounded daily

C++ Programming Language

```
// program to compute future value of $1,000

#include <iostream.h>
#include <iomanip.h>
#include <math.h>
main( )
{
    double di,n,nd,a,r;
    cout << " Enter the number of years the investment is held \n";
    cin >> n;
    cout << " Enter the annual interest rate (as a percent) \n";
    cin >> r;
// Calculations
    di=r/36500;
    nd=n*365;
    a=1000*pow(1+di,nd);
// Output
    cout << "\n";
    cout << "\n";
    cout << " An investment of $1,000 held for " << n << " years\n";
    cout << " will grow to " << a << " at an interest rate\n";
    cout << " of " << r << "% compounded daily\n";

    return 0;
}
```

OUTPUT

Enter the number of years the investment is held 8
Enter the annual interest rate (as a percent) 10.2

An investment of $1,000 held for 8 years
will grow to 2261.18 at an interest rate
of 10.2% compounded daily

continued

Exhibit 4.1 Continued

Pascal Programming Language

```
program INVTMENT (input, output);
var
   di,n,nd,a,r:real;

begin
   writeln (' Enter the number of years the investment is held');
   readln (n);
   writeln (' Enter the annual interest rate [as a percent] ');
   readln (r);
   di := r/36500;
   nd := n*365;
   a := 1000*exp(nd*ln(1+di));
   writeln;
   writeln;
   writeln (' An investment of $1000 held for ', n:4:1, ' years');
   writeln (' will grow to ', a:10:2, ' at an interest rate');
   writeln (' of ', r:6:1, '% compounded daily');
   end.
```

Output
Enter the number of years the investment is held 8
Enter the annual interest rate [as a percent] 10.2

An investment of $1000 held for 8.0 years
will grow to 2261.18 at an interest rate
of 10.2% compounded daily

Fourth-Generation Programming Languages

Whereas third-generation languages require specific step-by-step instructions on how the solution to a problem is to be obtained, fourth-generation languages (4GL) allow the user to focus on a description of the problem itself. The computer, in turn, then determines the appropriate sequence of operations necessary to obtain the desired solution. As a result, some might suggest that writing a new program need no longer be an activity restricted to professional programmers or technically trained individuals.

Two key features associated with 4GL languages are (see, for example, Stair 1996, 123):

1. query and database abilities that simplify the task of retrieving information from a database; and
2. code generation abilities that produce programming statements.

In addition, 4GLs often have graphics abilities that simplify the creation of illustrations compared to using third-generation languages. An example of a 4GL used to query databases is the Structured Query Language

(SQL). Fosdick (1996) reviews client/server versions of SQL from two leading software publishers. A 4GL with code-generation capability is Forté Version 1.1, a product of Forté Software Inc., Oakland, California. A review of this product is offered by Tumminaro (1995).

A wide spectrum of categories can be used to classify 4GLs (see, for example, Laudon and Laudon 1994, 218). These categories range from the programming capabilities built into spreadsheets and database managers (discussed later in "Application Software") to sophisticated application development software. While it is reasonable to assume that healthcare executives might begin to make increased use of application software programming capabilities, it is quite doubtful that they will ever be personally involved in the use of development software.

Fifth-Generation Programming Languages

The notion of a fifth generation of programming languages might be described as more of a concept than a reality. Languages that would fall into this category are sometimes called *natural languages* and have the property that the user is able to utilize the language as easily as he or she communicates with other people. A translator program would have the capability of converting these natural language statements into the binary number commands intelligible to the computer.

One would assume that healthcare executives (or physicians) would have a greater inclination to make "hands-on" use of a computer if the question to be answered or problem to be solved could be described orally to the computer with the same ease that words are currently spoken into a dictating machine. Of course, the technology necessary to recognize the spoken words, interpret their content, transform them into a set of procedures, and translate this sequence into machine commands is quite complex and currently not completely perfected. Perhaps, however, this is the model that the evolution of programming languages is moving toward, and the model that will make computer utilization even more widespread than it currently is.

The preceding discussion has presented an overview of the evolution of programming languages from the earliest machine languages to the notion of natural languages. Across the entire spectrum of these languages the objective of the user is quite simple: communicate with the computer in some prescribed format so that useful output can be generated. For the nonprogrammer user, the satisfaction of this communication process lies in the output created, not in the communication process itself. For many users, the communication process can only be described as a major source of frustration and inconvenience.

In fact, this communication process is often more than just a source of inconvenience. It is expensive, both in terms of time and money. The introduction of newer generations of programming languages represents one trend that helped to make the creation of software a more efficient process. Two other approaches to software development that the healthcare executive should be aware of are: computer-aided software engineering (CASE) tools, discussed in Chapter 8; and object-oriented approaches, which offer the advantages of lower development costs and faster development times by integrating previously developed modules into the current project (see, for example, Martin 1993).

Language Translators

Because computers are only capable of "understanding" instructions written in machine language, any program that is written in a language that is second-generation or higher must first be converted to machine language before it can be executed. This conversion is performed by software known as language translators.

The set of instructions comprising the program to be translated is known as *source code*, and these instructions comprise the *input data* to the language translator. The machine level equivalent to which the source code gets translated is known as *object code*, and this code constitutes the translator's *output data*. Three types of language translators are in common use: *assemblers, compilers*, and *interpreters*. In addition, *code-generation* software, which produces as output higher-level language code, might also be viewed as a language translator. Each will be briefly described.

Assemblers

A language translator capable of converting assembly language program code into machine language code is known as an *assembler*. The translation process involves substituting binary operation codes and memory addresses, respectively, for the mnemonics and label names that comprise the assembler language instructions. In many cases this process requires two passes through the assembly language program. Each source statement gets translated into one object statement.

Compilers

A *compiler* is a language translator that generates the necessary machine-language code to carry out the instructions contained in a program written in a high-level language. Unlike assemblers, a single source statement can generate several machine code instructions. This process of generating object code is known as *compilation*, and can be broken down into four major steps (Englander 1996, 592–594): *scanning*, which breaks down the source statements into the smallest possible meaningful language components; *syntax analysis*, which assesses whether source code statements have been written correctly so that object code can be created unambiguously and generates error messages as required; *code generation*, which creates the actual object code; and *optimization*, which analyzes whether it would be possible to reduce the amount of object code.

Two points about compilers bear mention. First, the optimization stage is quite important. The size and execution time of the object code created by the compiler depend on the quality of the optimization process. Second, whereas changes in the source code associated with a given application are easy to make, it is relatively difficult to make changes in object code. When application software is purchased, the product is typically delivered in object code format. Executives need to be sure that the source code for the application is being held in a secure location and will be available even if the vendor goes out of business.

Interpreters

The compiler described in the previous section translates all of the source statements of a higher-level language to object form before any execution of the statements occurs. In fact, after the compilation process has been completed, the object code can be run as many times as needed. As an alternative, the source statements could be translated to object code format one at a time, and, following translation, each statement could be executed. A language translator that performs this step-by-step conversion process is known as an *interpreter*. A classic illustration of an interpreted language is BASIC.

Interpreted languages work well for applications scheduled to be run only a few times or subject to frequent changes, since the compilation process can be avoided. However, compiled languages are preferred for production runs since the translation process needs to be performed only once.

Code-Generation Software

Some of the fourth-generation languages include code-generation features that produce third-generation language code as output. This software can be viewed as a language translator, where the 4GL statements comprise the input and the 3GL code represents the output. Typically the output represents a significant percentage of the total code necessary for a given programming project. The rest of the code is then written by a programmer. The 3GL code, of course, must then be compiled in order to obtain the object module necessary to allow the application to be run.

System Management Software

System management software is the group of programs that manage the resources of a computer system and perform a variety of routine processing tasks. Unlike the role of application software, the function of system management software is often not obvious to the user. Thus, many computer users are unaware of the important functions being performed by the *operating system* and by *utility programs*. These functions are described in the following sections.

Operating Systems

Operating systems serve as the interface between the human user and the computer. It is these systems that allow the computer to run application programs by providing these programs with access to the resources that they require. The efficiency and functionality of an operating system determine how effectively a particular computer system is employed. Englander (1996, 395) describes three basic types of services provided by an operating system, including:

1. accepting and executing commands and requests from the user and from the user's programs;
2. managing, loading, and executing programs; and
3. managing the hardware resources of the computer.

The complexity of the operating system and the scope of services that it must provide depend on the complexity of the computing environment in which the operating system is installed. An environment that allows only one user to run one program at a time possesses the least complexity and places the fewest demands on the operating system. Examples include the early mainframe computers as well as the early PCs. While these computers create few problems for the operating system, they do not make optimal use of their computing power.

The computing power of a given computer can be more effectively utilized when multiple tasks can be run by either a single user or by multiple users. In such an environment the operating system plays a more essential role. Since the computer's central processor unit (CPU) is only capable of working on one instruction at a time, it is not possible to actually work on more than one program at the same time. Rather, a technique called *time-slicing* is employed where the CPU executes a few instructions from one program, then works on a few instructions from the second program, and so forth. The operating system assumes responsibility for overseeing this process in the most efficient manner possible. The speed involved in this technique makes it appear to the users that the programs are running simultaneously.

Three Representative Operating Systems. Three operating systems serve to illustrate the range of such systems across the micro-, mini-, and mainframe-computer lines. A more detailed discussion of these operating systems is provided by Englander (1996, Chapter 18).

Windows 95 illustrates a popular microcomputer operating system. It is intended to be a single-user system with multitasking capabilities. It incorporates a graphical interface (see discussion below), focuses on documents to be processed rather than application programs, and is designed to take full advantage of the hardware capabilities of the computers on which it runs.

UNIX is a multiuser operating system licensed by many manufacturers that runs on many microcomputers and minicomputers. It has a command set that is similar to DOS (the PC-based operating system that preceded Windows) in many ways but is more robust for multiuser applications. It supports preemptive multitasking, provides an interactive interface with simple commands, and allows users to exert control over allocation of resources.

MVS is touted "as the premier operating system for IBM mainframe computers." (Englander 1996, 608) It supports large complex computer systems, offers support for a wide range of input/output facilities, for CPU multiprocessing, and for system interconnection. Installations with large mainframe computers using the MVS operating system must be willing to commit to significant personnel to support the system operations.

Interfacing with the Operating System. Users can take advantage of the functional capabilities of an operating system by issuing a command that a particular function be performed. For example, if a given file is to be copied to another disk drive, the user must indicate which file is to be copied and where the copy is to be stored. Two general approaches for communicating with the operating system are typically used: a command-based user interface and a graphical user interface (GUI).

Command-based user interfaces consist of text commands that the user inputs into the computer. This type of interface is common in mainframe systems. The set of commands available to the user comprise a language of their own, known as *job control language* (JCL). In some cases the complexity of the syntax of these commands rivals that of the application programs themselves. Early PC operating systems also used command-based user interfaces.

Graphical user interfaces use icons (graphical symbols on the screen) to represent available operating system commands. The user simply clicks on a given icon with the computer's mouse in order to invoke the desired command. Early GUIs were actually *shells* that resided between the operating system and the user. *Windows 3.0* and *Windows 3.1* are examples of such shells, which actually worked in conjunction with DOS, a command-based operating system. Windows 95, on the other hand, is a complete operating system with a built-in graphical interface. Windows 95 does not require DOS. Similarly, Windows NT is also a complete operating system designed particularly for business users.

Utility Programs

Utility programs are software packages that perform generalized data processing or computational functions on computers. These functions are not specific to any particular computer application (e.g., patient billing, medical records), but rather they offer general utility and support to a variety of information-processing tasks. In some cases this support can be viewed as supplementing the role of the operating system. In others, the utility might be performing a function that supports an application program.

Utility programs fall into three general categories:

1. Programs that support computer operations—Examples include programs that save and provide backup copies of computer programs written by users and programs that perform operational housekeeping tasks such as disk formatting.

2. Programs that provide generalized file manipulation—Examples include generalized database management systems and programs that sort or merge records in files.

3. Generalized computational programs—Examples include packages of mathematical subroutines that perform complex operations that can be called by application software. In this way the application software developer does not have to be concerned with writing the programming code to perform these complex operations.

One might wonder why these utility programs are not simply included as part of the operating system. Varhol (1995) provides two reasons:

1. The need for the utility might not become obvious until the operating system achieves widespread use. For example, the need for a utility that allows the user to examine the structure of a compressed disk only became obvious after the operating system allowed users to do disk compression.

2. Most users might not need the utility. Thus, it might not make sense to include a particular feature in the operating system. As interest in the feature increases, it is not unusual to see the feature included in later versions of the operating system.

Some mainframe utility programs are purchased from the computer manufacturer as part of the operating system and are fairly extensive. Most microcomputer utility programs are purchased separately, often from vendors different from those providing the hardware.

Application Software

From the user perspective, the most important category of software is application software. After all, it is this software that accomplishes the useful tasks that justify the purchase of the information system. In fact, application software can be further classified as general purpose or application specific.

General Purpose Application Software

Many computer programs provide an environment in which a user can solve a particular class of problems rather than a single, narrowly defined problem. Examples include word processors, desktop publishing software, spreadsheet software, statistical packages, and database management software. These programs, known as general purpose application software, are most often run today on a microcomputer, although in some cases where large data sets are involved a minicomputer might be employed.

Word Processors. The preparation of manuscripts, letters, forms, manuals, or just about any material once completed on a typewriter is now made much easier with the availability of *word-processing* software. Older word-processing packages usually resided on bulky, dedicated hardware systems and had a limited set of rudimentary features. Modern word-processing programs have a variety of sophisticated capabilities and are available for most hardware platforms.

The power of word processing lies in its editing capabilities. The need to retype a page to make a simple correction is a thing of the past. This, of course, can have a negative side as people find it perhaps too easy to make "just one more refinement" to a letter or report. Other features that contribute to the power of word processing include: the merging of form letters with a list of addresses; the insertion of graphical images or figures into a document; the easy conversion of a document from one word-processing format to another; spelling and grammar checking; a thesaurus for determining synonyms; and the ability to create tables and perform basic arithmetic operations on the values in a table.

Many newcomers choose word processing as a good starting point for learning and gaining experience in the field of computing. Popular word-processing programs include Word for Windows, Word Pro, and Word Perfect for Windows. (Leonhard 1996)

Word processing is one of many office automation systems. See Chapter 12 for a discussion of these applications.

Desktop Publishing Software. Slightly more powerful than traditional word-processing software is *desktop publishing software* (although as word processors become more sophisticated the two types of software look quite similar). Desktop publishing software is designed to create camera-ready copy of newspapers, invitations, programs, bulletins, and other similar documents typically produced by typesetting just a few years ago. Professional results can be achieved quite easily with desktop publishing software running on a microcomputer and a laser printer.

An important feature of desktop publishing software is the ability to support a wide array of fonts so that the desired printed effect can be achieved. Also important is the ability to import photographs, diagrams, and other figures, as well as the facility to easily combine these with text to produce exactly the page layout that is desired. While these features continue to be refined in word-processing systems, they receive particular emphasis from developers of desktop publishing software.

Tietz and Tabor (1995) report that the availability of relatively inexpensive desktop publishing software has facilitated their developing a monthly newsletter. Through this medium information about CQI activities is being disseminated. A desktop publishing system was used in the design of anesthesia record forms. (Fisher, Bromberg, and Eisen 1994) The authors report that desktop publishing facilitated numerous revision cycles and an iterative convergence on the final design. Peters (1994) reports on the use of desktop publishing at Baylor University Medical Center to prepare a quarterly medical journal for publication. Popular desktop packages include Ventura Publisher, Adobe PageMaker, and QuarkXPress. (Kaufhold 1996)

Spreadsheet Software. Users can prepare, edit, and print a wide range of financial, administrative, and other types of tables with the use of *spreadsheet software*. Developed in the late 1970s, the electronic spreadsheet, like the word processor, provided the impetus for many purchases of microcomputers. VisiCalc, as the first spreadsheet program was called, clearly demonstrated that a computer could be used to perform functions useful to the organization without a need for in-depth programming skill.

On initiating (or "booting-up") a spreadsheet program, the user is presented with a rectangular array of cells. Numbers, formulas, functions, or clusters of instructions (called macros) can be entered into the cells.

All of the standard mathematical operations can be performed on the cell values, and the results of these operations change if the cell values involved in the computations change. Thus, skeleton spreadsheets, called templates, can be designed and then run after cell values have been filled in. For example, a department overtime report can be designed as a template, and a report can be generated when the labor hours for a given month are entered into the spreadsheet.

The spreadsheet formulas are written in terms of constant values and/or values located in other cells. If a cell value changes, all of the cells containing formulas involving that modified cell will also change. This property gives the spreadsheet much of its power. A user can systematically change the value of a given cell and observe the impact of this change on other cells in the spreadsheet. Such systematic investigation is known as "What-If" analysis. As an example, consider a spreadsheet that evaluates the income and expenses of three potential configurations of a hospital department. If one of the variables on the spreadsheet is patient volume, one can systematically change this value and observe the impact on each configuration. It is also possible to change the value of patient volume until expenses just equal income. This gives rise to the "break-even volume." (See, for example, Austin and Boxerman 1995, Chapter 2.)

Today's spreadsheet software has a number of additional features that greatly enhance its power. These features include: creation, insertion, and printing of sophisticated graphs into the spreadsheet; text enhancement, such as cell shading, outlining, underlining, and multiple fonts; WYSIWYG display (what you see is what you get); data import and export to and from other file formats; and print screen preview. In addition, the software can perform sophisticated statistical analyses, database functions, and optimization. Boxerman (1996) describes the use of a spreadsheet to perform a simulation study.

A number of healthcare-related applications of spreadsheet software have been reported. Jones, Culpepper, and Shea (1995) use a spreadsheet to develop a model that allocates cost components of a community health center–based residency program. Munro and Potter (1994) describe a program written for a spreadsheet to analyze and predict waiting times for radiotherapy. The breadth of computing power offered by spreadsheet software is illustrated by Bowen and Jerman (1995), who use spreadsheets to perform nonlinear regression analysis, and by Anderson (1995), who has used a spreadsheet to implement a method for computing sample size requirements for a clinical study of a new heart valve. Popular spreadsheet programs include Lotus 1-2-3, Quattro Pro, and Microsoft Excel. (Pepper 1996)

Statistical Packages. The analysis of data has been greatly simplified by the availability of a wide range of *statistical packages*. With this software, users can easily enter raw data, make changes as necessary, sort the values, create subsets of the data using a specified criterion, merge data sets, and perform a variety of analyses from obtaining the simplest descriptive statistics to developing the most complex multivariate models. Many of these packages also construct high-quality graphical presentations that allow the user to visualize the data in a specified format.

Although modern spreadsheets have excellent statistical capabilities, the term *statistical package* is usually applied to software specifically written to perform statistical computations. In all cases, the user begins the analytical process by building a "data set," which contains the raw data values and data names associated with each data field. These names make it easier for the user to refer to those data fields, which are to be used in a given analysis. Full-screen editing of this data set allows the user to add or delete records or change the contents of a given record.

There is no need for the user of statistical software to specify formulas for a given analysis. All of the mathematics for a given statistical procedure are built into the software. All that the user must do is to specify, by name, the particular statistical method to be applied along with the options to be used in the analysis. Herein lies the power, as well as the danger, of statistical software. Certainly the drudgery of statistical problem solving has been eliminated. But at the same time it is perhaps too easy for a naive individual to subject a set of data to extremely sophisticated methodology. The software cannot judge the appropriateness of the method being used. Therefore, the use of this software requires a healthcare executive with a reasonable background in statistics and/or collaboration with a functional expert in this area.

Finally, statistical packages report the results of the analyses in an easily read form without the user incurring the drudgery of specifying the output format. Descriptive statistics, which are well labeled; cross-tabulations of data; detailed output from complex regression analyses; and graphs are all produced with minimal effort. Popular statistical software packages include SPSS (Hackman 1996), SAS (Custer 1995), Statgraphics Plus for Windows (Coffee 1996), and StatView (Seiter 1996). With the availability of this software, healthcare executives certainly have little excuse for not employing statistical analysis as part of their decision-making process.

Dickson, Hodgkinson, and Kohler (1994), for example, report the use of statistical software to examine the profile of patients admitted to an inpatient rehabilitation unit. Their analyses allowed them to identify factors that produce a prolonged stay or failure of patients to progress in their recovery. Fassett and Calmes (1995) describe their use of statistical software in a study of anesthesia care teams in a public teaching hospital. Among their goals was the desire to identify practice modifications that could possibly lower costs. Harris and Conner (1994) indicate the important role of statistical software in their implementation of a quality improvement program at a large state psychiatric hospital. This implementation, part of the hospital's efforts to attain accreditation by the Joint Commission on Accreditation of Healthcare Organizations, helped them to develop the technical ability to conduct "state-of-the-art" quality improvement.

Database Management Software. Database management software allows users to easily interact with databases—organized collections of files that are designed to provide easy access to needed information. The software makes it relatively straightforward to enter data, edit the data, and create reports based on those data to answer specific questions of interest. The increasing presence of managed care makes it imperative that users are able to access data from all entities within the organization. The implications of this imperative on the organization's data management are discussed in Chapter 6.

In addition, however, individual users often find the use of database management software quite beneficial for small projects or studies. In this context the software is often described as a personal or end-user database management program, and it functions quite similarly to spreadsheet or statistical software. Once the user has created a database, the software supports a variety of functions including: data editing and printing; extraction of a subset of records based upon one or more criteria; creation of reports; data import/export to and from other file formats; and an easy-to-use file record query language.

Bielefeld et al. (1995) describe their development of a research database for a five-year prospective investigation of the correlates of chronic lung disease during the first three years of life. The database software was used along with a statistical software package to handle a variety of data functions. Ross (1994) describes a process for handling text data in qualitative research projects using a combination of word-processing and database programs. The method makes the information more readily available and enhances the coding and organization of the data. Personal database management software reviewed in the literature includes Alpha Five (Columb 1996), Lotus Approach for Windows 95 (Alwang 1996), R:Base for Windows (Dragan 1996), Paradox (Stearns 1996), and Personal Oracle7 (McClanahan 1996).

Integrated Software Programs. Integrated software programs consist of a series of menu-driven module programs, all in the same software package. Module packages may include word processing, spreadsheet, database, graphics, communications, and internet hooks among others. Frequently used integrated software packages include Lotus Smart-Suite 96, Microsoft Office for Windows 95, and Corel PerfectOffice. (Rigney 1996)

Application-Specific Software

The term *application-specific software* denotes a computer program that has been designed to solve a single, somewhat specifically defined problem. A good example is a payroll program, which is developed to accumulate labor hours, compute deductions, write payroll checks, post summaries to the general ledger, and complete the several forms that are required by federal and state governments. Although the files associated with this program contain a lot of information, the user has no access to the information unless the programmer specifically built in this capability. Table 4.3 displays the categories into which typical application-specific software employed in healthcare settings can be classified. Details of these application areas comprise the material in Part IV of the text. Ankrapp and Di Lima (1996) present a comprehensive listing of application software for the healthcare field.

Healthcare organizations have the option of developing application-specific software in-house or purchasing (or leasing) a "package" and simply installing it on their computer system (this process is not always as trivial as it might sound). Each approach has its advantages and disadvantages. With in-house development the software can be tailored specifically to the organization's needs and when changes are needed they generally are easier to make. Purchased (or leased) software, by comparison, is generally cheaper, requires less time to get running, and requires fewer in-house computer personnel. A third approach, modifying an existing package, attempts to integrate the advantages of both alternatives.

Table 4.3 Categories of Application-Specific Software in Healthcare

• Financial Management	• Radiology
• Managed Care	• Materials Management
• Decision Support	• Food Services and Nutrition
• Quality Management	• Clinical Services
• Case Management	• Clinic/Practice Management
• Clinical Information Systems	• Home Healthcare
• Patient Management	• Long-Term Healthcare
• Medical Records	• Administrative Support
• Laboratory Systems	• Office Automation
• Pharmacy Systems	• Systems Integration

In-house development of application software used to be a favorite choice of many healthcare organizations. Today most software is purchased (or leased). Most healthcare executives have decided that they are in the business of providing healthcare services, not developing software. These executives, however, must be knowledgeable participants in the process of purchasing (or leasing) software. In addition, it is very important to involve key users in software purchase decisions, especially when major systems are being acquired. Other factors that must be considered when choosing application software are the required staffing and equipment resources, the cost of maintenance, complexity of the operations being automated, the number of potential users, and data security issues. Complete details of evaluating and selecting systems are discussed in Chapter 9.

Integrated vs. Interfaced Systems

Two general approaches are available for acquiring and implementing application software in a healthcare organization. In the first, all of the modules required to satisfy the organization's computing needs are identified and purchased from a single vendor. Typically, these modules will have been designed to work with one another so that data transfer among modules proceeds smoothly. This type of system is known as an *integrated* information system.

By contrast, each of the required modules could be purchased from the vendor thought to be the leader in that particular application area. In some cases the decision might reflect the personal bias of influential members of a particular organizational department. In any event, while a given module might work quite well for its particular application area, connecting the module to other modules could cause a problem. For example the data contained in the module could be incompatible with the data format of other modules. The solution very often is the development of an *interface*, which acts as a bridge between the two modules and which, for example, translates the data format into one that the receiving module can handle.

The use of an *interfaced* approach is made somewhat simpler if the modules comprising the interfaced system have all been developed in accordance with a standard that makes their data formats compatible. An important standard that is followed by many system vendors is *HL7*. Hammond (1996, 58) provides a very concise historical overview of the development of this standard. "A group of interested users, vendors and consultants" met in March 1987 at the University of Pennsylvania to deal with the problems of interfacing departmental systems. In 1990

Version 2.1 was presented, and a large number of systems have been implemented adhering to that standard. Current work on Version 3.0 focuses on "an object-oriented model using standardized health care objects." The standards definition goes well beyond just data format and includes "standard structures for reports, envelopes for images and automated waveforms."

Advantages of an integrated system include compatibility among the modules, no "finger-pointing" by one vendor toward another, and the need to have only a single source for system support and maintenance. Interfaced systems, on the other hand, allow users to choose the leading system for a given module (the so-called "best-of-breed"), can sometimes result in lower costs by leveraging one vendor against another, and obviate the need to replace all existing modules.

A Final Note

It is interesting to ask one final question: What is the quality of the wide range of software described in this chapter? In fact, the quality is quite variable and in some cases software purchasers wind up with systems that fall short of their expectations. Perhaps knowledgeable and informed executives participating in the evaluation, acquisition, and implementation of software will help to ensure that high-quality systems are installed in their organizations.

Summary

Computer software includes programming languages, software development tools, language translators, operating systems, and application software. Application software, in turn, can be divided into two categories: general purpose programs, such as word processors, desktop publishing, spreadsheet, statistical, and database software, and a variety of application-specific software packages, which perform specific functions in administrative as well as clinic areas.

Programming languages have evolved up to a fifth generation, and range from binary instructions native to the computer to natural languages that are essentially English-language statements. While little, if any, in-house program development is being done, a knowledge of the role of programming languages helps the executive to better appreciate some basic concepts associated with the software in use within the organization.

In addition to application software, computers also require software that manages the computer's resources. The complexity of this software, known as operating systems, is dependent on the complexity of the computing environment. Modern operating systems have GUIs and are more user-friendly than early operating systems.

The healthcare executive must consider many factors in choosing computer software. Among them are: number of existing and potential users, hardware configurations available, security considerations, future computer applications growth, and functional requirements for individual applications.

Discussion Questions

4.1 List the five generations of programming languages and briefly describe the characteristics of each.

4.2 Briefly describe an important characteristic of the C programming language that led to its having been chosen as the language in which to develop the UNIX operating system.

4.3 Why are users doing so little in-house development of software today?

4.4 What are the major advantages of using a microcomputer graphical user interface program?

4.5 Explain the difference between interfaced and integrated systems, and state one advantage of each.

4.6 Explain the difference between word-processing and desktop-publishing software.

4.7 What is the difference between a compiler and an interpreter?

4.8 List three specific functions of an operating system.

4.9 Explain how computers can run multiple tasks at the same time when they only contain a single CPU?

Problems

4.1 Assume that an ambulatory care center is about to purchase word-processing software for its staff. Choose two different systems (e.g., WordPerfect and Word) and compare the price of each system as well as the functional features of each. Indicate your choice and explain the rationale for your decision.

4.2 Talk to the chief information officer of a local healthcare organization. Determine to what extent the support requirements for the accounts payable system depend on the language in which the program was developed. Questions to be answered include: (1) Does the vendor provide support? (2) Are there in-house programmers capable of making changes to the system? (3) Are there plans to replace the system within the next year? (4) To what extent did the language in which the software was developed influence the organization's decision to purchase that software?

4.3 Perform an inventory of the information systems in use in a local healthcare system. In particular, determine the operating systems under which the software applications are running.

4.4 Refer to Problem 4.3. As part of the inventory, determine whether independent departmental modules have been implemented. Determine whether these modules have been interfaced, and, if so (1) Who wrote the interfaces? (2) What was the cost of obtaining these interfaces? (3) Are there problems associated with data being smoothly passed from one module to another through the interfaces?

4.5 Assess the use of personal computers among the managerial staff of a local healthcare institution. (1) Determine the level of proficiency that the managers have. (2) What specific categories of software do they routinely employ (e.g., Word Processing, statistical, database)? (3) Are there standards operative within the organization directing specific software packages for which the information systems department of the organization offers support?

4.6 Consult a reference on object-oriented programming languages. Name and explain the three attributes that characterize such a language.

References

Alwang, G. 1996. "Lotus Approach 96 Edition for Windows 95." *PC Magazine* 15 (10): 138–45.

Anderson, W. N. Jr. 1995. "Spreadsheet Method for Determining Sample Sizes for Heart Valve Studies." *Journal of Heart Valve Disease* 4 (1): 95–98.

Ankrapp, B., and S. N. Di Lima, eds. 1996. *Health Care Software Sourcebook*. Gaithersburg, MD: Aspen Publishers.

Anonymous. 1995. "A Brief History of Programming Languages." *Byte* 20 (4): 121–22.

Austin, C. J., and S. B. Boxerman. 1995. *Quantitative Analysis for Health Services Administration*. Chicago: AUPHA Press/Health Administration Press.

Bielefeld, R. A., T. S. Yamashita, E. F. Kerekes, E. Ercanli, and L. T. Singer. 1995. "A Research Database for Improved Data Management and Analysis in Longitudinal Studies." *M.D. Computing* 12 (3): 200–5.

Bowen, W. P. and J. C. Jerman. 1995. "Nonlinear Regression Using Spreadsheets." *Trends in Pharmacological Sciences* 16 (12): 413–17.

Boxerman, S. B. 1966. "Simulation Modeling: A Powerful Tool for Process Improvement." *Best Practices and Benchmarking in Health Care* 1 (3): 109–17.

Clark, D. E., D. R. Hahn, R. W. Hall, and R. E. Quaker. 1994. "Optimal Location for a Helicopter in a Rural Trauma System: Prediction Using Discrete-Event Computer Simulation." *Proceedings of the Annual Symposium on Computer Applications in Medical Care*: 888–92.

Coffee, P. 1996. "Stat Package Reveals What Figures Really Mean." *PC Week* 13 (14): 91.

Collen, M. F. 1994. "The Origin of Informatics." *Journal of the American Medical Informatics Association* 1 (2): 91–107.

Columb, T. E. 1996. "Alpha Five." *PC Magazine* 15 (10): 119–28.

Custer, L. 1995. "SAS System 6.10 Brings Stat Muscle to the Mac: Industrial-Strength Solution for Information Management Lands on Mac." *MacWEEK* 9 (38): 86–88.

Dickson, H. G., A. Hodgkinson, and F. Kohler. 1994. "Inpatient Quality Assurance By Local Analysis of Uniform Data Set." *Journal of Quality in Clinical Practice* 14 (3): 145–48.

Donovan, J. 1993. "Careful Programming Lets C Replace Assembler in Fast Embedded Applications." *EDN* 38 (April 15): 81.

Dragan, R. V. 1996. "R:Base for Windows." *PC Magazine* 15 (10): 152–54.

Englander, I. 1996. *The Architecture of Computer Hardware and Systems Software.* New York: John Wiley and Sons.

Fassett, S., and S. H. Calmes. 1995. "Perceptions by an Anesthesia Care Team on the Need for Medical Direction." *AANA Journal* 63 (2): 117–23.

Fisher, J. A., I. L. Bromberg, and L. B. Eisen. 1994. "On the Design of Anaesthesia Record Forms." *Canadian Journal of Anaesthesia* 41 (10): 973–83.

Fosdick, H. 1996. "Two Directions for SQL Server." *InformationWeek* 584 (June 17): 89–96.

Grouven, U., F. Bergel, and A. Schultz. 1996. "Implementation of Linear and Quadratic Discriminant Analysis Incorporating Costs of Misclassification." *Computer Methods and Programs in Biomedicine* 49 (1): 55–60.

Hackman, G. 1996. "SPSS 7.0 for Windows." *PC/Computing* 9 (4): 186.

Hammond, W. E. 1996. "How Long Does It Take to Write A Standard?" *Healthcare Informatics* 13 (1): 58.

Harris, C. S., and C. B. Conner. 1994. "Building a Computer-Supported Quality Improvement System in One Year: The Experience of a Large State Psychiatric Hospital." *Joint Commission Journal on Quality Improvement* 20 (6): 330–42.

Heinila, J., J. Yliaho, J. Ahonen, J. Viitanen, and M. Kormano. 1994. "X Window System Based User Interface in Radiology." *Computer Methods and Programs in Biomedicine* 43 (1–2): 129–38.

Jones, T. F., L. Culpepper, and C. Shea. 1995. "Analysis of the Cost of Training Residents in a Community Health Center." *Academic Medicine* 70 (6): 523–31.

Kaufhold, G. 1996. "Desktop Publishing for Windows 95." *National Association of Desktop Publishers Journal* 8 (5): 64–70.

Kingma, J., E. TenVergert, H. A. Werkman, H. J. ten Duis, and H. J. Klasen. 1994. "A Turbo Pascal Program to Convert ICD-9CM Coded Injury Diagnoses Into Injury Severity Scores: ICDTOAIS." *Perceptual and Motor Skills* 78 (3 Part 1): 915–36.

Laudon, K. C., and J. P. Laudon. 1994. *Management Information Systems: Organization and Technology,* 3rd Ed. New York: Macmillan Publishing Company.

Leonhard, W. 1996. "Word Processor Superguide." *PC/Computing* 9 (5): 149–66.

Martin, J. 1993. *Principles of Object-Oriented Analysis and Design.* Englewood Cliffs, NJ: P T R Prentice-Hall, Inc.

McClanahan, D. 1996. "Oracle7 Gets Personal—The Personal Version Resides Comfortably on Windows Desktops. *Data Based Advisor* 14 (2): 44–45.

Munro, A. J., and S. Potter. 1994. "Waiting Times for Radiotherapy Treatment: Not All That Mysterious and Certainly Preventable." *Clinical Oncology (Royal College of Radiologists)* 6 (5): 314–18.

Pepper, J. 1996. "Crunch Those Numbers—We Make the Latest Spreadsheets Jump Through Business Hoops." *Small Business Computing* 14 (4): 82–88.

Peters, B. A. 1994. "Production of a Small-Circulation Medical Journal Using Desktop Publishing Methods." *Journal of Audiovisual Media in Medicine* 17 (3): 121–24.

Rigney, S. 1996. "The Webbed Suites." *PC Magazine* 15 (8): 134–35.

Ross, B. A. 1994. "Use of a Database for Managing Qualitative Research Data." *Computers in Nursing* 12 (3): 154–59.

Seiter, C. 1996. "StatView 4.5: Statistics and Graphing Package." *MacWorld* 13 (2): 81–82.

Stair, R. M. 1996. *Principles of Information Systems: A Managerial Approach*, 2nd Ed. Danvers, MA: Boyd & Fraser Publishing Company.

Stearns, B. 1996. "Borland Nails Upgrade—Paradox 7.0 Has New Features and 32-Bit Functionality." *LAN Times* 13 (10): 78, 81.

Tietz, A., and R. Tabor. 1995. "Communicating Quality Improvement Through a Hospital Newsletter." *Journal for Healthcare Quality* 17 (4): 11–12.

Tumminaro, J. 1995. "Forté Leads 3-Tier Pack." *InformationWeek* Issue 529 (May 29): 54–59.

Vandegriend, B., D. Hill, J. Raso, N. Durdle, and Z. Zhang. 1995. "Application of Computer Graphics for Assessment of Spinal Deformities." *Medical and Biological Engineering and Computing* 33 (2): 163–66.

Varhol, P. D. 1995. "Filling in Windows Blanks." *Byte* 20 (11): 103–8.

Additional Readings

Anonymous. 1996. "1996 Database Buyer's Guide and Client/Server Sourcebook." *DBMS* 9 (6): 3–96.

Blum, B. I. 1996. *Beyond Programming: To A New Era of Design*. New York: Oxford University Press.

Broida, R. 1996. "Word Processors to the Wise—We Put Eight Popular Windows, Mac, and DOS Writing Packages Through Their Paces." *Home Office Computing* 14 (3): 72–78.

Davis, W. S. 1992. *Operating Systems: A Systematic View*, 4th Ed. Redwood City, CA: The Benjamin/Cummings Publishing Company, Inc.

Frankenfeld, F. M. 1993. "Basics of Computer Hardware and Software." *American Journal of Hospital Pharmacy* 50 (4): 717–24.

Frenzel, C. W. 1992. *Management of Information Technology*. Boston, MA: Boyd & Fraser Publishing Company.

Halfhill, T. R. 1996. "Unix vs. Windows NT." *Byte* 21 (5):42–46, 48, 50, 52.

Johnson, C. C., and M. Martin. 1995. "Lowering Physician Hospital Resource Consumption Using Low-Cost Low-Technology Computing." *Proceedings of the Annual Symposium on Computer Applications in Medical Care*: 661–65.

Johnson, J., R. Skoglund, and J. Wisniewski. 1995. *Program Smarter, Not Harder: Get Mission-Critical Projects Right the First Time*. New York: McGraw-Hill, Inc.

Mander, R., K. M. Wilton, M. A. Townsend, and P. Thomson. 1995. "Personal Computers and Process Writing: A Written Language Intervention for Deaf Children." *British Journal of Educational Psychology* 65 (Part 4): 441–53.

Prosise, J. 1995. "Much Ado About Objects." *PC Magazine* 14 (3): 257, 261–62.

NETWORKING AND TELECOMMUNICATIONS

U NTIL RECENTLY, the overview of hardware and software concepts presented in the last two chapters would have been adequate background for healthcare executives to interact knowledgeably with computer specialists regarding their institution's information needs.

Concepts and Applications

As hospitals and healthcare systems become more complex, and located in different physical areas, more and more information will have to be transported from different places—and be available throughout the system.

Computer networks allow data to be stored in one central location and accessed from remote points throughout the system. A network can be either widely or locally available, and can be configured in different ways, depending on the user's and facility's needs and equipment.

On completion of this chapter, readers will be able to understand the role and function of computer networks, how they can be applied to healthcare, and which networks are ideal for their organizations. Readers will also be able to discuss the media involved in networks. In addition, readers will gain an understanding of the technology associated with the Internet.

However, today's clinicians and managers require information from a variety of sources within the organization. And when independent healthcare organizations combine to form healthcare systems, the problems of obtaining needed information from each of the organization's components become increasingly complex. Satisfying these needs typically requires implementation of computer networks and the use of telecommunications.

The field of data communications, defined as a subset of telecommunications where data are transmitted to and from computer systems, dates back to the early 1940s. (Stamper 1994, 5) But the expansion of data communications systems and computer networks occurred in the 1970s. The technology associated with this growth is relatively complex, involving the expertise of communications engineers, computer hardware specialists, and software experts. It is quite unreasonable for healthcare executives to be expected to gain total mastery of these highly technical areas.

Nevertheless, these executives will have increasing responsibility for overseeing the development of information systems networks capable of satisfying the information needs of an integrated healthcare system competing in a managed care environment. As was true in the areas of hardware and software, the executive will need sufficient understanding of networks and telecommunications to work intelligently with the functional experts in these fields. The objective of this chapter is to provide such an understanding. Topics include: a rationale for installing computer networks; alternative ways to distribute the processing function; what the components of a network do; how networks are configured; how data are interchanged electronically; the role of wireless communication; and how communication can take place via the Internet. The discussion is meant neither to be exhaustive nor to make the executive a networking or telecommunications expert, but rather to present an introductory overview of these subjects.

A Rationale for Installing Computer Networks

Early applications of computers in hospitals, as in many other industries, consisted of a variety of financial applications like billing, payroll, and general accounting. These programs were typically run on a large mainframe computer located in the organization's Data Processing Department. (In some cases a hospital might decide against owning a mainframe computer, choosing rather to have their computing performed by an outside vendor of data processing services.) The input data for these programs were contained in handwritten documents, such as charge slips, invoices, or time and attendance sheets. These documents were handed to a keypunch operator (or transferred electronically as described below) who entered the data into punched cards which were then read into the computer. The output consisted of printed reports that were distributed to the appropriate users.

Two parallel developments threatened the role of the mainframe system in the healthcare setting: the introduction of software systems designed to perform specific functions within hospital departments such as the pharmacy, radiology, or the laboratory, along with minicomputers capable of running the software; and the introduction of the personal computer (PC), which allowed managers to analyze a variety of operational and financial data themselves, rather than depend on the Data Processing Department to run a special report, often with considerable delay.

As department managers purchased new minicomputer-based systems and other managers became increasingly involved with personal computing, they soon realized that the programs they were running were not independent "stand-alone" modules. Rather, there is actually a high level of interdependence among these programs. For example, the laboratory, pharmacy, and radiology systems all need information gathered by the admitting system. Similarly, many of the reports that users generated on their PC operated on data contained in a printed report generated by a mainframe financial application.

The problem grows worse in a healthcare system since data on a given patient might be found in a number of locations and a single laboratory might serve widely separated patient care locations. Data must flow across a large area and managers often require input from many sources in order to arrive at a solution to a problem. It is clear that the disparate systems throughout the organization (and even beyond) needed to be tied together to facilitate the exchange of data and the sharing of resources.

The linkage needed to facilitate this exchange of data and sharing of resources is accomplished through the construction of a network, which " . . . can be anything from a simple link between two computers in an office to a complex installation joining thousands of computers at many sites around the world." (Lee and Millman 1995, 1013) When all of the components of the network are located within relatively close proximity of one another, perhaps within a single facility, the network is known as a *local-area network* (LAN). A network that extends into a broad geographical area is known as a *wide-area network* (WAN).

Distributing the Processing Function

One way in which networks can be classified is the way in which the processing function is distributed among the devices making up the network. This processing function can be totally concentrated in a mainframe computer, giving rise to a *centralized* computing environment, or it can be split among all of the users on the network, which represents a *decentralized* approach to computing. Other classifications correspond to intermediate configurations. Increasing decentralization of the computing function typically creates greater managerial challenges, a fact that is particularly relevant for the healthcare executive.

Central Computer with Dumb Terminals

The most centralized computing environment consists of a large central computer, typically a mainframe, that may have dumb terminals connected to it. This configuration is depicted in Figure 5.1. Depending on the level of sophistication of the program running on the mainframe, the terminals allow users to perform a variety of functions. These include: entering a set of data for a program to be run at some later time in *batch* mode (that is, as part of a sequential stream of programs from several users); the *real-time processing* of a program immediately on entering data and/or programming commands; or responding to a query, such as a patient account balance. The important feature of this computing environment is that all computing is taking place on the mainframe.

An important subset of this computing configuration is *remote job entry* (RJE) where dumb terminals might be located at considerable distance from the mainframe computer. Several major companies have specialized in providing computing services to hospitals on an RJE basis. Hospitals enter their data (typically financial) into a dumb terminal (or a computer operating in a mode that emulates a dumb terminal) for

Figure 5.1   Central Mainframe Configuration

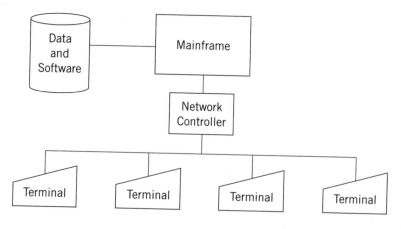

processing at a remote location. Results are mailed back to the hospital or received on their own remote printer.

Central computers with or without dumb terminals constitute the most centralized form of computing and thus are the easiest configuration for managers to control. All of the resources are close at hand and users have little potential to disrupt either program software or data files.

Client/Server Computing

It was not hard for users of dumb terminals connected to a mainframe computer to recognize the advantage that would result from their terminals having computing capability. Data could be edited, preliminary computations could be made, and other processing could be done that did not require the power of the mainframe or any of its data files. This early conceptualization was predictive of today's client/server computing configuration, which is characterized by less centralization than a mainframe installation. (See Figure 5.2.)

Client/server architecture divides applications into two components: client, or *front-end* functions, which include user interface, decision

Figure 5.2 Client/Server Computing

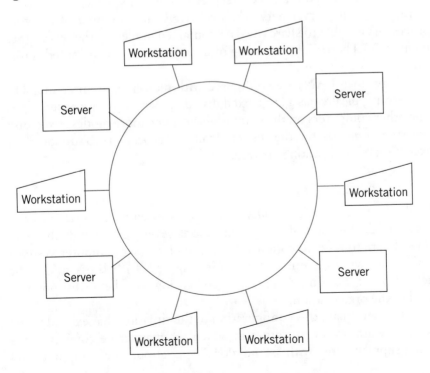

support, and data processing, and server, or *back-end* functions, such as database management, printing, communication, and applications program execution. The servers can be personal, mini-, or mainframe computers, and multiple servers can often be found in a client/server network.

When all back-end functions are performed on a single server, the configuration is known as a *two-tier* client/server architecture. The trend today is moving to a *three-tier* architecture. (Smith 1997, 32; Chin 1997, 79) In this configuration, the user interface resides on the client, the relational databases reside on one server, and the application programs reside on a second server. This configuration is easier to manage and offers faster information processing and distribution.

An example of a healthcare institution with a major client/server installation is Brigham and Women's Hospital in Boston. Dunbar (1994, 30) describes this system of 50 servers, 3,800 clients, and 50 gigabytes of online information as "one of the largest enterprisewide client/server environments in the world." The system is touted as "one hardware platform with one operating system and one language, completely integrated." (Dunbar 1994, 32)

File/Server Architecture

Even less centralized than client/server installations is file/server architecture. In a file/server network, a relatively large number of network processors are able to share the data contained in files on the server. (See Figure 5.3.) The actual processing of data, however, is distributed across the network machines.

Many small LANs are configured with file/server architecture. The file server typically has a large fixed disk drive with fast disk access time. The other computers on the network have much more modest fixed disk drive requirements, but they benefit from fast processors to support their execution of application software.

Distributed Data Processing

While the term *distributed data processing* is often used to refer to any degree of deployment of computing among several processors, the term is used here to refer to completely independent user computer systems with their own programs and files. (See Figure 5.4.) It is essentially the delegation of the computing responsibility down to the lowest possible level in the organization.

One can equate this configuration to the situation that existed in the typical healthcare organization in which the mainframe computer was being supplemented with "stand-alone" special-purpose computers and

Figure 5.3 File/Server Architecture

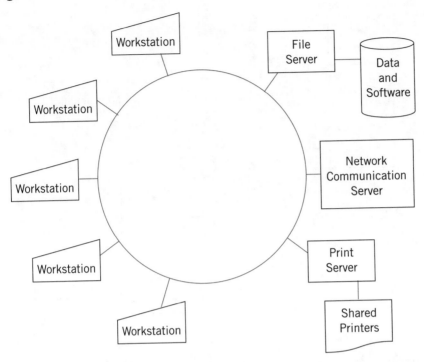

managers were beginning to bring their home PCs into the office. Each computer functioned independently, and no electronic communication took place between computers. As mentioned earlier, users quickly began to recognize the need for these computers to share data and, in some cases, application software. The first approach to supporting this sharing was the development of *interfaces* to allow the transfer of data from one computer to another.

Organizations comprised of a set of totally independent functions can often benefit from distributed data processing. In highly complex and interrelated fields like healthcare, however, some degree of centralization of the computing function is necessary. And the evolution of the field toward integrated healthcare systems and managed care makes information system integration even more vital.

In fact, the debate between advocates of mainframe computing and client/server technology continues in the literature. On the one hand a behavioral health group converted their information technology infrastructure to a client/server paradigm in order to enable their vision of operational excellence. In searching for their new system, a "key selection

Figure 5.4 Distributed Data Processing

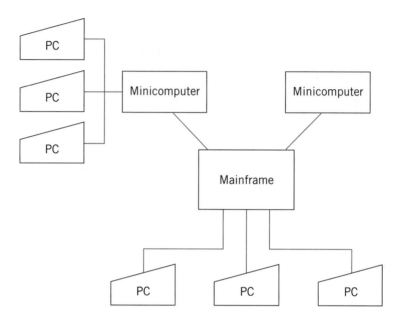

criterion was the soundness of the client-server architecture in terms of work distribution, performance, support of 24×7 up-time, tool set, etc." (Whyte and Matsumoto 1996, 36) By contrast, others have suggested that "many of the potential advantages of client/server architecture have yet to be proven." (Anonymous 1996, 3) They suggest that compared to more centralized systems, client/server applications require more hardware and support, the architecture generally has slower processing times, the number of terminals supportable is reduced, and the architecture provides less security.

Healthcare executives are well advised to monitor closely the architecture being chosen by their functional specialists in order to be sure that the information system function is moving in a direction that appropriately supports the organization's strategic direction. Chapter 7 discusses the need to match the information system plan to the organization's strategic plan.

Network Components

Creating an information network requires the assembly of a variety of hardware and software components. This section presents an overview of these components.

Transmission Media

Early in the process of designing a network, a decision must be made regarding the transmission medium to be used. This decision is more important than might be initially presumed since "the cabling system, if not done properly, can account for as much as 70 percent of all network problems." (McFarland 1994, 112) The transmission medium can be defined as "the means used to carry the signal being transmitted from one location to another. Data may be transmitted using electrical signals on wires, with optical signals on fiber-optic cable, or without wires, using radio waves. . . ." (Englander 1996, 681) Each transmission medium is discussed below.

Wired Media. Wired media consist of one or more strands of metal, which are excellent conductors of electricity. A commonly used metal is copper. Data are transmitted along these conductors in the form of changing electrical voltages and may be represented as either a *digital* or *analog* waveform. Digital transmission involves the representation of data with binary digits, or bits. Analog transmission represents data by varying the amplitude (height), frequency, and/or phase of a waveform. Traditional telephone lines carry signals in an analog format, while Integrated Services Digital Network (ISDN) lines, as well as the cable in a LAN, carry signals digitally.

Two types of copper media are in common use. (Longo and Lockhart 1996) The first, *Unshielded Twisted Pair* (UTP), is similar to telephone cable and can be classified (category 3, 4, or 5) according to speed and application. UTP installations will generally use category 5 cable because of its ability to handle voice, video, and data.

The second type of copper media in general use is *Shielded Twisted Pair* (STP). The shielding consists of a special conducting layer located within the insulation, which makes the cable less susceptible to interference. In addition, this shielding helps to keep the cable from emitting energy that would interfere with other nearby equipment.

Coaxial cable is a third type of copper media capable of transmitting high-speed digital signals and wide-bandwidth analog signals. Unlike UTP and STP cables, however, coaxial cable is not recognized by the Commercial Building Telecommunications Cabling Standard, which sets minimum requirements for telecommunications cabling within a commercial building. (A copy of the standard, known as ANSI/TIA/EIA-568-A, can be obtained from Global Engineering, [800] 854-7179.) A grandfather clause allows the maintenance, updating, or changing of existing coaxial systems.

Copper is a cost-effective, easily installed medium. It "can carry data at speeds of 100 million bits per second for short distances" (less than

100 meters) and "10 million bits per second or less" for distances up to 2,500 meters. (Rhodes 1996, 52) Drawbacks include susceptibility to electromagnetic interference and possibility of rust and corrosion.

Fiber-Optic Media. Data are carried in a fiber-optic medium in the form of light pulses. The electrical data signal is used to turn a light source (laser or light-emitting diode) on and off very rapidly. At the receiving end of the cable, an optical detector converts the light signal back to an electrical signal. There are two generic types of fiber-optic cable. The first, *single-mode cable*, uses lasers as its light source, carries more information than multimode cable, and incurs a lower loss of signal over the length of the cable. The second, *multimode cable*, uses light-emitting diodes (LEDs) as a light source. It carries less information than single-mode cable, but it is typically adequate for most LAN functions.

A number of advantages make fiber-optic cable an attractive medium. Because information is transmitted with light pulses traveling through a glass core, rather than electrical signals, interference is not a problem. In addition, "a single fiber can carry information at rates of hundreds of millions of bits per second." (Englander 1996, 682) These advantages of "fiber optics over electrical media and the inherent advantages of a ring design" (discussed in "Network Topologies" below) "contribute to the widespread acceptance of FDDI" (fiber distributed data interface) as a standard. (Sadiku 1995, 34) Disadvantages include a higher cost and greater difficulty to install.

Radio Media. Unlike copper and fiber media, radio media utilize radio waves of different frequencies to transmit data through the air. *Broadcast radio* is used to support paging devices and cellular technology. *Microwave radio* is capable of higher data rates than broadcast radio and is used in wide-area networks as well as wireless LANs. *Satellite radio* can use both land-based stations as well as orbiting stations. Typically, signals from a land-based station are sent to an orbiting *transponder*, which receives the signal and then transmits it to another land-based station. The use of a transponder can be leased from a commercial provider, making expansion of a data network relatively easy.

Some disadvantages of radio media bear mention. First, the savings resulting from not having to install cable can often be offset by the cost of microwave and satellite transmission equipment. Second, microwave transmissions are subject to interference from adverse weather conditions as well as any objects that might interfere with its *line-of-sight* travel from transmitter to receiver. Finally, all communication using radio waves is subject to *electronic eavesdropping*, thus resulting in special security issues that must be addressed.

Transmitters/Receivers

The general process of communication consists of a transmitter sending information (or in some cases "raw data") through a transmission medium to a receiver. (See Figure 5.5.) When two people have a conversation, at a specific point in time the person speaking plays the role of the transmitter and the person listening has the role of the receiver. During the course of the conversation these roles alternate many times.

Similarly, in an information systems network, at any given time, some network component is acting as a transmitter while a second component has the role of a receiver. And, like personal conversations, the roles of these components can change frequently. The devices used to connect transmitters and receivers to the transmission media depend on the media type and data format. These devices are briefly defined below.

Network Interface Cards. A network interface card (NIC) serves as an adapter to allow a microcomputer to connect to a high-speed LAN. The specific card that is required depends on the architecture of the microcomputer and the protocol of the LAN.

Modems. A modem (MOdulator DEModulator) is a device capable of changing signals from one format to another and then back again. Two types are available: copper-based and fiber optic. The copper-based modem converts a device's digital signals to analog signals appropriate for copper media. It can take the form of a card located inside the computer (internal modem) or a separate component connected to, but located outside of, the computer (external modem). Fiber-optic modems convert a device's digital signals to optical digital signals, which can then be carried over a fiber-optic network.

Multiplexers. Several devices (computer, printer, and scanner) can be connected to a multiplexer. The output of the multiplexer serves as the input to a modem, which in turn connects to the transmission medium. A multiplexer at the receiving end of the transmission medium separates the signals. Thus the devices appear to have their own line, when in fact they are sharing the transmission medium. Figure 5.6 graphically represents the function of a multiplexer.

Bridges. Bridges are interfaces that connect two or more networks that use similar protocols (rules or conventions governing the communication process).

Figure 5.5 Communication Process

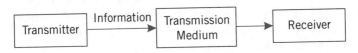

Figure 5.6 Function of a Multiplexer

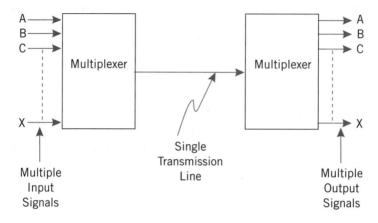

Gateways. Gateways represent the interface between two networks that use dissimilar protocols to communicate. This allows the users to access data and programs outside of their own region. Gateways play an important role in the interconnection of the many disparate networks that comprise the Internet (discussed briefly below and in Chapter 16).

Network Controller/Servers

A network controller is used in networks consisting of a number of terminals connected to one or more mainframe host computers. The function of this controller, which can be a minicomputer or microcomputer, is to "direct" the communications traffic between the host and the terminals and peripheral devices.

Local-area networks do not have a network controller. Rather, communication traffic is directed by a defined protocol that depends on the network topology (described later in this chapter). The network may have one or more *servers* that provide network users with a variety of services, including access to files (file servers); help with passing files over the transmission medium (database servers); and a connection to network printers (printer servers).

Network Control Software/Network-Operating Systems

Like network controllers, network control software is also associated with mainframe-based telecommunications networks. The software resides on the host (mainframe), on a small computer (front-end processor) connected to the host and dedicated to communications management, as well as on other processors in the network. Its purpose is to:

1. provide for the sharing of data and files;
2. facilitate the accessing of common applications and utility programs on the host computer;
3. regulate data transmission to and from the terminals and computers (workstations) on the network;
4. control access to common host databases and other files;
5. allow users to print to network printers; and
6. perform diagnostic and data transmission optimization features to improve network efficiency.

Local- and wide-area networks employ network-operating systems that coordinate and support the operation of the network. The list of services provided by these operating systems typically includes some or all of the following (Englander 1996, 706–8):

- support for several different communication protocols;
- support for locating files on the various computers of the network;
- support for handling print requests that allows users to share the printers connected to the network;
- support that allows users to pass messages from one to another;
- support for managing the security of the network; and
- support for logging in to another system on the network in order to use its facilities for processing.

Some network operating systems serve as supplements to the computer's existing operating system, adding the network support outlined above. Others, like Windows NT, constitute comprehensive computer operating systems where the networking capabilities have been integrated into the operating system.

The healthcare IS manager, when choosing network software, must therefore consider several factors, such as the number of existing or potential users, what type of network hardware is available, what type of applications software programs are needed, available resources (human and equipment), and network configuration costs.

Network Topologies

The configuration used to connect the computers and peripheral devices in a LAN is known as the network *topology*. Three alternative configurations are available to network designers: bus, ring, and star topologies. (See Figure 5.7.) These topologies, which can be used singly or in combination with one another to form a hybrid network, are described in this section.

Figure 5.7 Network Topologies

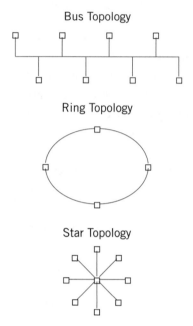

Source: Longo and Lockhart 1996. Figure 1, p. 60.

In addition, four important technologies will be introduced. The first, FDDI, has been mentioned earlier in the discussion of fiber-optic transmission media. The other three are asynchronous transfer mode (ATM), fast ethernet, and switched ethernet.

Bus Networks

In a bus network, a single circuit, or bus, is used to link the computers and other devices comprising the network. The medium employed for this single circuit can be twisted wire, coaxial cable, or fiber-optic cable. A hardware device known as a terminator is used at either end of the bus.

A device wishing to send a message listens first to see if the bus is "busy." The message is then sent out and received by every other device. Only the intended recipient, however, pays attention to the message. If by chance two devices send out messages at the same time a "collision" will occur, which will be detected. The problem is resolved by having the two devices involved wait for a random length time interval and then send the message out again. This protocol controlling how devices send and receive messages is known as *Carrier Sense Multiple Access with Collision Detection* (CSMA/CD). (A trade name for this protocol is Ethernet.)

Advantages of a bus network are the relative ease of wiring the network and the relatively fast communication rate. Disadvantages are limitations of length of the bus due to signal attenuation and the fact that if a break in the bus were to occur then all of the devices beyond the break are disconnected from the network.

Ring Networks

A ring network can be conceptualized as a group of devices (nodes) arranged in a circle with a connection between adjacent devices so as to form a closed loop. Data travels in a single direction around the ring, and each device on the network retransmits the signal it receives from the previous device to the next device in the ring.

A protocol often used with ring networks is known as the *token-ring* protocol. Under this protocol, an electronic token is continually passed along the loop. Only the node computer that holds the token at a given time can place a message on the network. The token is then passed on to the next node. The message passes from node to node until it reaches its destination. Since only one node can access the network at a time, the collisions that are possible with the CSMA/CD protocol cannot occur here.

Ring networks offer the advantage of facilitating the construction of high-speed networks that operate over large distances. This is accomplished through the use of a fiber-optic transmission medium for the connection between adjacent nodes along with the use of an amplification device (repeater) at each node. In addition, the operation of the network is not affected by removal of a node from the ring. Disadvantages include difficulty in troubleshooting the network and adding new nodes to the ring.

Star Networks

In a star network each of the nodes has a single point-to-point connection to a center node, called a *hub*, or *concentrator*. When a given node wants to send a message to a second node, the message must first travel through the center node. How the message gets properly routed to its intended destination depends on the nature of the central hub.

The simplest hub, known as a *passive hub*, simply serves as a connector for the several wires coming from the various nodes. A message sent from a given node goes to every other node. The intended "recipient" node is responsible for claiming its own messages. If the hub serves not only as a connector but also regenerates message signals before sending them on to the other nodes, then the hub is known as an *active hub*. The message signal still goes to all of the nodes, and the appropriate node claims its own messages. Finally, hubs that have "reasoning" capability are able to determine the destination address for a particular message and to route the message to that address. These hubs are known as *intelligent hubs*.

Advantages of a star network include the ease with which they can be initially wired and repaired and the relative ease with which nodes can be added to an existing network. One disadvantage of a star network is the fact that a malfunctioning hub can bring the entire network "down." The use of backup hubs can help to address this difficulty. Additionally, star networks can require more cabling than networks using other topologies. Nevertheless, this topology is in wide use in many network installations.

Hybrid Networks

Two or more of these network topologies are often combined into a single network known as a *hybrid network*. One example is a WAN formed by linking several LANs having different topologies. Another example is the Internet (discussed briefly later in this chapter and in Chapter 16), which consists of an interconnection of a variety of network types.

Four Important Network Technologies

As greater demands are placed upon networks, such as multimedia communication, transmission of larger volumes of data, and larger numbers of users, new technologies are being introduced. In some cases several alternative options are available from which the network designer or manager can choose. The following discussion introduces the healthcare executive to four technologies having an important role in the networks that health institutions and systems are developing.

FDDI. Fiber Distributed Data Interface (FDDI) has been previously introduced as a network having a token-ring topology with two rings, using fiber-optic cable, and operating at a minimum of 100 million bits per second. Edlin (1996, 13) describes the use of "a 144 fiber-count FDDI network backbone, connecting nine campus subnets . . ." at the City of Hope Medical Center in Duarte, California. The network is expected to "offer ample capacity for transporting data, images and video using a variety of transport protocols and hardware platforms."

ATM. Asynchronous Transfer Mode (ATM) refers to a networking technology that segments data to be transmitted into small packets called *cells*, directs the cells through switches to the appropriate destination node, and then reassembles the data. It allows voice, data, and video to be mixed over the network, and Englander (1996, 704) indicates that "ATM is capable of data rates in excess of a billion bits per second." Smith

(1996) describes a clinical information system installation at ProMedica Health System, Toledo, Ohio, which uses an ATM wide-area network. ProMedica felt that "ATM technology was going to be the emerging environment that would offer the capability . . . to integrate voice, data and image in a wide area environment." (Smith 1996, 16)

Fast Ethernet and *Switched Ethernet.* Recall that Ethernet is a protocol in which many users share a line's bandwidth, just like people used to share a telephone party line. Fast Ethernet and Switched Ethernet represent two proposed solutions for the problem of bottlenecks caused by a large number of users on an ethernet network.

Fast ethernet simply uses a higher quality line and associated network components capable of operating at 100 million bits per second, ten times the speed of traditional Ethernet. It "costs less per port than FDDI and is beginning to see use as a 'fat pipe' to servers and power users. . . ." (Ford 1996a, 45) Switched Ethernet "gives smaller segments of users access to the full bandwidth—much like today's dedicated telephone lines." (Cupito 1997, 18) "Children's Hospital in Philadelphia uses many types of networking technologies to meet the growing demand on its computer networks." (Anonymous 1997, 20) This includes fast ethernet installed on servers and some switched 10 megabit Ethernet. "When the load on the network becomes too great, network administrators use faster networking solutions, such as fast Ethernet, ATM or eventually gigabit Ethernet, to handle the traffic." (Anonymous 1997, 20)

Electronic Data Interchange

The networks described in this chapter can serve as the medium for transferring structured information from one computer to another without human intervention. Such a transfer is known as *electronic data interchange* (EDI). It is important that this process incorporate standards and procedures so that the "receiving" computer will be able to interpret the output of the "sending" computer. The fact that the information is structured serves to differentiate EDI from electronic communication such as e-mail in which unstructured text is transferred in the form of messages.

The use of EDI dates back to the 1980s when it was employed in a number of settings such as the shipping and automotive industries. The technology provides a cost-effective and efficient alternative to the processing of paper-based transactions or the exchange of computer tapes or disks. (Dombkowski, Charles, and Uren 1996)

While early applications in the healthcare field involved the electronic processing of health insurance claims, Bigley (1995) suggests even broader EDI applications for the future, including: automated pharmacy transactions; electronic enrollment; check and collection services; advanced claim systems; and electronic survey techniques. Siwicki (1996a) adds materials management to the list of applications in which EDI systems play a large supportive role. He describes how EDI is used for the electronic ordering of supplies and materials from vendors and indicates that EDI plays a key role in the implementation of stockless inventory and procedure-based delivery systems.

As Girton and Haupert (1996) indicate, the increase in prevalence of managed care has created increasing demands for a variety of information. Payors demand more and more information from providers. Governmental payors are also increasing their informational demands. Physicians must provide managed care organizations with increasing amounts of information to document cost and quality. EDI is seen as an effective way of providing this information while reducing costly paper processing.

Wireless Communication

In each of the computing configurations described earlier, users interact with the information system at a fixed location, often called a *workstation*. But healthcare practitioners deliver their expertise at the site of the patient, and it is there that they must be able to retrieve needed information and record newly acquired patient data. Mobile computing and wireless communication make this flow of data at the point of care possible.

Mobile computing and wireless communication are in fact two separate concepts. *Mobile computing* refers to the use of a portable computing device such as a laptop, notebook, or palmtop computer (introduced in Chapter 3). For example, home health care nurses can download the records of their patients for a given day from a central database into their laptop computer's hard disk, enter new data and notes into their laptop computer over the course of the day, and then upload the newly acquired information back to the central system at the end of the day.

While this procedure is workable, it creates the very difficulty that led hospitals to adopt networking technology. Because the laptops function as stand-alone computers, the information in the central database is not current until data collected by the portable devices are uploaded back to the central system. If a second provider, say a physical therapist, calls on the patient later in the day, the nurse's notes, collected earlier but not yet uploaded, will not be available to the therapist.

Even within an inpatient setting similar problems result when independent mobile computers are used. Until newly acquired information within the hard disk of the mobile computer is transmitted back to the central database, there will be a discrepancy between two or more databases relative to a given patient. The severity of this "mismatch" depends on the particular application.

The combination of mobile computing and *wireless communication* enables portable computers to be connected to an established information systems network. In this way the computing activities performed on the portable devices will be *real time*, and the central database will always be current. The application of two wireless communication technologies is described below.

Spread Spectrum. Spread spectrum is a type of radio frequency (RF) technology that is widely used in healthcare today for wireless communication between devices on a network. An adapter card is added to each portable computer and to the fixed server(s) to provide the needed radio equipment. Ongoing improvements in the technology have resulted in lower power requirements, improved antenna design, and decreased radio interference. (Grimm 1996)

This technology serves as the basis for several wireless LANs described in the literature, including the wireless and paperless system installed in 11 of the 19 multispecialty healthcare clinics comprising the Austin Regional Clinic (Nudd 1995); the "fifty carts with wireless enabled notebooks . . . allowing nurses to go room-to-room . . . and input information or access records on the hospital network" at St. Joseph Hospital in Denver (Hahn 1996, 49); and the wireless LAN in the 45-bed emergency room of Methodist Hospital in Indianapolis that allows patient information "to be recorded while the patient is being transported or even when the patient is being treated." (Braly 1996, 17)

Healthcare executives overseeing wireless LAN installations should be aware of the three capabilities of spread spectrum equipment that were considered by Methodist Hospital personnel during their evaluation (Braly 1996, 70):

- Range—distance covered by the transmitted signal; this will determine the number of *access points* into the network that are required;
- Frequency—the goal is to avoid interference problems with other systems in the hospital; spread spectrum equipment typically operates at a frequency of 2.4 gigahertz (1 gigahertz = 10^9 hertz); and
- Aggregate Throughput—the rate with which data can be transferred by the wireless medium; the equipment at Methodist Hospital had a data rate of 1.6 million bits per second (Mbps).

Cellular Digital Packet Data (CDPD). CDPD is a WAN architecture whose systems and communications protocols "make the transmission of data across cellular networks possible." (Wu et al. 1996, 178) CDPD network users are "serviced by the same cell sites as cellular telephone users and their calls are handed off just like the calls of cellular telephone users. The difference is that the CDPD user is transmitting or receiving data rather than a voice message . . ." and data are "transmitted in well-defined packets of information rather than a continuous . . . voice signal." (Wu et al. 1996, 179)

Mathis et al. (1996) describe an ongoing pilot study by Emory University System of Health Care in Atlanta, Georgia, and two other companies involving the implementation and evaluation of CDPD technology campuswide and beyond. The three-phase project began with the installation of an in-building cellular system on a single hospital floor, expanded to provide cellular coverage for a campuswide network, and then went on to evaluate the CDPD technology as a support for the wireless connection between the mobile devices and the host system. The third phase had not been completed at the time of the authors' report, so the final results of their evaluation remain unknown.

In fact, Grimm (1996, 40), in summarizing the state of wide-area wireless communication suggests that "for now, at least, health care will only be piloting wide-area wireless applications." He indicates that "most of the health care pilots that tried wide-area wireless communication technologies did not move forward to implementation." Nevertheless, most healthcare executives have very likely discovered the value of mobile voice communication through their cellular telephones. Certainly they will eventually support the adoption of technology that makes data available with the same degree of mobility.

Communicating via the Internet

The LANs described in this chapter can be connected to form larger networks, known as internets (observe the use of a lowercase *i*). For example, the LANs within each institution comprising an integrated delivery system can be linked to form an internet known as an enterprise computer network. These enterprise networks can, in turn, be interconnected to create another internet, known as a *community health information network* (CHIN), which links the networks of all of the healthcare delivery institutions and/or systems in a given region. Enterprise systems and CHINs are discussed in Chapter 15.

The largest interconnection of networks in the world today is known as the Internet (note the uppercase *I*). "The Internet originated in obscurity in 1969 as a project by the Defense Department and was originally built to connect various government laboratories and contractors. However, as the Net began to be used, it was soon recognized that a data link between researchers was indispensable, and in the last few years, the Internet has become readily available to the general public." (Kramer and Cath 1996, 833) The World Wide Web (WWW), developed in 1991, is a collection of electronic resources distributed over the Internet that combine text, graphics, sound, and video.

Not only have individuals found the Internet and the WWW to be valuable tools, but a wide spectrum of businesses has also developed numerous applications utilizing these resources. The healthcare field is no exception, and Chapter 16 is devoted to a survey of the applications on the Internet directly applicable to healthcare organizations. This section provides an overview of the technology issues associated with communication on the Internet, including how one connects to the Internet, the concept of a Web site, the role of an intranet, and the notion of a network computer.

Connecting to the Internet

Except for the very few institutions with a staff of in-house engineers, computer specialists, and networking experts, who are capable of connecting directly to the Internet, the majority of health organizations will obtain their Internet services through an intermediate provider. This provider can be an *online service connection* (OLSC) such as Prodigy, CompuServe, or America Online, which provides an array of information services, or an *internet service provider* (ISP) whose function is to provide users with a link to the Internet. A list of these ISPs can be obtained on the Internet at http://www.thelist.com. As of early 1997 there were more than 4,400 ISPs listed.

These providers can be reached using a *dial-up connection* or a *direct network connection.*

Users of dial-up services typically have a high-speed modem (33.6 kilobits per second) connected to a standard telephone line, or they make use of an Integrated Services Digital Network (ISDN) line with an appropriate card to connect their computer to the line. The data transfer rate is typically 64 or 128 kilobits per second.

"A direct connection is the fastest and best way to connect to the Internet." (Kramer and Cath 1996, 835) This approach uses dedicated digital telephone lines that go directly from the computer to the ISP. They can be fractional T-1 lines (about 1 megabit per second) or T-3 lines (45 megabits per second).

With either means of connection, software is needed to manage the Transmission Control Protocol/Internet Protocol (TCP/IP), which is a set of protocols "for internetwork file transfers, electronic mail transfer, remote logons, and terminal services." (Stamper 1994, 594) Other software accesses text, reads mail, and browses the World Wide Web.

The Concept of a Web Site

The connection to the Internet described above is sufficient if one's goal is to simply utilize the array of information available on the Internet. Many organizations (and individuals), however, want their own "presence on the Web," known as a Web site. This presence enables them to provide other Internet users with a variety of information—typically some combination of text, graphics, and perhaps even audio or video (see Chapter 16). Achieving this "presence" requires a home page file along with an appropriate combination of hardware, software, and technical support. (Bazzoli 1996)

There are several approaches available to assemble these resources. Jaquet (1996) outlines the process followed by a Florida hospital in weighing its options for developing a Web site. A work group quickly realized that a relatively powerful server and related hardware would have to be installed and maintained. In addition, software would be required to create the *home page*, or information presented to Internet users connecting to the Web site, and to update its contents. Capable people dedicated to this task would be needed. The work group's recommendation called for using the local telephone company to provide access to the Internet and to house the hospital's Internet site. The telephone company handles all of the necessary server maintenance and lets the hospital update its Web site as needed. The hospital then hired an additional staff member to build and maintain its home page.

Two points about Web pages bear mention. First, Web pages use *hypertext links*. This means that if the user "clicks" on a particular word or image in a document (such as the home page), the display will transfer to another document or image. For example, by clicking on "Women's and Infants' Services" on a hospital's home page, the user will be shown a new document describing these services. Second, each Web site is identified by a unique *Uniform Resource Locator* (URL). For example, the URL for the American College of Healthcare Executives (ACHE) is

http://www.ache.org

The *org* is the "domain" name of this Web site and indicates that ACHE is a nonprofit organization. Other domain names are *com* (commercial organization), *gov* (government organization), and *edu* (educational institution). A press release from the International Ad Hoc Committee (whose URL is http://www.iahc.org) in early 1997 described a plan to add seven new domain names.

The Role of an Intranet

Once the technology necessary to allow employees to access the Internet is in place, the healthcare executive might wonder why that infrastructure couldn't support communication *within* the organization. In fact it can, and this use of the Internet technology is known as an intranet. "An intranet is basically a Web-based corporate network." (Claridge 1996, 144) It has the same "look and feel" as the Internet, but the "major difference is that an intranet is primarily a closed system—it can be kept as private as the host organization wants." (Claridge 1996, 144)

Siwicki (1996b) indicates that a "handful of basic components" make up an intranet: a web server, a browser (software to allow searching of the network), a formatting language for Web-based documents, and appropriate (TCP/IP) communication protocols. A major advantage of using an intranet is cost savings that result from using "the standard languages and protocols developed for the Internet" rather than a "proprietary system that you have to modify and redistribute every time you include new data elements." (Siwicki 1996b, 37)

One concern among intranet users is security. By including access to the Internet as a feature of the intranet design, healthcare organizations create potential security risks. Protection against unauthorized outside users is provided by a *firewall*, which consists of a combination of hardware components placed between the organization's network and the Internet. The role of these components is to serve as a filter against unauthorized access.

While some information specialists wonder whether intranets are a fad, "their growth cannot be stopped. With organizations like Eli Lilly to the Mayo Clinic to Columbia/HCA implementing Internet-derived technologies, intranets definitely have come into the mainstream." (Siwicki 1996b, 47)

Network Computers

Among the benefits that a healthcare organization can realize from an investment in Web technology is the ability of the Web to facilitate the use of inexpensive *network computers* (NCs). "Network computers are similar to the old 'dumb' terminals in that information displayed on these devices is not stored locally, but in a central data center which distributes everything from software programs to the data itself out to the individual NC users." (Wheeler 1997, 24–25) Network computers have a lower purchase price and cost much less to maintain and support.

In addition to offering cost savings, NCs offer a second advantage. Because there is no disk storage on the NC, users will obtain Web software from a central source. "This will allow for central control of software, eliminating software and database 'anarchy,' such as end-users installing non-approved software on their own PC's." (Wheeler 1997, 25)

"It's not clear that the NC will eventually succeed the PC . . . will users be willing to abandon their nifty gizmo-packed machines for a plain, pared-down box that is entirely dependent on the network?" (Schneider 1997, 42) In this area, like all decisions concerning information systems acquisition and installation, the healthcare executive is well-advised to be aware of all alternatives and select the one best suited for his or her organization.

Summary

The trend toward the creation of integrated health systems and other environmental changes have made the information needs of healthcare organizations increasingly complex. Among the strategies necessary to respond to these changes is the development of computer networks and the use of telecommunications. A network can be a LAN or a WAN according to how narrowly or broadly dispersed are the components that comprise the network.

Networks can also be classified according to the manner in which the processing function is distributed among the devices comprising the network. Four alternative configurations are: a mainframe computer that does all of the processing and may have dumb terminals connected to it; a client/server network that divides the computing function between two or more machines; a file/server configuration in which most processing takes place on the user's computer and the server is used to store the files; and a distributed processing configuration where the computing responsibility is delegated down to the lowest possible level in the organization. Each alternative has its own strengths and weaknesses, and the appropriate configuration is dependent on the organization's strategic direction.

A variety of components comprise an information network. Transmission media include wired media, fiber-optic media, and radio media. Transmission and receiving components include network interface cards, modems, multiplexers, bridges, and gateways. Network controllers and protocols associated with the network servers help to direct the communication traffic on the network. Finally, network software and operating systems control the accessing and use of network resources and help to improve network efficiency.

The configuration with which devices are connected to form a network is known as the network topology. Three alternative configurations, each with pros and cons, are a bus, ring, or star topology. Two or more topologies can be combined to form a hybrid network. Other important network technologies include a Fiber Distributed Data Interface (FDDI), asynchronous transfer mode (ATM), and Fast or Switched Ethernet.

The transfer of structured information between computers is known as electronic data interchange (EDI). The healthcare field employs EDI for a number of important applications including claims processing, pharmacy transactions, electronic enrollment, electronic survey techniques, and materials management.

Wireless communication and mobile computing make information available at the point of care. Spread spectrum technology serves as the basis for wireless LANs. Cellular digital packet data (CDPD) is a WAN architecture that makes data transmission across cellular networks possible.

The Internet is evolving into an important resource for healthcare organizations. It provides access to a wide range of information, allows the organization to achieve a presence on a worldwide information network, and provides an infrastructure for communication within the organization.

Networking and telecommunications are highly technical and rapidly changing areas. Gaining a basic understanding of these areas, staying abreast of the changes, and knowledgeably interacting with the technical specialists in the field, are ongoing challenges for the healthcare executive.

Discussion Questions

5.1 Describe how the development of integrated healthcare systems has created an impetus for installing computer networks.

5.2 Name and describe the computer environment that offers the highest degree of centralization.

5.3 Explain the difference between two-tier and three-tier client/ server architecture.

5.4 What is the difference between digital and analog waveforms?

5.5 Name and describe the two types of copper media in common use.

5.6 What are the advantages of fiber-optic media compared with copper media?

5.7 Describe the function of a modem.

5.8 Describe the functions of a network-operating system.

5.9 Name and describe the three network topologies.

5.10 Describe some important applications of EDI in the healthcare field.

5.11 Explain the notion of a wireless LAN.
5.12 Define the concept of cellular digital packet data.
5.13 Explain the difference between internet and Internet.
5.14 What is meant by the term *Web site?*
5.15 Explain the role of an intranet.

Problems

5.1 The executive suite of your hospital is contained in a contiguous space on a single floor. It has a total of 12 computers currently functioning independently. Each is a 160 Mhz Pentium machine with 16 Mb memory, and a 2 GB hard drive. All of the computers are running under Windows 95. The furthest distance between any two machines is about 70 feet. Discussions are under way to link these computers into a LAN. Determine the specific additional hardware and software required and the approximate cost of this hardware and software (assume that the building has been prewired with appropriate cabling and that each computer is no more than six feet from a cable connection).

5.2 Use the Internet to obtain a list of the Internet Service Providers in your zip code. Contact at least one of these providers to obtain details about available Internet service and the associated cost. Recommend an appropriate level of service for a three-physician medical office wishing to have access to the Internet for medical research purposes.

5.3 Interview one or more hospital CIOs in your area in order to find one who has evaluated taking their institution from a mainframe configuration to a client/server architecture. Indicate whether they decided to keep their mainframe and/or to install a client/server system. Describe clearly the logic they used in order to reach their decision.

5.4 Contact the telephone company in your area to determine their cable offerings for data services into your home. For each type of cable, indicate the transmission speed and the price. Suppose you are an independent healthcare consultant operating from your home and that access to the Internet is important for your work. Specify the cable option that would seem to make the most sense.

5.5 The CFO of your hospital has just returned from a conference where healthcare claims clearinghouses were discussed. She wonders if the use of such a clearinghouse would be beneficial for your institution. Using the library, interviews of CFOs, and other appropriate sources, do sufficient research to determine the following:

- what a claims clearinghouse is;

- the scope of services provided;
- the relationship between claims clearinghouses and EDI;
- any hardware and/or software requirements to utilize the services of a claims clearinghouse; and
- the financial viability of utilizing a claims clearinghouse.

Write a report to your CFO describing your findings.

5.6 The areas of mobile computing and wireless communication are dynamic fields. You have been hired by a home health agency to investigate the feasibility of equipping their home health nurses with laptop computers capable of utilizing CDPD technology. They want you at a minimum to determine:

- whether new technology (if any) exists that should be considered as an alternative to CDPD technology;
- what specific benefits result from the real-time transmission of data;
- the feasibility of the home health nurse transmitting the data back to a central computer from a fixed telephone location after each home health visit; and
- any additional information relevant to the question of whether to adopt the CDPD technology.

Write a report to the CEO of the home health agency describing your findings and documenting your recommendation(s).

References

Anonymous. 1996. "The Architecture Decision: RIMS Client/Server Direction." *RIMS Online* 2 (7): 3–4.

Anonymous. 1997. "At Children's Hospital of Philadelphia, the 'Layered Look' in Networks is in Style." *Health Management Technology* 18 (1): 20.

Bazzoli, F. 1996. "The Ins and Outs of Internet Outsourcing." *Health Data Management* 4 (2): 19–20.

Bigley, J. 1995. "The Electronic Data Interchange: Avoiding Potholes to Add Value & Power for Payors & Providers." *Infocare* (August): 34–37.

Braly, D. 1996. "Methodist Hospital's Wireless POC Network Strategies." *Health Management Technology* 17 (3): 17, 70.

Chin, T. L. 1997. "Payers Begin the Migration to a New Architecture." *Health Data Management* 5 (1): 78–79, 81.

Claridge, A. 1996. "Harnessing Intranet Technology." *Healthcare Informatics* 13 (6): 144.

Cupito, M. C. 1997. "Widening the Pipe: Plain Talk About Fast and Switched Ethernet." *Health Management Technology* 18 (1): 18, 21–22.

Dombkowski, K. J., M. Charles, and R. L. Uren. 1996. "Using Electronic Data Interchange in Managed Care Performance Measurement." In *Proceedings of the 1996 Annual HIMSS Conference, March 3–7, 1996, Atlanta, Georgia, Volume 1.* 159–76. Chicago: Health Care Information and Management Systems Society.

Dunbar, C. 1994. "It's Not the Goal . . . It's the Journey." *Health Management Technology* 15 (11): 28–30, 32, 34.

Edlin, M. 1996. "HOPENET Puts Center on Path for Year 2000." *Health Management Technology* 17 (11): 13–14, 16.

Englander, I. 1996. *The Architecture of Computer Hardware and Systems Software: An Information Technology Approach*. New York: John Wiley and Sons.

Ford, J. 1996a. "Switched Networks Extend Life of Today's Internetworks." *Health Management Technology* 17 (10): 45–46, 69.

Girton, T. A. and Haupert, C. S. 1996. "EDI Helps Group Practices Manage Costs." *Health Care Financial Management* 50 (6): 50, 52, 54, 56, 58.

Grimm, C. B. 1996. "Moving Ahead With Wireless and Mobile." *Healthcare Informatics* 13 (11): 38, 40, 42, 44, 46.

Hahn, D. 1996. "Going Wireless at the Point of Care." *Healthcare Informatics* 13 (4): 49–50.

Jaquet, G. J. 1996. "Building a Web Site Strategy." *Health Data Management* 4 (9): 75–76.

Kramer, J. M., and A. Cath. 1996. "Medical Resources and the Internet: Making the Connection." *Archives of Internal Medicine* 156 (8): 833–42.

Lee, N., and A. Millman. 1995. "ABC of Medical Computing: Hospital Based Computer Systems [Education & Debate]." *British Medical Journal* 311 (7011): 1013–16.

Longo, M. C., and P. Lockhart. 1996. "Structured Cabling: Foundations for the Future." *Health Care Information Management* 10 (4): 59–77.

Mathis, J. L., M. Killian, D. Cohen, J. M. Dunbar, and P. Mathews. 1996. "Case Study: A Health Care System's Use of Wireless Technology." In *Proceedings of the 1996 Annual HIMSS Conference, March 3–7, 1996, Atlanta, Georgia, Volume 2*. 89–97. Chicago: Health Care Information and Management Systems Society.

McFarland, B. 1994. "Wire Today for Tomorrow." *Healthcare Informatics* 11 (6): 112.

Nudd, A. 1995. "Texas Clinic Goes Wireless and Paperless." *Healthcare Informatics* 12 (5): 48, 50.

Rhodes, P. D. 1996. *Building A Network: How to Specify, Design, Procure, and Install a Corporate LAN*. New York: McGraw-Hill, Inc.

Sadiku, M. N. O. 1995. *Metropolitan Area Networks*. Boca Raton, FL: CRC Press, Inc.

Schneider, P. 1997. "Emerging Technologies: From Fascination to Application." *Healthcare Informatics* 14 (1): 39–44.

Siwicki, B. 1996a. "EDI Enables Hospitals to Trim Inventories." *Health Data Management* 4 (6): 50–52, 56.

———. Siwicki, B. 1996b. "Intranets in Health Care." *Health Data Management* 4 (8): 36–38, 41–42, 44, 47.

Smith, L. 1996. "Preparing for Health care in the Next Century." *Health Management Technology* 17 (10): 15–16, 18, 65.

Smith, L. 1997. "Putting the Servers in Client-Server." *Health Management Technology* 18 (1): 32–34.

Stamper, D. A. 1994. *Business Data Communications*, 4th Ed. Redwood City, CA: The Benjamin/Cummings Publishing Company, Inc.

Wheeler, M. 1997. "The Healthcare Enterprise Web and the Future of Clinical Information Systems." *Health Management Technology* 18 (1): 24–26.

Whyte, L., and K. Matsumoto. 1996. "Client/Server Allows Faster Addition of New Members and Benefits." *Health Management Technology* 17 (12): 36, 38.

Wu, J. B., J. Colon, J. Lauer, and J. Kromelow. 1996. "Wireless Data Transmission: How to Implement Remote Data-Access." In *Proceedings of the 1996 Annual HIMSS Conference, March 3–7, 1996, Atlanta, Georgia, Volume 2*. 175–87. Chicago: Health Care Information and Management Systems Society.

Additional Readings

Anonymous. 1996. "Electronic Data Interchange." *Health Management Technology* 17 (1): 26, 28.

Berson, A., and A. Anderson. 1995. *Sybase and Client/Server Computing*. New York: McGraw-Hill, Inc.

Bird, D. 1994. *Token Ring Network Design*. Wokingham, England: Addison-Wesley Publishers Ltd.

Bysinger, B. 1996. "Client/Server: Minefield or Garden Path?" *Health Data Management* 17 (11): 42–43, 46.

Ford, J. 1996b. "Network Architectures and Configuration Choices." *Health Management Technology* 17 (12): 34–35, 55.

Ford, J. 1997. "Network Migration Requires an Understanding of Real-Life Needs." *Health Management Technology* 18 (1): 50–52.

Pesicka, J. 1995. "EDI Gives Central Plains Competitive Edge." *Healthcare Informatics* 12 (4): 106.

Ramos, F. 1997. "Client/Server System: The Answer in a Distributed Environment." *Healthcare Informatics* 14 (1): 34, 36.

Siwicki, B. 1995. "Will Paper Ever Go Away? Document Imagers Bet It Won't." *Health Data Management* 3 (8): 49–50, 52, 54–55.

6

DATA MANAGEMENT

T
HE APPLICATION of information technology to the healthcare field is characterized by a high degree of complexity and interdependence among users and applications. The formation of healthcare systems and growth in managed care have served to add to this complexity. As a result, multiple users often require access to the same data; data collected in one institution are often needed by a user in another location; and newly acquired data must be merged into existing data. Recall from Chapter 5 that providing a linkage to facilitate the exchange of data was cited as a key rationale for the installation of computer networks.

However, even when computers have been networked, users will not be able to easily access the data they need unless care has been given

Concepts and Applications

Information is only useful to system users when it is accessible, and a database management system (DBMS) helps to make it available. A DBMS can store data in different ways and manipulate it using a query language, which can take different forms.

This chapter will allow readers to list the types of database models and explain how data are stored in them and how they are retrieved and manipulated. Readers will also be able to discuss issues related to database management such as security of information, viruses, and information backup.

to the organization of the data and to the development of software for storing, modifying, deleting, and disseminating the data. A collection of data carefully organized to be of value to the user is called a *database* and the associated software used to manipulate the database is commonly known as a *database management system* (DBMS). The development of database technology has provided much improvement over previous data storage methodologies.

Because the healthcare field is so dependent on the timely availability of data, the appropriate implementation of database technology is particularly important. Healthcare executives must have sufficient understanding of this technology in order to oversee its implementation. This chapter is designed to help the executive develop this understanding. Specific topics that are covered include a review of computer files as a data storage approach; the improvement offered by databases; an overview of database models; the notion of database management systems; issues surrounding data security; developments in database technology; and the role of data warehouses in healthcare.

Computer Files: A Brief Review

Long before electronic computing and storage devices were introduced, organizations maintained data in paper files. Filing cabinets containing one or more drawers were designed to "hold" the data in file folders, which were arranged alphabetically, numerically, or according to some predefined sequence. By placing a document or other "piece" of data into the proper folder when the data item was received, the user could be sure of being able to retrieve the item when it was needed.

The secondary storage devices described in Chapter 3 provide an electronic alternative to the filing cabinet. Recall that these devices can be either sequential devices or direct-access storage devices, and the type of storage device has an impact on the format of the files maintained on it.

Sequential Computer Files

The tape drive allows users to create one or more tape *files*. Each file, roughly equivalent to a file drawer, contains a series of *records*. The record is essentially equivalent to a file folder, and each record consists of a number of *fields* corresponding to the data items stored within the file folders of a paper-based system. As an example, an early hospital personnel system typically utilized a tape file in which each record stored information on a given employee. Within the record were multiple fields containing specific data about the employee—date of hire, Social Security number, date of birth, address, foreign language skills, etc. Figure 6.1 depicts the hierarchy of a field, a record, and a file for this application.

Figure 6.1   Hierarchy of a Field, Record, and File

	Employee Name	Date of Hire	Social Security No.	Language Fluency
FILE	Ken L. Watt	03/03/86	111-23-3223	None
	Jane Sargent	11/10/90	356-29-0588	German
	Mary Smith	05/05/97	334-44-9876	Spanish
	⋮	⋮	⋮	⋮
	Robert Cardin	09/12/92	056-88-4848	French

	Employee Name	Date of Hire	Social Security No.	Language Fluency
RECORD	Mary Smith	05/05/97	334-44-9876	Spanish
FIELD	Mary Smith		(Employee Name Field)	

The hospital either developed or purchased software that was capable of adding new employees to the file, modifying one or more fields in an employee's record, or deleting an employee from the file. This software might also produce one or more reports, such as an alphabetical listing of the employees, a list of employees in descending order of years of affiliation with the hospital, or a list of employees fluent in Spanish.

The fact that a tape drive is a *sequential* storage device creates challenges for the software developer. The simple task of changing an employee's address requires reading through the entire file in order to find the employee's record. Adding several new employees to a file maintained in alphabetical order requires sorting the employees to be added, creating a transaction file containing the new employees, reading the old employee file, merging the records from the transaction file where applicable, and writing a new employee file. Computer code had to be developed to accomplish these tasks.

Direct-Access Computer Files

When disk files, which are *direct-access* storage devices (DASD), were introduced, a major difficulty was addressed. In order to update a given employee's record, it was no longer necessary to read through the entire employee file. Rather, the program could "go directly" to that employee's record and make the necessary corrections.

In fact, the ability of the file maintenance program to directly access a given employee's record depends upon the program's "knowing" the *record number* containing that employee's data. That is, it was the software developer's responsibility to create a system for keeping track of the location of each employee's record within the file. One approach commonly used was to develop an algorithm that converted the employee number to a unique record number. Alternatively, an index file could be maintained whose records contain either employee name or number along with the number of the record in the employee file containing that employee's data. If no means is provided for determining the record number associated with a given employee, then the file could only be processed sequentially.

Problems of Computer Files

The need for the programmer to design a means for identifying the number of a desired record in a direct-access file is just one of several problems associated with traditional computer files. Other problems include program/file dependence, data redundancy, and data inconsistency. Each of these problems is briefly described below.

Program/File Dependence. The notion of program/file dependence refers to the fact that a given computer-based data file is typically associated with a specific application program. Thus, when developing a hospital billing system using, for example, COBOL, a programmer would also design and implement the related data file using the same language.

This dependence has several implications. First, a second application program written in another language, for instance, Pascal, could not practically access the billing system file. Second, even when another application program is written in COBOL, its developer needs detailed information about the file structure in order to be able to use the file for the second application. And finally, even though the billing file contains valuable detailed information about the resources consumed by all of the inpatients, retrieving this information can be a very difficult task requiring development of a custom program. The impact of this difficulty on the development of decision-support and executive information systems will be discussed in Chapter 13.

The close linkage between a given application program and its associated data files is easy to understand within the healthcare field. Each application was often developed independently of other applications, taking the form of a stand-alone module. Thus, an admissions/discharge/transfer (ADT) program, an order entry and results reporting program, a radiology program, and a laboratory program all have data files that could potentially be shared, but instead function independently. This situation is portrayed graphically in Figure 6.2.

Figure 6.2 Linkage between Application Programs and Associated Data Files

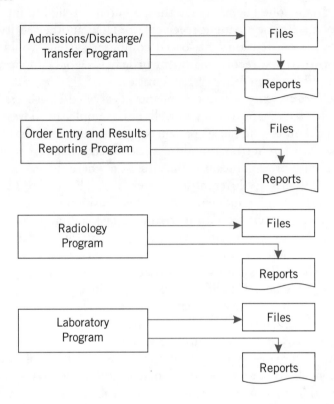

Data Redundancy. As its name implies, data redundancy refers simply to the situation in which the same data item appears in several files within the health organization's computer system. (The same data item can also occur redundantly within a single data file.) For example, the files used by the ADT program contain the name, address, telephone number, and other patient demographic data. But it is quite likely that the computer program used by the radiology department will have associated files whose fields include similar patient demographic information. Patients are all too familiar with the fact that they are typically asked for the same demographic information by multiple persons during their inpatient stay or outpatient encounter.

Similarly, the results of laboratory tests will be stored in a file associated with the laboratory computer system and will also be sent back to the patient floor. There it will be added either to a computer record (if one is in place) or filed in the patient's paper chart. In any event, the same patient information will be stored in multiple locations.

This duplication of information wastes resources—personnel, time, and computer storage. As healthcare organizations expand into large health systems, one begins to see the potential for significant data redundancy. Each time a patient receives care from another entity within the system, a conventional file-based computer system would require the creation of a new record, many of whose fields would duplicate those existing in files within other system entities.

Data Inconsistency. The redundancy described above creates the potential for data inconsistency as well. For example, an address change between encounters can cause a patient to have an address in the file of one entity that is different from the address contained in another entity's file. Perhaps even more significant is the situation where the patient's name appears differently in different computer files. This can result from a typing error, use of a middle initial on one occasion but not another, or a name change associated with marriage. A task as simple as searching for all of the records associated with a specific patient can become quite difficult when there are patient name inconsistencies.

Data redundancies can also lead to data inconsistencies when changes are made in a file field. Consider the patient billing system. Suppose that the pharmacist has discovered that the wrong price has been quoted on a given pharmaceutical item. All of the fields recording the dispensing of that pharmaceutical item must now be changed in order to correct the error. Failure to change *all* of the fields will lead, of course, to inconsistencies. If it were possible to store the price of the item in a single location to which reference would be made as the statement is generated, this chance of data inconsistency would be greatly reduced. The database technology discussed below provides such a possibility.

Databases: An Improvement over Files

A number of difficulties associated with the use of traditional computer files were described in the previous section. Database technology does an excellent job of addressing these difficulties. Among the benefits offered by using the database approach (see, for example, Date 1995, 14–17) are the following:

1. Redundancy can be reduced. Although not all data redundancy is eliminated, the redundancy is *controlled*. This results in efficient data storage as well as data processing.

2. Inconsistency can be avoided. This is accomplished either by storing a given data item only in one place or by making the system aware of redundancies so that they can be properly handled.

3. Data can be shared. An important benefit of the database approach is the ability to make data available to many applications, both existing

as well as new applications. Thus, the sharing of data allows a decision-support system (discussed in Chapter 13) to utilize data generated by a number of the applications running within the organization. When data are shared, careful attention must be paid to how the information resource is managed, such as the development of standards.

4. Standards can be enforced. The centralization of the information resource affords the opportunity to enforce standards. (Of course it is the centralization itself that is responsible in part for the need for standards.) Three important areas of standardization are:

- data representation;
- naming of variables; and
- documentation.

5. Security restrictions can be applied. Again, this benefit is also something made necessary by the centralization of the information resource. Users can be required to use a password in order to gain access to data, and security levels can be defined so that data are made available only to users having a legitimate "need to know."

6. Data integrity can be maintained. The reduction in inconsistencies increases the users' confidence in the integrity of the data. In addition, the administrator in charge of the centralized data resource can define rules, which are imposed when the database is updated. Adherence to these rules will also help to maintain data integrity.

7. Conflicting requirements can be balanced. The centralization of the data resource will result in a system that attempts to globally optimize the value of that resource enterprisewide. This is in contrast to a noncentralized configuration that works well for one department but not for any others.

8. Data independence. The tight coupling between the data file and the application program no longer exists. Thus, changes in the structure of the data file or of techniques for accessing the file do not impact the application program. This independence is of course related to the benefit of sharing data.

An Overview of Database Models

Healthcare executives will typically use databases whose logical structure follows one of three models: hierarchical; network; or relational. To better understand each of these models, consider the following simple database application: A large medical center has many departments, each of which has a variety of equipment. Technicians from the biomedical engineering department are assigned the task of providing scheduled maintenance on this equipment as well as servicing the equipment when it breaks down. The medical center wishes to develop a database system to support this equipment maintenance process. The database will maintain a profile of the equipment as well as the employees in each department, the technician assigned to each piece of equipment, and a detailed description of each maintenance procedure performed on the equipment.

Hierarchical Data Model

The hierarchical data model stores data as nodes in a *tree* structure. Figure 6.3 illustrates the application of this model to the equipment maintenance process. The node "Department" is called the *root*, a special node always drawn at the top of the diagram. "Department" has two *child nodes*, "Employees" and "Equipment." Similarly, "Equipment" is the *parent node* of "Technician" as well as "Maintenance Records." Thus, each node can have only one *parent node*, but it may have multiple *child nodes*. This property is referred to as a "one-to-many" relationship, a characteristic of the hierarchical database model. A node having no branches leaving it is known as a *terminal node*. "Employees," "Technician," and "Maintenance Records" are terminal nodes.

Network Data Model

The network data model, as its name suggests, stores data as nodes in a network. The parent nodes and children nodes defined in the hierarchical data model become *owners* and *members*, respectively, in the network data model. The model uses links, called *pointers*, to connect the owners and members, forming a relationship called a *set*. Unlike the hierarchical

Figure 6.3   Hierarchical Data Model—Equipment Maintenance Database

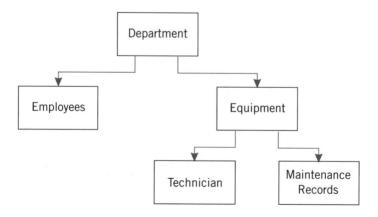

model where a node can have only one parent, in the network data model a member can have more than one owner. As a result, "many-to-many" relationships are possible, which result in reduced data redundancy. The network data model for the equipment maintenance process is shown in Figure 6.4.

Relational Data Model

The relational data model stores data in individual files, or *tables*, with data items arranged in rows and columns. The application of this model to the equipment maintenance process is illustrated in Figure 6.5. The two-dimensional tables are also known as *relations* (from which the name *relational model* derives).

Each row, or *tuple*, normally includes data for a single data *record* (e.g., a department), with each column, or *field*, of the table containing one piece of data. The fields in the department relation, for example, are DEPT_NO, DEPT_NAME, and DEPT_MGR. (See Figure 6.5.) At least one field of the table should be a key field used for searching and retrieving records, with each record having a unique value. An example of a key field in a department record is the department number, DEPT_NO.

A Comparison of the Three Data Models

There are advantages and disadvantages associated with each of these three data models. Both the hierarchical and network models have pre-defined links, or pointers, that define *explicit* relationships. These links provide efficient processing in high-volume applications so long as the search follows a path through the data that was specified in advance.

Figure 6.4 Network Data Model—Equipment Maintenance Database

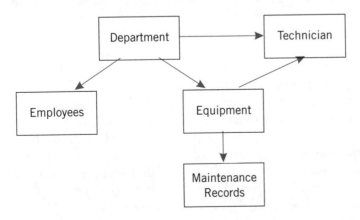

Figure 6.5 Relational Data Model—Equipment Maintenance Database

DEPTABLE:

DEPT_NO	DEPT_NAME	DEPT_MGR
15	Radiology	Jones
18	Nursing	Smith
23	Admitting	O'Riley
⋮	⋮	⋮
37	Physical Therapy	Krusher

EMPTABLE:

EMP_NO	EMP_NAME	DEPT_NO
3021	Lynn Francis	19
3034	Harry Kildare	23
3049	Michael Cruse	22
⋮	⋮	⋮
3812	Fran Simmons	17

EQTABLE:

EQUIP_NO	EQUIP_NAME	DEPT_NO
803	Pocket Pager	12
844	Laptop Computer	19
850	Cart	20
852	Portable X-ray	15
⋮	⋮	⋮
879	Respirator	28

However, although the network structure is somewhat more flexible than the hierarchical structure, both models tend to be limiting with respect to the searches that can be easily performed. Thus, for ad hoc inquiries the relational model is preferred.

Network data models appear to have achieved little popularity in healthcare management computer applications or among personal computer (PC) users. Two research applications have been reported. Knuppel et al. (1994) suggest that the network model possesses particular advantages for data management of a complex structure. They have used this model as part of a retrieval program to make data on DNA sequences accessible. Nicolosi (1995) describes a system designed to support researchers in epidemiology. The nodes of the network model database consist of text, graphics, and executable procedures and correspond to windows on the screen. The network structure allows the user to follow the links between the nodes and locate desired information.

The hierarchical model is appropriate in applications where the data form a natural hierarchy. Frank and Berge (1995) describe the implementation of several hierarchical databases in a radiology department to provide online access to a variety of information including protocol manuals, emergency procedures, and telephone and pager numbers. Tomioka (1995) proposes a radiology reporting system based on the concept of a hierarchical structure.

The Decentralized Hospital Computer Program (DHCP), a hospital system implemented by the Department of Veterans Affairs (VA), provides a third example of the use of a hierarchical data model. Its structure results in a database that "is optimized for retrieval of information about individual patients, not about groups of patients." (Graber et al. 1996, 149) Thus, although the database plays a "critical and central role in the day-to-day management of VA patients . . . (it) is difficult to use for epidemiologic analyses." For example, the simple question " 'how many patients with diagnosis of tuberculosis within the past year are having their prescriptions for antituberculosis drugs regularly filled and have had timely chest x-rays' would require considerable effort to answer using the DHCP database." (Graber et al. 1996, 149)

The relational data model, the newest of the three database models, seems to be emerging as the most popular and widely used. Among respondents to a survey conducted by the College of Healthcare Information Management Executives, about half currently use this model in a production environment, while the others indicated a position ranging from "interested in the technology" to "conducting a pilot." (Ream 1996) The strengths of this model lie in its ability to handle ad hoc queries, the ease with which it can be created and maintained, and its ability to easily interface with a variety of systems in the organization. (Sherr 1995) A disadvantage of the relational data model is the relatively slower processing time compared to the other two models, a result of the relational model's greater flexibility and ad hoc query capability.

The importance of query capabilities in a database system can be seen in the Managed Care Workstation developed by the VA. (Levy, Beauchamp, and Hammond 1995) Recall that the VA's Decentralized Hospital Computer Program (DHCP) utilizes a hierarchical database. This data model makes it difficult for staff interested in managed care and outcomes assessment to obtain needed information "which is based on elements that cross services and hospital functions, populations of patients, or summary information grouped by providers and clinics." (Levy, Beauchamp, and Hammond 1995, 388) To address this difficulty, the authors developed a workstation in which the DHCP data elements are mapped into *relations* or *tables* that can then be queried by the workstation user. Pilot studies demonstrated the feasibility of this mapping and clearly showed the advantages that relational databases have over hierarchical databases for ad hoc queries.

A variety of applications using relational database models has been reported in the literature. A database developed from Tennessee Medicaid files and described by Chyka et al. (1996) supports retrospective drug-use review. Computer queries can be used to create profiles of physicians' or pharmacies' experiences from claims data and other Medicaid data. Balfour (1996) describes the use of a relational database to store information on clinical cases involving a microbiologist. Once constructed, the database yields information on the clinical involvement of the microbiology department within the hospital, providing a reference point from which further research and audit can be based. Finally, Borok (1995) emphasizes the importance of relational databases in the coming generation of healthcare information systems, suggesting that the relational model will support complex utilization review requirements and provide a foundation for the operational demands of large managed care networks. The role of relational databases in decision-support systems is discussed further in Chapter 13.

Database Management Systems

The discussion thus far has focused on the advantages of databases over traditional files and an overview of three alternative database models. But it is not enough to merely conceptualize about the data elements that will support the operations and management of a healthcare institution. One must be able to actually build and maintain the database as well as to easily extract desired information from it. These tasks are accomplished with a *database management system* (DBMS). Recall that such a system was defined earlier as the software used to manipulate the database. This section provides more detail about the specifics of this software. In particular, two languages and a special file are introduced: the *data definition language* (DDL) used to define and describe the data in the database; the *data manipulation language* (DML) used to access, edit, and extract information from the data contained in the database; and the *data dictionary* used to store a detailed description of the data in the database.

The Data Definition Language

The computer views data stored on a secondary storage device as a given number of bytes located at a specific location on the disk. This perspective, known as the *physical view* of the database, may be appropriate for the computer, but it is anything but satisfactory for the user. The healthcare executive prefers a *logical* or *user* view of the data in which a data item is known by some "logical" name, typically one that suggests the quantity being stored. The DDL is used to create the link between the user view and the physical view of the database.

The user begins the process by defining his or her view, or schema, of the database. In those cases where multiple users will be accessing portions of the same database, each user's view would be known as a *subschema*. The schema can be stored as part of the database or in a separate file. Among the items included in the schema (or subschema) are: a description of the file; a description of the record; and information about the data fields, including field name, type of quantity stored in the field (numeric, logical, text, etc.), and length of the field. In addition, the DDL is used to define relationships among the records, allow relationships among data to be defined, and establish data security access.

The Data Manipulation Language

Because programming skills are typically required in order to extract information from a traditional file, managers have generally been unable to easily interact with this form of data storage. A major benefit of database technology is that interaction with the data does not require a high level of computer programming proficiency. This ease of interaction with data results from the inclusion with the DBMS of a *data manipulation language* (DML).

"The term 'data manipulation language' refers broadly to the mechanism used for retrieving data stored in a database." (Gillenson 1990, 92) The DML allows users to perform a variety of operations including adding new data; sorting, deleting, editing, or displaying data; and generating reports. Two basic methods for interacting with the database are available: (1) "embedded statements," which can be added to an application program to instruct the database to find certain data and return it to the program; or (2) the user can issue a command through a workstation in a special language to find a certain data item and return it to the screen. Use of the DML for direct interaction with the database gives rise to the notion of a *query language*.

To illustrate a direct query to a database, consider a user who wants to generate a list of the name and number of all pieces of equipment associated with department number 15. There are at least three ways such a query might be handled.

Natural Language Queries. Perhaps the ultimate way for a user to query a database is in simple English words. For this approach, the sample query might be:

> "Please give me the name and number of all pieces of equipment that are associated with the department having the number 15."

Notice that the use of a natural language query requires very little new vocabulary to be learned. The computer processes the request by looking for key words in the sentence. If a key word cannot be found, the user might be asked to rephrase the request.

Even better than typing natural language requests into the computer would be the ability to make English language requests verbally. Such a system would combine natural language query with voice recognition technology as discussed in Chapter 3. The practical implementation of such a system would undoubtedly be well received by the community of database users.

Query-by-Example. A very common and easy to use query method is known as query-by-example (QBE). Many microcomputer database systems employ this method, in which the user makes appropriate entries into selected fields of a table displayed on the screen. Figure 6.6 illustrates the use of QBE to obtain the name and number of the equipment in department 15. The "P." placed in the EQUIP_NAME and EQUIP_NO fields indicates that these fields are to be printed, while the "15" in the DEPT_NO field indicates that only records having a department number of 15 are to be included in the output.

Structured Query Language. Structured query language (SQL) is a query language that combines elements of both a data definition language and a data manipulation language. It was developed in the 1970s and adopted as a standard relational language in 1986. Because it is a standard, programmers familiar with the language can use it on a number of hardware platforms from microcomputers to mainframes. As with other data manipulation languages, a user can invoke SQL statements either interactively or from within an application program.

Many of the language statements consist of verbs like "Create," "Update," "Select," or "Delete," along with appropriate modifiers describing the nature of the desired action to be taken. For example, in order to

Figure 6.6   Illustration of Use of Query-by-Example

EQUIP_NO	EQUIP_NAME	DEPT_NO
P.	P.	15

accomplish the sample inquiry (obtaining a list of the name and number of the equipment in department 15), one might issue the following SQL command:

> SELECT EQUIP_NAME, EQUIP_NO
> FROM EQTABLE
> WHERE DEPT_NO=15

where EQUIP_NAME, EQUIP_NO, and DEPT_NO are the "logical" names for the name of the piece of equipment, the number of the piece of equipment, and the department number, respectively (refer to Figure 6.5).

A number of database applications described in the literature specifically indicate the use of SQL. Examples include the formulation of queries in a pathology information system (Miaoulis et al. 1993), in a large, integrated hospital information system (Hooymans et al. 1995), and in a managed care workstation (Levy, Beauchamp, and Hammond 1995).

The Data Dictionary

The data dictionary is a file that stores detailed information about the data elements used in a database. This information includes such things as the name of the data element, the type of element (numeric, alphanumeric, logical, etc.), the amount of storage allocated to the data element, the person in the organization authorized to change the element, the date the element was last changed, the programs that use this element, and the reports that use this data element.

There are a number of benefits provided by the data dictionary (see, for example, Gillenson 1990, 311–12), including:

- assisting in the design of new databases by making available the database structure of earlier applications;
- avoiding changes to a database that will impact an application using that database;
- helping to avoid data redundancy and promote data standardization by indicating that a given data element already exists; and
- providing a natural vehicle for documentation so that programmers will be less likely to skip this important documentation process.

Data dictionaries can be *passive* or *active*. A passive data dictionary simply provides documentation about the data elements within the database in the form of a report. When changes are made to an active data dictionary, these changes are able to be automatically used by the applications that utilize the database.

Data Security

Healthcare information systems typically contain data that are highly critical and sensitive. Therefore, data security becomes a particularly important issue in this environment. In fact, "data handling has become a hospital accreditation issue, and part of that requirement is making standardized, accurate data available for clinical decision making and comparative analysis while ensuring that confidentiality and security are not breached." (Lafrance 1995, 58) The healthcare executive must ensure that at least three areas of data security have been addressed: privacy/confidentiality protection; virus protection; and data backup/recovery procedures. Each is briefly outlined below.

Privacy/Confidentiality Protection

Patient data privacy is a very important concern. In addressing that concern one quickly realizes that "access and confidentiality frequently represent opposing forces as one creates policies and systems for electronic record storage and retrieval." (Aikins, Leavitt, and Skinner 1997, 42) At least two levels of confidentiality issues will need to be considered by healthcare organizations implementing database technology: individual patient records used by healthcare providers and aggregate databases used by planners and managers.

In the clinical setting, user access codes and password procedures must be established and enforced so that only users with a legitimate "need to know" can obtain specific patient information. For example, the financial portion of the database might be made available to billing personnel, demographic information to a registration clerk, and full clinical data to physicians for their own patients.

An interesting question arises regarding allowing physicians to access data on a patient who is not recorded in the database as being under that physician's care. (This can arise from the common situation where a physician encounters a colleague in the hospital corridor and asks her to "look in" on a particular patient.) One large Midwest healthcare system has chosen to address this question by allowing the colleague to access the patient's record. However, the healthcare system has made its physicians aware that in such cases a permanent log will be recorded so that the exact queries that the colleague makes will be known. (Weiss 1997) This serves as a deterrent to users gaining access to unauthorized information.

In addition to supporting clinical care, patient data serves as the basis for a variety of analyses such as outcomes research, resource planning, and managed care contracting. For the most part, these analyses are based on aggregate patient data so that the identity of individual patients is not really necessary. In these cases, it is important to mask all patient identifiers including, of course, name, patient number, Social Security number, and any other field that would allow the researcher or analyst to identify the patient.

A typical approach is to scramble the patient number so that there is a unique identifier associated with each patient record. This will allow the analysts to link data on a given patient obtained from several databases. The scrambling procedure should of course be known by only a limited number of people. In a similar fashion, when patient data are used to develop profiles of physicians with regard to outcomes achieved, resources consumed, etc., the confidentiality of the physician is frequently maintained. The physicians know only their own code, so they are able to compare their performance against that of their peers.

Further discussion of data security policies can be found in Chapter 7.

Virus Protection

Computer users and IS staff must also protect software from computer viruses, programs that intentionally try to alter or destroy data, programs, or operating system files on computer hard drives or floppy disks. A virus may be unintentionally passed from one computer to another by floppy disk or through a network. The healthcare IS manager must have security procedures to prevent viruses from infecting computers, including not allowing the use of any bulletin board or other unauthorized software that hasn't first been checked out with an antivirus program; employing and enforcing effective security codes and passwords for users on networks; and purchasing, installing, and periodically running antivirus software programs on network servers and other computers.

O'Connor (1997) suggests that an organization's information network becomes increasingly vulnerable to computer viruses through accessing the Internet. Downloading information and software from an Internet source can introduce a virus into the organization's entire network. "To combat this risk, the network provider organization should implement Internet-specific policies, including equipping all network terminals with antivirus software, installing firewalls, and regularly auditing the network and deleting all unauthorized files and software." (O'Connor 1997, 30–31)

Data Backup/Recovery Procedures

The healthcare executive should make sure that effective data backup and recovery procedures are implemented on a regular basis across the organization. At the central processing site, daily, weekly, and other periodic backups to removable disk packs or tape must be performed. Duplicated data should be secured and stored in a separate location away from the central site, preferably in a different building if possible.

Individual sites also need to have regular and effective backup procedures, especially for microcomputers and workstations. (Jones 1995) Access codes, passwords, audit trail boards, and software may be used in conjunction with physical cable-lock systems to protect hardware and software. Disk or tape backup and software should be used to automate data backup and recovery. Also, data at individual sites that also reside on the main processor or at other individual sites must be correctly updated at all locations. The IS manager must weigh the needs of individual departments and sites to have specific data versus efficient data integrity and updating.

The IS manager must also be able to trace data transactions on distributed systems in case of data corruption, loss, or tampering. These transaction traces, or audit trails, will allow the IS manager to recover data in a timely and effective manner. Transaction auditing procedures must be an integral part of the database management system design. IS and other authorized personnel must maintain accurate, up-to-date, secure transaction logs, both at the central IS site as well as at individual sites.

Developments in Database Technology

The information demands of the healthcare field often require database technologies beyond those discussed thus far. Three additional technologies offer potential advantages that the healthcare executive should understand: *object-oriented databases* and *hypermedia databases*, both of which are capable of storing multimedia data; and *distributed databases*, which allow data to be stored in multiple physical locations.

Object-Oriented Databases

Recall that the relational databases described earlier contain text fields stored in rows and columns. Many of these databases have a feature known as binary large objects (BLOBs) that allows them to link to graphic images. However, such linkages are somewhat clumsy, cannot be "searched" to locate records having certain defined properties, and do not support other media, such as audio or video, which are gaining increasing importance in today's medical record. One approach to addressing these deficiencies is object technology.

Introduced in the late 1980s, Dyck (1996) defines object-oriented databases as "an information retrieval system that manages complex objects containing both data (referred to as properties) and procedures for manipulating this data (called methods). Although early implementations have failed to live up to expectations, developers are actively working to incorporate object support into their products for at least three reasons:

- Object-oriented databases turn out to be effective at modeling and storing complex business objects such as document archives, personnel records, and World Wide Web pages.
- Object-oriented databases will allow faster retrieval of complex objects than is possible with relational databases, at least in theory.
- Object-oriented databases promise faster development and easier maintenance of database applications. (Dyck 1996)

Applications of object-oriented database technology have been reported in the healthcare literature. Combining data with query routines (Gray et al. 1990) or with algorithms for creating genetic and physical maps (Kochut et al. 1993) in a single database highlights an advantage of object technology over traditional relational models. Object-oriented databases can also be an important part of decision-support systems, supporting, for example, diagnosis and patient alerting (Frost and Gillenson 1993) or health resource planning and allocation (Rafanelli et al. 1995).

Hypermedia Databases

To understand the concept of a hypermedia database, one needs first to be familiar with a *hypertext database*. A hypertext database consists of a network of *nodes*, each of which stores text. The *links* between the nodes are defined by the user. Users of the World Wide Web are familiar with this database structure. As the reader scans a paragraph of text on a particular topic, certain words are observed to be highlighted in a different color from the rest of the text. By clicking the cursor on one of these highlighted words, the user can cause the program to branch to another node where text on this new topic can be accessed.

In a *hypermedia database*, the *nodes* can store a variety of media—text, graphics, motion pictures, audio, or programming code. As in the hypertext database, the nodes in the network are connected by *links* that can be defined by the user. In this way, a multimedia patient record can be constructed in which text fields can have audio or video fields linked to them. For example, associated with a brief textual summary of the results of a cardiac catheterization procedure could be a video of the actual procedure. By clicking on the text of the report, the user could "branch" to the video and see the actual catheterization displayed on the screen.

Applications of hypermedia systems to computer-assisted instruction (CAI) have been reported. Chen, Hoffer, and Swett (1989) describe a hypermedia textbook of nuclear medicine that contains text, graphs, tables, figures, literature citations, and an image database. Mankovich et al. (1991) have also developed a hypermedia system that integrates text, graphics, and image information in an introductory CAI course for nuclear medicine. In addition, Michael and Foxlee (1992) report on a prototype hypermedia-based workstation designed for the practicing radiation oncologist in which demographic, clinical history, presentation, staging, course, laboratory, and treatment data are linked.

Distributed Databases

Recall from Chapter 5 that the processing function within a computer network can be concentrated in a single computer, often a mainframe, or it can be split among all of the network workstations, typically microcomputers. The former approach represents a *centralized* computing environment while the latter is known as *distributed processing*. In a similar fashion, an organization can choose to store its data in a single, centralized database, or to spread the data across several smaller databases. This latter data storage configuration is known as a *distributed database*.

Distributed systems allow extensive data storage and processing at multiple departments within the same building, in several buildings on a single campus, or on several campuses separated by significant distances. In a modest-sized, stand-alone healthcare facility, it is frequently possible to maintain a single database to support all of the organization's data needs. However, in today's large, integrated healthcare systems this single database concept becomes impractical for at least two reasons:

- the use of distributed databases within each of the geographically dispersed entities comprising the system is more practical than the use of a single centralized database; and
- the use of a single database to support both clinical operations as well as database searches results in unacceptable time delays for users of the information system.

Berson and Anderson (1995, 146) cite the following benefits associated with distributed databases:

- Data reside closer to their source.
- Single point-of-failure of critical data is eliminated since multiple copies of critical data reside at different locations.
- Data access is more efficient since no network communication is required.
- Applications are more balanced so far as data access is concerned.

- The easier access to data facilitates growth in applications and satisfaction of end-user demands.

Chueh and Barnett (1994) discuss a computer-based healthcare record system designed to meet the needs of the patients and providers of a homeless population. They propose combining client/server technology and distributed database strategies to produce a common medical record for this population.

Of course, the use of distributed databases has disadvantages as well. As Berson and Anderson (1995, 146) indicate, the management of distributed databases is more complex, and a relatively significant potential for loss of data synchronization among the various databases exists. Therefore, it is very important that provisions have been made for maintaining the overall integrity of the organization's data, including specific details for sharing and controlling the data.

One final challenge resulting from the use of distributed databases bears mention. While users in a particular entity can more easily interact with the databases located within their facility, gaining access to information distributed among databases in several entities of an integrated system can be difficult. This same difficulty presents itself to corporate executives wishing to do systemwide planning or to a physician wanting to gather information about a patient who has received treatment in several of the system's facilities. This challenge is being addressed through the development of data warehouses.

Data Warehouses

As noted, there are many occasions when executives and physicians have need for an aggregate view of the data contained in the distributed databases of their system. Constructing such a view on an "as-needed" basis can be time-consuming and inefficient. A better approach is to maintain this aggregate view in one or more databases called *data warehouses*. A data warehouse "enables the collection and organization of disparate data sources, both internal and external, to an enterprise and provides users with a common, integrated subject-oriented view for decision-making." (Ladaga 1995, 26)

Clinicians use this aggregate view to obtain a profile of past data for a given patient. For example, a physician might want to compare a current blood pressure reading with those obtained over the past three years. Investigators use the data warehouse to perform outcomes research, evaluating alternative treatment modalities to see which have better results. And executives need aggregate patient and financial data to support a variety of planning, marketing, contracting and decision-making activities. More details of the uses of data warehouses are given in Chapter 13, and computer-based patient records (CPRs) are discussed in Chapter 11. The databases themselves are discussed below.

Clinical Data Repository

"A clinical data repository is a database that brings together information from various venues of care and various departments within hospitals to make patient information available where it's needed." (Bazzoli 1995, 51) The data in the repository can include details of inpatient stays, outpatient visits, tests ordered and their results, immunizations, emergency room visits, home health care (Rainey, Bailey, and Scott 1996), and even stays in a long-term care facility. It truly represents longitudinal descriptions of individuals' healthcare.

Bazzoli (1995, 52) describes three components of a clinical data repository:

- the database itself, which typically stores vast sums of information;
- a loader program, which supports the "uploading" of data from entity systems and external sources into the repository; and
- a user interface, which makes it easy for clinicians and executives with no technical computer skills to extract the information they seek.

The physical structure of the data repository is subject to discussion. Since the goal is to make aggregate data from across the system available in a single location, it would appear that a single database would be most appropriate. However, the transactional needs of clinicians and the research needs of investigators can often be a source of conflict. As a result, performance issues will often cause "providers to add a second database when they begin research efforts with their repository. Having day-to-day clinical data in one database and research data in another will prevent a repository system from slowing down." (Siwicki 1996, 58)

Successful implementation of a data repository, like any systems development and implementation project, is not an insignificant task. However, two specific challenges bear brief discussion: development of a *master patient index* to facilitate tracking of patient information; and standardization of terminology and format to facilitate transfer and comparisons of data from diverse sources.

Master Patient Index. Since each of the entities within an integrated system frequently use a different patient numbering system, it can be difficult to link data on a given patient uploaded from the various entity computer systems. Because of spelling errors, omission of middle initials, or legal name changes, even the use of the "Name" field may not totally solve the problem. One possible solution is the use of a *master patient index* (MPI), a relational database containing all of the identification numbers that have been assigned to a patient anywhere within the system.

The MPI "assigns a global identification number as an umbrella to all patient numbers. Database queries go through the master patient index so that all appropriate data in the repository is retrieved." (Siwicki 1996, 58) The global identification number must be matched to all of the records associated with the given patient, a process made particularly difficult because the match must be made in real time.

There are three additional qualities that master patient indexes should have in order to be able to handle the rapid changes occurring in the healthcare field:

- They must be flexible enough to incorporate patient numbers as integrated delivery systems add new providers with a variety of legacy systems.
- To accommodate changes in the network or in identification parameters, they must be easily configurable without requiring extensive programming.
- They must be scalable to fit any size organization and to accommodate growth in an integrated delivery system. (Bazzoli 1996, 62)

Standardization of Terminology and Data Format. In addition to differences in a patient's name, variations can also be found in the format and terminology within the various computers of an integrated delivery system. As a result, one could experience difficulty uploading data from these computers to a data repository as well as using the data in the repository to draw comparisons among the entities of the healthcare system. One resolution of this dilemma is the development of standards to guide both the format and substance of the data. A number of such standards exist, two of which are described below.

Health Level-7 (HL7) "is designed to standardize the exchange of data among disparate systems within a health care organization. . . . HL7 is now routinely used in health care to tie systems together." (Anderson and Bunschoten 1996, 42) The HL7 standard is supported by most system vendors and is used in the majority of large hospitals in the United States. Thus, each of the health system entities can implement the software of their choice and can transfer data from one system to another so long as the software is HL7-compliant.

Of course, even when the system entities adhere to the HL7 standard, the system still "must tackle the challenge of making sure all users use the same terms the same way. This is a particularly important issue for integrated delivery systems attempting to share clinical data among multiple sites." (Anderson and Bunschoten 1996, 41) One standard vocabulary that is proposed by a number of electronic records experts is the Systematized Nomenclature of Human and Veterinary Medicine (SNOMED). SNOMED is the "most comprehensive vocabulary system available and provides the best framework for terminology. . . . SNOMED could serve as the framework for a new broader vocabulary that all medical specialties could use." (Anderson and Bunschoten 1996, 41)

The success of the HL7 and SNOMED standards clearly requires the cooperation of the entities. In a health system with a large number of legacy computer systems and a heritage of "independent thinkers," enforcing a policy requiring adherence to these standards could be difficult. An alternative approach is to feed the output of the entity systems to a translator interface, which standardizes the content before passing the information to the data repository. The translator might even be capable of recognizing non-HL7-compliant data from the existing systems, and only future systems would be required to adhere to HL7 standards.

The "Clinical Data–Financial Data" Interface

The literature suggests that the ultimate survival of healthcare organizations depends heavily on their ability to interface clinical and financial data. While the clinical data repositories described in the previous section have received a great deal of attention in the literature, little discussion of the development of financial data repositories has appeared. This dearth of discussion is particularly puzzling since the collection of financial data has always been an important role of computer systems in the healthcare setting. In fact, many early installations were justified on the basis of their ability to significantly reduce the loss of charge slips.

One explanation might be the fact that today's increasing managed care market creates a need for accurate cost data. While there appears to be multiple approaches that could be taken in order to compute these costs, the need for an accurate and detailed accounting of the resources consumed by a given patient would seem to be clear and unambiguous.

This need for accurate data on patient resource consumption creates an additional role for the clinical data repository as well as additional criteria for its design. Developers of these repositories must be sure that sufficient details and descriptions are included regarding each component of care that is delivered to the patient, no matter what setting the care is delivered in. In addition, the charges typically assigned by the institution to these resources could also be stored to serve as a surrogate indicator of the value associated with these resources. Decision makers can then apply an appropriate algorithm for determining the cost of the care delivered.

Finally, steps should be taken to be sure that outcome data is also included in the repository. Not only must decision makers know what care was given, the value traditionally placed on that care, and how much the care cost, but they also need to associate an outcome, or "benefit," with the episode so that the healthcare system can demonstrate a cost benefit for the care offered by their delivery system. More details on the role of the clinical data repository in decision analysis is provided in Chapter 13.

Summary

As healthcare computer systems increase in complexity, the IS manager must choose new DBMSs with care, taking into account patient data security and privacy vs. user access to data, distributed or centralized systems, and data accuracy and quality. These DBMSs offer a number of advantages over traditional file storage methods.

The three main database models are the hierarchical, network, and relational models. The model most used today is the relational, although the hierarchical model is also used for some applications. Network data models appear to have achieved little popularity in healthcare management computer applications.

Database Management Systems allow users to fully utilize the power of databases. These systems consist of: a DDL used to define and describe the data in the database; the DML used to access, edit, and extract information from the data contained in the database; and a data dictionary used to store a detailed description of the data in the database.

Use of the DML for direct interaction with the database gives rise to query languages, which allow the database user to easily and efficiently extract data records and fields. These queries can take the form of a natural language query, a query-by-example, or a structured language query. The database designer must decide how data will be used in designing a good DBMS.

Data security is an important issue and one that database designers and users must constantly address. At least three areas to be considered are privacy/confidentiality protection, virus protection, and data backup/recovery procedures. Only users with a genuine "need to know" should have access to individual patient data where the identity of the patient can be determined. In other cases, aggregate data with scrambled identifiers should be used. Passwords should be implemented that help to ensure that only authorized users can gain access to the system. Deliberate steps should be taken to reduce the potential impact of viruses on the database, particularly in light of the increased vulnerability created by greater use of the Internet and other external data sources. Backup and recovery procedures are an essential component of data security, including the use of audit trails.

Healthcare executives will find increasing use of object-oriented, hypermedia, and distributed technologies, and they are well advised to become familiar with how these approaches can benefit their database applications. In fact, distributed systems are now used at many healthcare units with multiple processing sites. The IS manager must take into account several factors in deciding to use distributed systems, including the type of data to be distributed, data security and quality, protection and privacy of patient data, and user security training procedures.

Although distributed systems are being increasingly used, executives and physicians in integrated delivery settings require aggregate views of data distributed throughout the system. As a result healthcare organizations are building data warehouses to serve as clinical data repositories to support clinical care, outcomes research, and managerial decision making.

Good audit procedures are needed to ensure patient and other data integrity and security. Two types of auditing include user control and transaction tracking. To be effective, audit controls must be communicated to users and enforced. To be successful, these repositories require adoption of data standards, for example, the HL7 and SNOMED standards.

Without question, healthcare delivery has been and continues to be a data-driven endeavor. The skill with which healthcare executives lead the process of developing and managing database technology within their enterprise will have a great influence on the ultimate quality of the healthcare services offered.

Discussion Questions

6.1   Name and explain three problems associated with traditional computer files.

6.2   Name and describe the three most widely used database models.

6.3   Define *schema* and name the items typically included within a schema.

6.4   Explain the function of a data manipulation language.

6.5   Describe three ways of handling a direct query to a database.

6.6   What is a *data dictionary file*?

6.7   Explain how security issues dealing with accessing aggregate patient data differ from security issues associated with accessing individual patient records.

6.8   How does accessing the Internet impact the security of an organization's information network?

6.9   Describe a hypermedia database.

6.10 Define the concepts of distributed databases and centralized databases, and indicate the strengths and weaknesses of each.

6.11 Explain the function of a master patient index.

6.12 Why is standardization of terminology so important in developing a data repository within integrated delivery systems?

Problems

6.1   Set up a sample patient record with pertinent data fields using both a relational and hierarchical database model.

6.2   Obtain a copy of the schema that is employed in an electronic medical record system. Prepare a brief presentation that outlines how the schema supports the query capability of this system.

6.3   Identify an integrated delivery system that has developed, or is developing, a data repository. Determine the data fields that comprise this database, the composition of the committee who decided on the structure of the database, and the mechanism by which the decision regarding the structure was made. In addition, determine who has access to the data, and what specific security measures are in place. Write a brief report of your findings.

6.4   Interview a chief information officer (CIO) in a nearby healthcare organization or system. Determine the role that data standards such as HL7 and SNOMED play in their selection and purchase of software. Summarize your findings in a memo.

6.5   Prepare an annotated bibliography of articles from the literature that describe the use of SQL in application software written for the healthcare field.

References

Aikins, R., M. Leavitt, and R. I. Skinner. 1997. "Confidentiality, Access, and Security: An Integrated Delivery System's Experience." In: *Proceedings of the 1997 Annual HIMSS Conference, February 16–20, 1997, San Diego, California, Volume 3.* 37–48. Chicago: Health Care Information and Management Systems Society.

Anderson, H. J., and B. Bunschoten. 1996. "Creating Electronic Records: A Progress Report." *Health Data Management* 4 (9): 36–38, 41–42, 44.

Balfour, A. 1996. "Review of Clinical Activity by Microbiologists." *Journal of Clinical Pathology* 49 (5): 429–31.

Bazzoli, F. 1995. "Repositories Promise to Quench Growing Thirst for Health Data." *Health Data Management* 3 (9): 50–54, 56.

Bazzoli, F. 1996. "Providers Point to Index Software as Key Element of Integration Plans." *Health Data Management* 4 (9): 61–62, 64–65.

Berson, A., and G. Anderson. 1995. *SYBASE and Client/Server Computing.* New York: McGraw-Hill, Inc.

Borok, L. S. 1995. "The Use of Relational Databases in Health Care Information Systems." *Journal of Health Care Finance* 21 (4): 6–12.

Chen, C. C., P. B. Hoffer, and H. A. Swett. 1989. "Hypermedia in Radiology: Computer-Assisted Education." *Journal of Digital Imaging* 2 (1): 48–55.

Chueh, H. C., and G. O. Barnett. 1994. "Client-Server, Distributed Database Strategies in a Health-care Record System for a Homeless Population." *Journal of the American Medical Informatics Association* 1 (2): 186–98.

Chyka, P. A., T. D. Holimon, J. T. Tepedino, and H. Petersen. 1996. "Relational Database for Drug-Use Review of Tennessee Medicaid Claim." *American Journal of Health-System Pharmacy* 53 (2): 164–66.

Date, C. J. 1995. *An Introduction to Database Systems*, 6th Ed. Reading, MA: Addison-Wesley Publishing Company, Inc.

Dyck, T. 1996. "Relational Model's Limits Fuel Move to Object Databases." *PC Week* [http://www.pcweek.com/archive/1345/pcwk0078.html] 11/11/96.

Frank, M. S., and R. E. Berge. 1995. "Value of On-Line Informational Databases in a Radiology Department." *AJR. American Journal of Roentgenology* 164 (6): 1537–39.

Frost, R. D., and M. L. Gillenson. 1993. "Integrated Clinical Decision Support Using an Object-Oriented Database Management System." *Methods of Information in Medicine* 32 (2): 154–60.

Gillenson, M. L. 1990. *Database Step-by-Step*, 2nd Ed. New York: John Wiley and Sons.

Graber, S. E., J. A. Seneker, A. A. Stahl, K. O. Franklin, T. E. Neel, and R. A. Miller. 1996. "Development of a Replicated Database of DHCP Data for Evaluation of Drug Use." *Journal of the American Medical Informatics Association* 3 (2): 149–56.

Gray, P. M., N. W. Paton, G. J. Kemp, and J. E. Fothergill. 1990. "An Object-Oriented Database for Protein Structure Analysis." *Protein Engineering* 3 (4): 235–43.

Hooymans, M.P., H. Liefkes, J. A. Schipper, and A. R. Bakker. 1995. "Retrieval From a Large, Integrated HIS-Database Through Formal Descriptions and SQL." *Medinfo* 8 (Part 1): 478–81.

Jones, K. 1995. "Contingency Planning in LAN/WAN Environments." *International Journal of Network Management* 5 (2): 77–81.

Knuppel, R., P. Dietze, W. Lehnberg, K. Frech, and E. Wingender, E. 1994. "TRANS-FAC Retrieval Program: A Network Model Database of Eukaryotic Transcription Regulating Sequences and Proteins." *Journal of Computational Biology* 1 (3): 191–98.

Kochut, K. J., J. Arnold, J. A. Miller, and W. D. Potter. 1993. "Design of an Object-Oriented Database for Reverse Genetics." *ISMB* 1: 234–42.

Ladaga, J. 1995. "Let Business Goals Drive Your Data Warehouse Effort." *Health Management Technology* 16 (11): 26, 28.

Lafrance, S. 1995. "Security is Achievable Even in Today's Complex Networks." *Health Management Technology* 16 (11): 58.

Levy, C., C. Beauchamp, and J. E. Hammond. 1995. "A Managed Care Workstation for Support of Ambulatory Care in Veterans Health Administration Medical Centers." *Journal of Medical Systems* 19 (5): 387–96.

Mankovich, N. J., R. C. Verma, A. Yue, D. Veyne, O. Ratib, and L. R. Bennett. 1991. "NMINT—Introductory Courseware for Nuclear Medicine: Database Design." *Proceedings of the Annual Symposium on Computer Applications in Medical Care*: 757–61.

Miaoulis, G., E. Protopapa, G. Skarpetas, C. Skourlas, and G. Delides. 1993. "Information Retrieval for Pathology Information Systems." *In Vivo* 7 (4): 373–77.

Michael, P. A., and R. H. Foxlee. 1992. "HyperOncology: Demonstration of an Evolving

Hypermedia-Based Workstation for the Radiation Oncologist." *Proceedings of the Annual Symposium on Computer Applications in Medical Care*: 841–42.

Nicolosi, A. 1995. " 'Hyperstat': An Educational and Working Tool in Epidemiology." *Medinfo* 8 (Part 2): 1697.

O'Connor, K. J. 1997. "Information Technology Policies for Integrated Delivery Systems." In: *Proceedings of the 1997 Annual HIMSS Conference, February 16–20, 1997, San Diego, California, Volume 2.* 23–32. Chicago: Health Care Information and Management Systems Society.

Rafanelli, M., F. Ferri, R. Maceratini, and G. Sindoni. 1995. "An Object Oriented Decision Support System for the Planning of Health Resource Allocation." *Computer Methods & Programs in Biomedicine* 48 (1–2): 163–68.

Rainey, M., M. Bailey, and H. Scott. 1996. "Enabling Information Technologies for Home Care." *Journal of the Healthcare Information and Management Systems Society* 10 (2): 43–48.

Ream II, T. E. 1996. "Technology Watch: Relational Database Management Systems." *Healthcare Informatics* 13 (2): 140.

Sherr, B. 1995. "Flexibility, Access Give RDBMS the Edge." *Health Management Technology* 16 (9): 38.

Siwicki, B. 1996. "Data Repository: Early Users Learn Valuable Lessons, Reap Benefits." *Health Data Management* 4 (10): 57, 58, 60, 61.

Tomioka, K. 1995. "[Radiology Reporting System Based on the Concept of Hierarchical Structure] [Japanese]." *Nippon Igaku Hoshasen Gakkai Zasshi—Nippon Acta Radiologica* 55 (9): 690–96.

Weiss, D. 1997. Private communication to author. BJC Health System, St. Louis, MO. 63110.

Additional Readings

Barry, D. K. 1996. *The Object Database Handbook: How to Select, Implement, and Use Object-Oriented Databases.* New York: John Wiley and Sons.

Connolly, T., C. Begg, A. Strachan. 1996. *Database Systems: A Practical Approach to Design, Implementation and Management.* Harlow, England: Addison-Wesley Publishing Company, Inc.

Costaridou, L., N. Sphiris, T. Pitoura, G. Panayiotakis, and N. Pallikarakis. 1993. "An Educational Hypertext System Supporting Radiographic Image Quality." *Medical Informatics* 18 (4): 331–38.

Date, C. J., with Darwen, H. 1997. *A Guide to the SQL Standard*, 4th Ed. Reading, MA: Addison-Wesley Longman, Inc.

Delobel, C., and C. Lécluse. 1995. *Databases: From Relational to Object-Oriented Systems.* London, England: International Thomson Computer Press.

Elmasri, R., and S. B. Navathe. 1994. *Fundamentals of Database Systems*, 2nd Ed. Menlo Park, CA: Addison-Wesley Publishing Company, Inc.

Helms, R. W., and I. McCanless. 1990. "The Conflict Between Relational Databases and the Hierarchical Structure of Clinical Trials Data." *Controlled Clinical Trials* 11 (1): 7–23.

Markou, S. A., D. Koukouras, T. Pimenidis, and J. Androulakis. 1995. "Using Hypertext Software to Develop Computer-Assisted Instruction in Oncology for Medical Students." *Journal of Cancer Education* 10 (3): 141–43.

Mattison, R. 1996. *Data Warehousing: Strategies, Technologies, and Techniques*. New York: McGraw-Hill, Inc.

Ross, S. 1995. "Is It Security or Disaster Recovery? Who Cares?" *International Journal of Network Management* 5 (4): 193–97.

Shimada, M., K. Akazawa, H. Higashi, Y. Watanabe, Y. Hayashi, S. Moriguchi, K. Fujisawa, and Y. Nose. 1990. "Development of an Automatic Medical Summary Report System." *Japan-Hospitals* 9 (July): 49–54.

PART

III

Information Systems
Planning and Management

STRATEGIC INFORMATION SYSTEMS PLANNING

STRATEGIC INFORMATION systems (IS) planning is the process of identifying and assigning priorities to a set of computer applications that will assist an organization in executing its business plans and achieving its strategic goals and objectives. As health services organizations grow in size and complexity and information technology becomes increasingly sophisticated, the need for careful system planning is paramount. Managers must take responsibility for an orderly planning

Concepts and Applications

Information systems and an organization's strategic plan must be closely linked. A healthcare executive interested in implementing a new information system must take several factors into account, including defining the system's purpose, determining hardware and software requirements, and setting key dates and schedules for implementation.

The planning process should be guided by an enterprisewide information system steering committee with representation from the major clinical and administrative units of the organization.

At the conclusion of the chapter, the reader will be able to discuss the importance of a master plan for an organization's information system development and implementation, and describe the ways the system and its software can be developed or acquired.

process to insure that information systems are supporting the strategic priorities of the organization.

As the 21st century approaches, information systems priorities are changing to focus on integration of systems across multiple facilities, automation of patient records, and improved decision support for clinicians and managers. Achieving these complex objectives requires a careful planning process to develop a flexible information architecture that facilitates data exchange and provides remote user access to information from all locations.

Unfortunately, many information systems in health services organizations have evolved in a piecemeal fashion rather than from a carefully controlled planning process. Specific requirements for capturing, storing, and retrieving data when needed are often developed on an ad hoc basis as new programs and services are added. As a result, the same data are captured repetitively; files are duplicated needlessly; information is not always available when needed; and numerous other gaps and inefficiencies are commonplace.

Lacking an information systems planning process, priorities for development of individual computer applications often are established by the exigencies of the moment: which operational "crisis" has the current attention of management, or which department complains the loudest. In such an environment, *strategic* use of information to serve *institutional priorities* is often ignored.

According to a recent survey of leaders in healthcare computing, their greatest frustration was the lack of strategic IS planning within their organization. Thirty-five percent of the survey respondents indicated that their healthcare organizations did not have a strategic IS plan. (HIMSS/HP 1996)

This chapter presents an overview of the process of IS planning in health services organizations. Topics covered include the purposes of planning, organization of a planning effort, the elements of a strategic information systems plan, and the development of enterprisewide standards and policies.

Purposes of Strategic IS Planning

Strategic IS planning serves multiple purposes in the health services organization. The most important of these are listed in Figure 7.1 and discussed briefly below.

Strategic Alignment with Organizational Goals and Objectives

Information systems should support the strategic goals, objectives, and priorities of the organization they serve. As healthcare organizations

Figure 7.1 Purposes of Strategic Information Systems Planning

- To align information systems goals with strategic goals and objectives of the organization
- To define specific information requirements and priorities
- To define the information technology infrastructure of the organization
- To develop a budget for resource allocation

become more sophisticated in IS planning and management, they will use information more effectively in strategic positioning within the environment in which they operate. (Austin, Trimm, and Sobczak 1995, 27) The strategic IS plan should address such questions as:

- How can information technology be used to generate new services in response to market demands?
- How can information technology be used to distinguish among services provided by the organization from those of competitors?
- Which computer applications and supporting technology are needed to make the new strategy work? (Tan 1995, 306)

Historically, hospitals and other health services organizations have employed information technology to support day-to-day operations. Increasingly, executives are recognizing the role of information systems in increasing marketshare, supporting quality assessment and improvement, and adding value to the organization. In order to accomplish these strategic objectives, the IS plan must be closely aligned with the strategic plans of the organization. Since these objectives change over time, the information technology plan should be reviewed frequently to be sure it remains in alignment with current organizational strategy.

Definition of Information Requirements and Priorities

Given limited resources and pressures for cost containment, healthcare organizations must make choices and set priorities for their information systems. Consequently, the IS plan should identify the major types of information required to support strategic objectives and establish priorities for installation of specific computer applications for the time period covered by the plan (normally about five years).

Definition of the Information Technology Infrastructure

The third essential purpose of strategic IS planning is more technical in nature. In order to meet strategic objectives and develop high-priority applications, the health services organization must develop blueprints for its information technology infrastructure. This involves decisions about hardware architecture, network communications, degree of centralization or decentralization of computing facilities, and types of computer software required to support the network.

A 1995 survey of healthcare executives (Morrissey 1995a, 66) identified the following information technology infrastructure priorities:

- client/server network architecture;
- optical disk storage and data warehouses for clinical records;
- interface engines for linking the information systems of members of integrated delivery systems;
- wide-area fiber-optic networks;
- relational databases; and
- multimedia workstations.

Budgeting and Resource Allocation

The final purpose of strategic IS planning is to provide data for estimating resources required to meet the objectives and priorities established through the planning process. Planning will provide the basis for development of operating and capital budgets for information systems in the organization.

Organizing the Planning Effort

The development of information systems in a modern healthcare organization is a complex task involving major capital expenditures and significant manpower commitments if the systems are to function properly. The development of an overall master plan for IS development is an essential first step in the process. To exclude this critical planning activity would be analogous to beginning a major construction project without functional specifications for the new building. And yet, many organizations have moved directly into the development of computer systems without any kind of master plan.

The chief executive officer (CEO) should take direct responsibility for organizing the planning effort. An IS steering committee should be formed with representatives from major elements of the organization, including the medical staff, nursing staff, financial management, human resources management, planning and marketing, facilities management, and clinical support services, The steering committee should be directed by a knowledgeable member of executive management, preferably the chief information officer (CIO), if such a position has been established. Strategic information planning is primarily a managerial function, not a technical one.

A suggested organizational chart for the planning effort is shown in Figure 7.2. Steering committee members should serve as chairs for the subcommittees; additional personnel from the organization and technical consultants can be appointed members of specific subcommittees as needed.

Consideration also should be given to the use of outside consultants, if additional technical expertise is needed. However, outside consultants should be chosen carefully. They should possess technical knowledge of systems analysis and computer systems and should be well-informed about healthcare organizations. It is essential that consultants be truly independent practitioners and not associated with any equipment manufacturer or firm that sells software. Finally, consultants should be familiar with the latest technological developments but able to resist the temptation to push for applications that are too close to the leading edge.

Lohman (1996) suggests that the following factors be considered in selecting an information systems consultant:

Figure 7.2 Organizing the Planning Effort

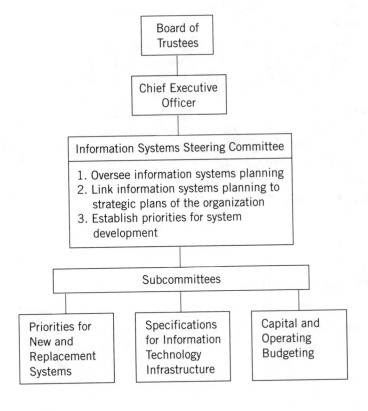

1. Independence and objectivity—exclusive focus on interests of the client
2. Healthcare expertise—understanding of healthcare business and clinical issues
3. Resources—sufficient breadth and depth of resources to complete the assignment without "on-the-job training"
4. Effective personality—appropriate mix of character traits and skills

Consultants should be used as sources of technical information and as facilitators of the planning process. They should *not* be employed to do the planning; this must be the responsibility of knowledgeable managers and users of information within the organization itself. Before using a consultant's "off-the-shelf" planning product, be sure that the planning methodology is compatible with the organization's culture and strategic priorities.

The CEO should ensure that staff members participating on the steering committee are provided sufficient released time from their normal duties so that they can participate fully in the planning efforts. Released time estimates should be drawn up in advance, and formal written notification of this should be provided to all involved. The administration and board of trustees should be prepared to spend a significant amount of the institution's manpower resources on carrying out this important task.

As stated, the organization's CIO should chair the steering committee if the CIO position has been established. Reporting directly to the CEO or chief operating officer (COO), the CIO serves two important functions: (1) assisting the executive team and governing board in using information to support strategic planning and management, and (2) providing management oversight and coordination of information systems and telecommunications throughout the organization. The CIO's role is further discussed in Chapter 10.

Elements of an IS Master Plan

Figure 7.3 lists the major elements that should be included in the strategic health IS master plan.

Goals and Objectives

The plan should begin with a review and concise statement of major organizational goals and objectives for the planning period (usually two to five years). Information systems goals and objectives should be aligned with the strategic objectives of the organization. For example, if CQI is a major organizational priority, then this goal should be reflected in the

Figure 7.3 Elements of the Information Systems Strategic Plan

1. Statement of corporate/institutional goals and objectives
2. Statement of information systems goals and objectives
   a. Management information needs
   b. Critical success factors
   c. Information priorities
3. Priorities for the applications portfolio
   a. Clinical
   b. Administrative
   c. Decision support
4. Specification of overall systems architecture and infrastructure
   a. Level of distribution (centralized to decentralized)
   b. Network architecture
   c. Data location (central data warehouse to total data distribution)
   d. Database security and control requirements
5. Software development plan
   a. Commercial packages
   b. In-house development
   c. Tailor-made applications through contracting
   d. Combinations of the above
6. IS management plan
   a. Central IS staffing
   b. Outsourcing
   c. Limited central staffing in support of department level IS staff
   d. Combinations of the above
7. Statement of resource requirements
   a. Capital budget (hardware, software, network communications equipment)
   b. Operating budget (staff, supplies, consultants, training, etc.)

priorities for IS development—with particular attention paid to medical records; clinical protocols; incident reporting; and measures of patient, physician, and employee satisfaction. If diversification and expansion of the market service base are strategic objectives, then information systems should focus on utilization analysis and forecasting, analysis of changes in the demographic profile of the service market, and analysis of resource requirements for new service development. If an urban medical center has placed priority on expansion of ambulatory care services but information system priorities continue to focus on inpatient services, then the organization has a serious problem of goal displacement.

In a classic *Harvard Business Review* article, Rockart (1979) proposed that critical success factors (CSF) be used in defining information requirements and IS goals during the planning process. Top executives need to define these requirements but often have difficulty describing their needs for management information. By specifying those critical areas where things must go right for the organization to flourish, executives assist the IS planning team in determining information requirements and setting priorities for system development.

Information systems objectives should be as specific as possible and should flow from a review of strategic priorities as well as an analysis of deficiencies and gaps in current information processes. Avoid general statements of objectives such as, "Information systems for Metropolitan Health System should be designed to improve the quality of care and increase the efficiency of system operations." Such statements are self-evident and nonfunctional as far as planning is concerned. Rather, a detailed list of objectives should be established that will provide specific targets against which future progress can be measured and systems evaluated. Examples of specific objectives might include:

1. Information systems should be designed such that all records from the master patient index file are available online to all physicians in the plan.

2. Information systems should be designed such that all diagnostic test results are available within two hours after the tests have been completed.

3. Information systems should be designed so that information on inpatient and outpatient activity by major diagnostic categories is reported to corporate management on a monthly basis with reports indicating the health system's share of the total services provided in the market area.

Applications Priority List

Health services organizations will not be able to acquire all the systems they need in any given year. The statement of IS objectives will aid the steering committee in preparing a priority list of individual computer applications for design and acquisition. The applications priority list, in turn, will be essential in planning how limited resources can be used to have the greatest impact on strategic priorities.

The applications list should consider the needs of all major functional areas of the healthcare organization for clinical, administrative, and decision-support systems. Applications should be rank-ordered in the recommended sequence for systems development. For example, the steering committee might determine that financial control is the most pressing problem and direct that development of a financial information system take top priority.

Moriarty (1992, 89) states that the applications priority list should be cross-referenced to specific organizational strategies. For example, if a hospital is stressing prenatal compliance as part of a strategy to develop a center of excellence in women's health, then the applications priority list might include an information system for obstetrical clinic appointment scheduling, tracking, and follow-up.

Many healthcare organizations have initiated programs of *business process reengineering* (BPR) to achieve operational efficiency through dramatic improvement in core processes used in the organization. Many of these reengineering projects involve development of new information systems and these should be considered by the IS steering committee in developing the applications priority list. "The primary philosophy of BPR is that information technology enables dramatic adjustments to work processes and thus the achievement of significant improvements in operational performance." (Kratz and Feldbaum 1995, 54)

After these steps have been completed, the steering committee should report preliminary results back to the CEO and board of trustees. The statement of objectives and priority lists should be carefully reviewed and modified, as necessary.

System Architecture

Specification of overall system architecture is a critical task in the planning process. The plan must specify an overall system architecture and infrastructure to include:

1. the degree to which computing will be centralized or decentralized throughout the organization;
2. the network architecture that specifies how computers and work-stations will be linked together through communication lines and network servers;
3. the manner in which data will be stored and distributed throughout the organization, including database security and control requirements; and
4. the manner by which individual applications will be linked so that they can exchange information. Options range from a multivendor approach with interfaces developed to link the various applications to a single-vendor approach in which applications are already integrated.

There are differences of opinion about the degree to which computing should be centralized or decentralized in health services organizations. Proponents of centralization argue that this approach facilitates system integration and provides better control over the organization's costs of hardware and software. Central control may reduce unnecessary duplication of data entry and storage. In addition, technical staff expertise can be maximized by concentrating IS professionals in one central unit.

Proponents of decentralization argue that this approach places control of IS back where it belongs, in the hands of users. It fosters innovation in system design and develops increased user interest and support. Local flexibility is maintained and the frustrations of lengthy programming and processing backlogs at a central facility are avoided.

Chapter 5 includes a detailed description of alternative network architecture configurations including:

1. central mainframe architecture;
2. client/server architecture;
3. file/server architecture; and
4. distributed processing architecture.

Data distribution plans will help determine which type of network architecture should be employed by the health services organization. Alternatives range from creation of large, centralized (enterprisewide) "data warehouses" to complete distribution of data in which each organizational unit on the network maintains its own database. Many healthcare organizations, particularly integrated delivery systems (IDS), are moving toward a combination of approaches to data distribution. For example, the IDS might develop a centralized data warehouse containing a master patient index and computerized records for all patients in the system. Individual organizational units (hospitals, ambulatory care centers, etc.) might maintain their own data files for patient appointments, employee records, inventory control, budgeting, and financial management. The telecommunications network supporting the system would be designed to facilitate electronic exchange of information so that patient records would be accessible at all treatment sites, and financial information could be transmitted to corporate offices on a periodic basis. Policies for maintaining data security and protecting confidentiality of information are discussed later in this chapter.

In addition to network architecture, the plan should specify how the infrastructure will support data, voice, document imaging, radiographic imaging, full motion video, cellular phones, intercom, paging, and wireless communications. (Spitzer, 1993)

The subcommittee that reviews systems architecture (see Figure 7.3) must include competent technical staff and/or consultants working closely with representatives of management, the medical staff, and other major system users.

Software Development Plan

The IS plan should also specify procedures for software development. In the early days of healthcare computing (1960–1980), most hospitals and other health services organizations employed a large staff of computer analysts and programmers to develop computer applications in-house. Today, most healthcare organizations rely primarily on software packages purchased form commercial vendors. A wide array of software products are available. (See, for example, *Health Care Software Sourcebook* [Ankrapp and Di Lima, 1996] and the Annual Market Directory issue of *Health Management Technology* (1996).

Many large health services organizations and integrated delivery systems will use combinations of software development procedures. Commercial software will be combined with tailor-made programs developed by in-house staff, particularly programs that support database management and electronic communications across the network. Software evaluation and selection procedures are described in Chapter 9.

Information Systems Management Plan

The IS plan should also specify the IS management structure for the organization. Most health services organization still employ an in-house staff for system operation and management, even if all or most software is purchased from commercial vendors. Decisions must be made on the extent to which technical system management staff will be centralized or distributed among the major user departments of the organization. An increasing number of organizations are *outsourcing* all or some of their information processing functions to contractors who provide on-site system implementation and management services.

Centralized staffing offers the advantages of economies of scale and reduction in the number of technical personnel to be employed. Decentralized staffing brings systems management closer to the user and offers the potential for increased support and user involvement in system development and operation.

Outsourcing of IS functions allows the health services organization to get out of the information technology business through contracting with experts in the field. However, the costs of outsourcing may be high and may tend to generate too much distance between users and technical systems specialists. A more detailed discussion of information resource management issues is found in Chapter 10.

Statement of Resource Requirements

The final element of the IS plan specifies resources required to carry it out. A capital budget should include five- to ten-year projections for the cost of computer hardware, network and telecommunications equipment, and software. The operating budget should include costs for staff, supplies and materials, consultants, training programs, and other recurring expenses. Both budgets should be updated annually and the timing for their preparation should be coordinated with the overall organizational budget cycle.

No general level of expenditures can be specified since each healthcare organization has its own set of requirements for IS development. Morrissey (1995b, 60) reported that integrated healthcare delivery systems were making major investments in upgrading their information systems: Sharp Healthcare in San Diego investing $30 million over four years; Inova in northern Virginia investing $35 million over five years; and Allina Health System in Minnesota investing $75 to $80 million over three years.

The final section of the IS plan should also specify an overall schedule and target dates for implementation. Although cost estimates and target dates will be preliminary at this point, they will aid management and board members in evaluating the magnitude of organizational commitment required to implement the recommended set of alternatives.

Review and Approval of the Plan

After the IS steering committee has approved the plan, it should be presented to executive management and the governing board for review and approval prior to implementation. The written plan should be submitted to management in advance of a formal presentation and discussion session.

As with any plan, the strategic plan for IS development must be a dynamic instrument that is reviewed periodically and updated. At least once a year, the steering committee should review progress in meeting the original criteria set forth in the plan, and the plan should be changed as necessary.

End-User Computing

A problem that many healthcare organizations face is what to do about dissatisfaction among organizational units whose IS needs are not identified as priorities in the strategic IS plan. End-user computing strategies offer one potential solution to this problem.

Reynolds (1995, Chapter 13) points out that workers in many organizations have become increasingly sophisticated in the use of computers. In addition, powerful microcomputer systems with user-friendly software and end-user-oriented programming tools have helped to facilitate end-user computing that does not require the services or resources of the central information systems department.

End-user computing most often involves use of departmental software packages purchased from vendors (e.g., laboratory, pharmacy, radiology systems). In some cases, computer-literate users may write programs to meet specialized needs in their departments. An example would be the creation and maintenance of a database of companies who provide medical supplies for an outpatient clinic in a large medical center, where the clinic developed its own programs to create and update the database.

End-user computing offers the potential to expand the base of IS development and overcome problems of low priority assigned to certain applications that are viewed as important to units within the organization. However, end-user computing must be approached cautiously. Most activities in health services delivery are interrelated, and computer applications must be able to exchange information if operations are to be efficient. If a departmental system is completely independent of all other activities in the organization and can stand alone, then there should be no problem with the department developing the system on its own if it has the resources available to carry out the project. However, if the system will need to interact and exchange information with other user departments, then central control and planning is needed before the end-user department should be authorized to develop the system itself. Particularly critical is *data compatibility*, common codes and data definitions that will allow information to be exchanged electronically across the organization. The subject of data standards is discussed in more detail in the next section.

Organizationwide Information System Standards and Policies

In order to implement the strategic IS plan, the IS steering committee should oversee the development of a set of enterprisewide policies that govern the design, acquisition, and operation of information systems throughout the organization. This section includes a brief description of four important sets of policies that every organization should develop: data security policies; data definition standards; policies governing the acquisition of hardware, software, and telecommunications network equipment; and policies on use of the Internet.

Data Security Policies

Health services organizations must establish enterprisewide standards to maintain data security and protect the privacy and confidentiality of information, particularly patient records. Data security involves two essential elements: (1) protecting against system failures or external catastrophic events (fire, storms, and other acts of God) where critical information could be lost and (2) controlling access to computer files by unauthorized personnel.

The IS steering committee must insure that effective data backup and recovery procedures are implemented at all processing sites throughout the organization. Critical data files should be copied to removable disk packs or tapes and stored in a secure location, away from the processing sites, preferably in a different building if possible. The CIO should develop a data backup plan for approval by the steering committee. The plan should specify which files require duplication and how frequently backup procedures should be conducted. Recovery procedures in the event of catastrophic events should also be included.

Data can also be lost through computer viruses, which have become increasingly prevalent. Each software program should be inspected by virus-identifying programs every time the application is run. Hammond (1992, 5) states that " . . . a strict institutional policy must be enforced related to the acquisition of software, particularly free software obtained over networks. . . . Wherever possible, such programs should not be permitted on the medical center backbone, where they can spread to unsuspecting users."

Protecting data confidentiality is an even more difficult task. A comprehensive information security policy should include three elements: (1) physical security; (2) technical controls over access; and (3) management policies that are well-known and enforced in all organizational units. (See Figure 7.4)

Physical security includes such elements as using keys or badges to unlock computer terminals and using dial-back procedures to determine that a request to access data has come from a specific terminal and modem.

Figure 7.4 Information Security

Physical Security
- Hardware
- Data Files

Technical Safeguards
- Passwords
- Encryption
- Audit Logs

Management Policies
- Written Security Policy
- Employee Training
- Disciplinary Actions for Violations

A number of technical controls to data access can be built into operational information systems. Passwords are the most common. Each user is assigned a password that is known only by that individual and the data security manager. Users should be warned never to share their passwords with anyone else, and passwords should be changed periodically. Passwords should allow access only to those portions of the organization's database appropriate to the individual user and his or her departmental affiliation. For example, personnel in the purchasing department would have access restricted to materials management data files only, and they could not use their terminals to access patient records.

Encryption is a method of coding or altering information such that it is unintelligible if obtained by unauthorized users. Encryption is used with very sensitive information such as lists of passwords or diagnostic information on mental health or sexually transmitted diseases. It is not a practical method for providing general data protection. The data security manager should be the only one able to decode encrypted information.

The most important technical safeguard may be the maintenance of audit logs that track every transaction associated with use of critical data files. The logs will identify the user and/or terminal, the date and time of access, and the type of transaction carried out (simple access, addition, changes, or deletions to the record). If employees are aware that all transactions are being monitored for violations, they will be deterred from seeking unauthorized use of sensitive information.

Management policies must support the physical safeguards and technical controls that protect data confidentiality. Training of all users is essential to be sure they understand the importance of data confidentiality and the procedures in place to protect privacy of records. Every employee should be required to read the organization's privacy protection policy and sign a statement indicating that he or she will not violate provisions of the policy. Strict disciplinary measures, including termination, should be followed when employee violations occur.

Data security issues are particularly complex for multiple-facility integrated delivery systems. These issues include questions such as who will have ownership of data on computer networks, what criteria will be used to determine who should have access to member and patient data, and who will be legally liable for guarding the confidential patient and financial data that resides on the network. (Work, Pawola, and Henley 1996)

Data Standardization

As mentioned previously, system integration is an important element of strategic IS planning in healthcare organizations. Most computer applications must include the ability to share information with other systems. For example, a laboratory test results reporting system must be able to transfer information for storage in the computerized medical records system operated by the organization.

Electronic data exchange cannot occur without some level of standardization of data structures used in computer applications. For this reason, healthcare organizations should consider developing a data dictionary that specifies the format of each data element and the coding system (if any) associated with that element. For example, the data element "Date of Birth" might be defined as follows in the organization's data dictionary:

Date of Birth: Eight digit numeric field with 3 subfields:
Month—two digits ranging from 01 to 12
Day—two digits ranging from 01 to 31
Year—four digits ranging from 1850 to 2050

Notice that the range of the subfield for year in this example is designed to accommodate historical records of patients with birth dates back to the mid-19th century and accommodate future records through the mid-21st century. Many organizations are facing major costs in changing dating systems for the new millennium as the year 2000 approaches since most current systems use a two-digit coding system for year.

In addition to data compatibility among information systems within the healthcare organization, there is growing need to facilitate extra-organizational exchange of information among health systems, insurance companies, medical supply and equipment vendors, etc. A number of projects have been initiated to develop industrywide standards for electronic data interchange in the healthcare field. Examples of these projects include:

1. the American National Standards Institute (ANSI) X.12 Group working on specifications for transactions involving the processing of health insurance claims;
2. Health Industry Bar Code Supplier Labeling Standard (HIBC) for common coding of supplies, materials, and equipment;
3. Health Level-7 (HL7) Standard for Healthcare Electronic Data Transmission; and
4. MEDIX, the Institute of Electrical and Electronics Engineers (IEEE) Committee for Medical Data Interchange.

The latter two projects (HL7 and MEDIX) are complementary efforts to develop a comprehensive set of data standards for sharing clinical information within and across healthcare organizations. The HL7 project was initiated in 1987. It is a voluntary effort of health services providers, hardware and software vendors, and professional organizations with the goal of developing a cost-effective approach to system connectivity. (Hettinger and Brazile 1994) HL7 has had solid success in developing standards for interfacing departmental computer applications in hospitals, and more recently has expanded efforts to develop standards for exchange among different types of organization (e.g., physician offices and hospitals).

As part of the strategic IS planning process, the IS steering committee should study the need for data interchange and should develop a policy on data standardization for the organization. For example, many hospitals and integrated delivery systems are specifying that all software purchased from vendors must meet an industry standard protocol such as HL7.

Hardware and Software Standards

A number of technical policies related to information systems need to be developed by health services organizations. Most of these are highly technical and should be developed by the CIO or director of IS. However, the IS steering committee should oversee the development of a broad set of policies related to the acquisition of computer hardware, software, and networks communications equipment for the organization.

The committee must determine whether or not the organization will require central review and approval of all computer hardware and software purchases. As the costs of personal computers (PCs) and related software packages have come down, they are often within the budgetary authority of individual organizational units. However, there are some compelling reasons for requiring central review and approval, regardless of costs. These include the following:

1. Central review will help ensure compatibility with enterprisewide data standards such as HL7.
2. Central review of PC purchases can ensure that data terminals and workstations use a common operating system such as Windows.
3. Central review and purchasing of generalized software provides cost advantages through the acquisition of site licenses for multiple users of common packages (word processing, spreadsheets, database management systems, etc.).
4. Central review will ensure that hardware and software will be of a type that can receive technical support and maintenance from the IS staff.
5. Central review can help to prevent illegal use of unlicensed software within the organization.

The IS steering committee should also approve the network communications plan for the enterprise. A variety of network configurations are possible, and it is important that the network plan be compatible with the overall IS development plan for the organization.

Policies on Use of the Internet

As discussed in Chapter 5, healthcare applications on the Internet are increasing rapidly, and the World Wide Web has become an important tool for many healthcare organizations. However, the Internet is a very open communications system and management policies are needed to ensure that the system is used effectively and not abused. These policies fall into four categories:

1. policies on creation of home pages;
2. policies related to security of information on the Internet;
3. legal protection of intellectual property on the Internet; and
4. policies on controlling employee use and potential abuse of the system.

Many healthcare organizations are using home pages on the Internet as a marketing tool to make information about programs and services widely available. In some larger organizations, such as university medical centers or complex integrated delivery systems, there may be multiple home pages created by individual departments or other organizational units. Central control and policies on home page development are needed. These policies should include items such as:

1. organizational units who are authorized to create home pages;
2. use of corporate information, logos, etc.;
3. responsibilities for maintaining the home page and keeping information current;
4. data security policies to be followed (see below);
5. guidelines for general graphic design and writing style to be used; and
6. procedures for obtaining central review and approval before the page is published on the Internet.

Data security policies and procedures are particularly important if the Internet is to be used for internal communications (intranet) or sharing of information among organizational units. This is particularly true if clinical or financial information is included. Since the Internet is such an open communications system, extraordinary security features such as encryption of highly sensitive information and creation of "firewalls" to screen information passing through network connections may be necessary.

Some healthcare organizations may be posting copyrighted information and other intellectual property belonging to individuals and/or the organization. This is particularly true of research institutions where publications, data files, and teaching material are made available on the Internet for use by colleagues. Organizations and individuals employing the Internet for these purposes should be aware of the elements of copyright law pertaining to the rights of authors and copyright owners. (Stern and Westenberg 1995)

Finally, policies are needed to regulate employee use of the Internet to avoid abuses that can easily develop. Of particular concern is potential employee misuse or abuse of electronic mail (e-mail). These policies should cover such items as prohibition of use of e-mail for personal communications not related to the business of the organization, the privacy of e-mail communications of others, and prohibition of messages that contain sexually explicit language or language that might be construed as disparagement of others based on race, sex, national origin, religious beliefs, and similar items. Employees should be reminded that e-mail differs from telephone conversations in that data is stored on the network and can be accessed long after a message has been sent.

Employees with web browsers on their computers need to be reminded that Internet access is being provided for business purposes. Internet browsing and web "surfing" can become addictive, and managers should control the amount of time spent by employees who may use the Web for personal reasons or to satisfy idle curiosity about the many subjects covered. Policies are also needed to control which employees are authorized to participate in "chat rooms" and other information-sharing mechanisms on the Internet.

Strategic IS Planning for Integrated Delivery Systems

Integrated delivery systems must consider the need for integration of information systems across institutions as well as within individual organizational units. Such integration is particularly critical in vertically integrated organizations where patients may progress and seek treatment at various organizational components including clinics, surgicenters, acute care hospitals, substance abuse centers, and skilled nursing home facilities. Information systems must be patient-centered in order to aggregate data from the various medical care units and track patients throughout the system. At the same time, corporate system management must recognize that different types of facilities within the organization (hospitals, ambulatory care centers and clinics, nursing homes, home health agencies) have their own distinct information requirements, and corporate policy must provide mechanisms for specialized information systems to meet the needs of individual units in the system.

Information systems for an IDS must also be able to provide comparative financial data in order for management to efficiently allocate resources to individual units. Such a capability is especially critical when healthcare costs are paid on a capitation basis. Corporate management will need to carefully monitor how patient care dollars are being spent across system units for actuarial risk analysis. The IDS will also have special information needs in market research and analysis of competitor services. Physician performance in various components of the system must be monitored as well.

At the technical level, information systems for an IDS may require standardization of coding and data definition for all organizational units—for example, a common chart of accounts for financial reporting. If such an approach is not possible, then complex data conversion tables will be required to facilitate electronic data exchange. In order to serve both corporate management information needs and the operational support requirements of each medical care unit, integrated delivery systems need to strike a balance between centralized data management and local control of data processing.

In recent years, the health services industry has been in a state of rapid change. Hospitals have merged to form corporate systems; medical centers have acquired community hospitals and brought them into their organizations; and some corporate systems have sold or divested some of their existing facilities. These mergers and changes in ownership can create special problems with respect to information systems at the individual facilities.

If the corporate system has highly centralized information processing through a corporate data center and a new facility is acquired, special planning will be required to bring the new unit into the central system while allowing it to continue to use its current hardware and software to support ongoing operations. If computing within the corporate system is decentralized at the facility level, the newly acquired facility may not have compatible hardware and/or software with other units of the system, and special conversion programs will be required in order to meet corporate reporting requirements. Unique information processing problems usually result from these mergers, acquisitions, and joint ventures. Management at both the corporate and institutional levels must be prepared to address these problems as the plans for organizational change are developed.

The American Health Information Management Association (AHIMA) has issued a position statement on "Managing Health Information in Facility Mergers and Acquisitions." The statement calls for patient records to be consolidated or linked in a master patient index. It goes on to state:

The compatibility and functionality of existing information systems should be assessed, and a plan should be formulated for integration of the systems to the extent possible. Such integration may be essential for the organization to successfully meet the demands of integrated delivery systems. Existing databases should be maintained in an accessible form to meet anticipated future needs. (AHIMA 1994, 1)

Jean Balgrosky, Vice President of Information Resources for Holy Cross Health System discussed the planning process within her multifacility system, which serves several healthcare markets across the country:

We are just now in the process of defining what needs to be standardized across the System and what can be dealt with uniquely in each marketplace that Holy Cross serves. Each hospital entity of Holy Cross Health System has a CIO. . . . We are defining ways, via a strategic I/S planning methodology and collaboration on various initiatives, to strike the balance of each CIO's orientation to the hospital entity with that of the multisystem. (Reavis 1992, 28)

Summary

Information systems development in the health service organization should begin with development of a master plan that is linked to the strategic plan of the organization. The plan should include (1) a statement of information system goals and objectives aligned with organizational goals and priorities; (2) a list of priorities for the computer applications portfolio (clinical, administrative, and decision support); (3) specification of overall system architecture and infrastructure; (4) a software development plan; (5) an information resources management plan; (6) a statement of resource requirements including projected capital and operating budgets; and (7) schedules and target dates for implementation of various elements of the plan.

The planning process should be guided by an enterprisewide IS steering committee with membership from executive management, medical staff, nursing staff, financial management, human resources management, planning and marketing, facilities management, and clinical support services. The CIO should chair the committee if the health services organization has established such a position.

System integration, that is, the ability of information systems to communicate with one another and share information, is essential. Integration can be achieved through a number of alternative information network architecture configurations including a central mainframe approach, client/server architecture, file/server architecture, and distributed processing.

End-user computing can supplement central planning in order to facilitate development of systems for users whose applications are not high on the priority list. However, caution must be exercised to insure that user-developed computer applications meet requirements of data compatibility with other information systems with which they will exchange information.

The planning process should include development of major institutional policies related to information systems. The IS steering committee should oversee policies related to data security, privacy, and confidentiality; data standardization; acquisition of hardware, software, and telecommunications network equipment throughout the enterprise; and policies on use of the Internet.

Information systems planning within integrated delivery systems must strike a balance between the need for central data management and data-processing requirements of individual organizational units. Health systems created through mergers, acquisitions, and joint ventures must deal with the problem of major investments already made in "legacy" systems in individual organizations with the need to exchange clinical and financial information across the system through a carefully planned telecommunications network.

Discussion Questions

7.1 Why is planning important in the development of health information systems?

7.2 Describe a typical organizational structure for oversight of information systems planning in a vertically integrated health delivery system.

7.3 Describe the elements of a master plan for information systems development.

7.4 What is meant by the term *information systems integration*? Why is it an important element of strategic IS planning?

7.5 Describe some of the alternatives available to healthcare organizations for system design and software development.

7.6 Discuss some of the special information planning requirements and problems of integrated delivery systems created through mergers and acquisitions.

Problems

7.1 Assume that you are the president of a healthcare corporation consisting of a medical group practice, 200-bed acute care hospital, day surgery center, and 75-bed skilled care nursing home. Develop an organizational plan for an information systems steering committee for the corporation.

7.2 Conduct an interview with the CIO of a health services organization in your community regarding IS planning practices in the organization. Obtain a copy of the IS strategic plan if possible. Prepare a summary of your interview and a critique of the planning process being followed.

References

American Health Information Management Association (AHIMA). 1994. "Position Statement,Issue: Managing Health Information in Facility Mergers and Acquisitions." Chicago: The Association.

Ankrapp, B., and S. N. Di Lima, eds. 1996. *Health Care Software Sourcebook*. Gaithersburg, MD: Aspen Publishers.

Austin, C. J., J. M. Trimm, and P. M. Sobczak. 1995. "Information Systems and Strategic Management." *Health Care Management Review*. 20 (3): 26–33

Hammond, W. E. 1992. "Security, Privacy, and Confidentiality: A Perspective." *Journal of Health Information Management Research*. 1 (2): 1–8.

Health Management Technology. 1996. Annual Market Directory. Atlanta, GA: Argus, Inc.

Healthcare Information and Management Systems Society and Hewlett Packard Co. (HIMSS/HP). 1996. *Seventh Annual Leadership Survey: Trends in Health Care Computing*. Chicago: Healthcare Information and Management Systems Society.

Hettinger, B. J., and R. P. Brazile. 1994. "Health Level Seven (HL7): Standard for Healthcare Electronic Data Transmission." *Computers in Nursing* 12 (1): 13–16.

Kratz, L. A., and E. G. Feldbaum. 1995. "Reengineering and Integration: Six Tales from the Health Care Front." *Journal of the Healthcare Information and Management Systems Society* 9 (1): 53–61.

Lohman, P. 1996. "Measure Consultant's Objectivity and Character before Contracting." *Health Management Technology* (July): 31.

Moriarty, D. D. 1992. "Strategic Information Systems Planning for Health Service Providers." *Health Care Management Review* 17 (1): 85–90.

Morrissey, J. 1995a. "Information Systems Refocus Priorities." *Modern Healthcare* (February 13): 65–67.

———. 1995b. "CIOs Use Outsourcing to Revamp Systems." *Modern Healthcare* (July 24): 60–68.

Reavis, M. 1992. "The Role CIOs Must Play in Multihospital Strategic Planning." *Computers in Healthcare* (May): 26–28.

Reynolds, G. W. 1995. *Information Systems for Managers*, 3rd Ed. Minneapolis, MN: West Publishing Company.

Rockart, J. F. 1979. "Chief Executives Define Their Own Data Needs." *Harvard Business Review* 57 (2): 81–84.

Spitzer, P. G. 1993. "A Comprehensive Framework for I/S Strategic Planning." *Computers in Healthcare* (May): 28–33.

Stern, E. J., and L. Westenberg. 1995. "Copyright Law and Academic Radiology: Rights of Authors and Copyright Owners and Reproduction of Information." *American Journal of Radiology* 164: 1083–88.

Tan, J. K. 1995. *Health Management Information Systems*. Rockville, MD: Aspen Publishers.

Work, M., L. Pawola, and A. Henley. 1996. "CHINs, IHD Systems Remain in Evolutionary State." *Health Management Technology* (March): 54–58.

Additional Readings

Bridgman, S. 1992. "HL7 Looks Beyond the Hospital Walls." *Computers in Healthcare* (November): 26–27.

DeFauw, T. D. and D. L'Heureux. 1995. "How to Strategically Align Information Resources with the Goals of an Integrated Delivery System." *Healthcare Information Management* 9 (4): 3–10.

Ferrand, D. J. and C. M. Lay. 1994. "Diagnosing Strategic Performance of the Hospital Information Systems Planning Cycle." *Health Care Management Review* 19 (3): 21–33.

Kurz, R. A. 1996. *Internet and the Law*. Rockville, MD: Government Institutes, Inc.

Lawrence, L. M. 1994. "Safeguarding the Confidentiality of Automated Medical Information." *Journal on Quality Improvement* 20 (11): 639–46.

Orens, J. 1996. "Strategic I/T Planning: A Four-Pronged Approach." *Health Management Technology* (March): 62–64.

Rushing, S., and J. F. Anderson. 1996. "When the Playing Field Changes, Rethink the Rules." *Health Management Technology* (February): 26–29.

Skok, R. 1993. "Patient-Centered Information Systems Planning." *Journal of the American Health Information Management Association* 64 (1): 54–56.

Stall, M., M. Brooks, and K. Pfrank. 1992. "Long-range Planning for Information Systems." *Healthcare Financial Management* 46 (6): 34–46.

SYSTEMS ANALYSIS

THE INFORMATION systems (IS) plan establishes overall parameters for the development of information systems in health services organizations including specification of general system architecture and priorities for the development of individual computer applications (see Chapter 7). Chapters 8 through 10 discuss IS project organization and management from initial systems analysis through operation and maintenance after a system is implemented.

Concepts and Applications

The type of system chosen by a healthcare organization should be carefully analyzed, with no factors being left to chance. The steps a healthcare leader should take when analyzing system requirements are clearly defined: The rationale for the system must be determined, along with determining the system's detailed requirements. This is **systems analysis**. Then, based on that information, a **design approach** can be determined.

This chapter will allow the reader to ask the pertinent questions that will determine which system should be used, determine how and where that system will be constructed, and how to design the optimal system.

The System Development Life Cycle

The process of IS development (often referred to as the life cycle for a system) involves seven major activities. (See Figure 8.1.) Each of these activities are described briefly below.

1. Systems analysis, the essential first step in any application development, is the activity in which current information practices are reviewed and functional system requirements are established. It is the process of collecting, organizing, and evaluating facts about information system requirements and the environment in which the system will operate.

2. Systems analysis serves as the basis for selection of a design approach for the proposed new information system. Alternative approaches available include use of predesigned or "packaged" software purchased from commercial vendors; design and programming of the system by in-house staff; use of contractual services for design and programming; and combinations of these alternatives. Most health services organizations are choosing to use predesigned or packaged software systems if a suitable package is available that meets organizational requirements as determined through systems analysis. Some in-house programming may still be required to modify the software packages or to build linkages with other systems.

3. System design is the process of converting functional information system requirements into a set of specifications for an application. If the system is to be implemented by in-house computer programming, detailed design specifications are required. If commercial software is to be used, a more general set of design requirements are developed to support the software selection process including possible development of a request-for-proposals (RFPs) to vendors (see Chapter 9).

4. System acquisition or construction involves evaluation, selection, and purchase of commercial software and/or writing of computer programs by in-house staff. In addition, it includes reengineering of processes and development of organizational policies and procedures associated with the new system.

Figure 8.1   Information Systems Development Life Cycle

1. Analyze functional requirements (systems analysis)
2. Select design approach
3. Specify system requirements (system design)
4. Acquire or construct system
5. Install system (implementation)
6. Operate and maintain system
7. Evaluate and improve system

5. System implementation includes ordering of new equipment (if needed), preparing space, training personnel to use the system, building databases and converting data files, and testing the system prior to operation. The importance of careful system testing cannot be overemphasized. Many catastrophes in healthcare IS projects could have been avoided if adequate testing had been carried out prior to putting systems into operation.

6. Operation and maintenance is the next step in the cycle. System maintenance is particularly important. Some organizations seem to believe that automated information systems, once operational, require no further attention. Nothing is further from the truth. No matter how good the original system testing, operational systems are subject to occasional breakdowns and trained personnel must be available to make quick corrections.

7. Health services organizations are dynamic, and the requirements placed upon information systems are subject to frequent change. All information systems should be evaluated periodically, with changes made to improve the effectiveness and efficiency of each system. Each major system should be formally evaluated to see if goals have been achieved and functional requirements met within reasonable costs. Postimplementation evaluation and quality improvement may result in the need to repeat some of the steps in the life cycle in order to make modifications to the system.

Activities 1 and 2 (systems analysis and selection of a design approach) are discussed in more detail in this chapter. Activities 3 and 4 (system design and evaluation and selection of software) are described in Chapter 9. Activities 5, 6, and 7 (implementation, operation and maintenance, and postimplementation evaluation and improvement) are discussed in Chapter 10.

Project Organization

Major IS projects should be carried out by an interdisciplinary team of user department personnel, management representatives, and information analysts. (See Figure 8.2.) If the system to be developed includes clinical components, a representative(s) from the medical staff should be involved as well. A senior systems analyst from the IS Department should serve as project leader. This individual should not be a narrow specialist in computer technology, but rather should combine technical knowledge with experience and understanding of the health services organization and its operations.

At least one representative from each department using information from or generating data for the system should be assigned to serve

Figure 8.2 Information Systems Project Organization

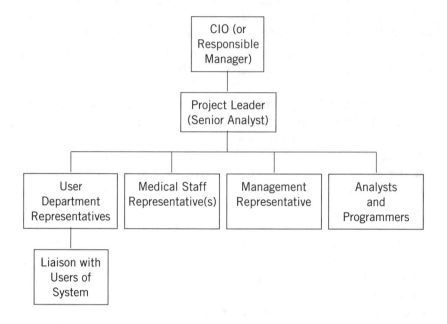

on the project team. Departmental representatives should be key staff members who understand departmental procedures and policies in their totality rather than individuals who are specialists in only one phase of departmental activity. Departmental representatives play a key role in liaison with employees in their departments, and they must be well accepted by their colleagues to lend credibility to the changes that will be necessary when the new system is implemented. Physician involvement is essential, particularly if the information system includes processing of clinical information.

Every major project team should include a representative of central administration who can interpret organizational policy and serve as a liaison with the chief executive officer (CEO) or chief operating officer (COO) as the new system develops.

Technical personnel (systems analysts and programmers) are assigned to each project as needed. Technical personnel requirements will be higher for systems to be developed in-house and lower when packaged software is to be purchased and installed. Actual staffing requirements will depend on who will have responsibility for installing the system and how much work will be required by in-house staff for building interfaces to other applications.

If a systems development project is to be carried out under contract, the contract specifications should call for a similar form of project organization. The contractor will provide the project leader and technical staff, but operating and clinical personnel should be involved in the same way as they would be for an in-house development effort. If this user involvement is not included, the result often is a system that is technically correct but out of touch with the realities of a particular organization, its culture, and environment. Early involvement of users in a contractor-developed system will aid immeasurably in system operation and maintenance after the new system is working and contractor personnel have departed.

Once the project team has been organized, agreement should be reached on a regular schedule of periodic meetings to assess progress and to report on various phases of the project. Estimates should be made of the time requirements for each team member, and these should be formalized in writing with approval obtained from the appropriate department manager and from top management. Formalizing a time commitment for each member of the team will help to ensure availability of key personnel when they are needed, particularly when other demands for their time compete with the system project, as inevitably they will. The best insurance against a poorly developed information system is the active and enthusiastic involvement of user personnel at all stages of the project.

Project teams should report to the CIO or other manager with responsibility for oversight of information systems in the organization. Further discussion of information systems staffing and the role of the CIO is found in Chapter 10.

Systems Analysis

Systems analysis is an essential first step in the development of any health information system. Guided by the principles and priorities set forth in the master plan for IS development, systems planners should conduct a careful study of functional requirements in advance of the design stage of a project. Technically trained staff (systems analysts and management engineers) and personnel who will be using the information system must join in this effort. Systems analysis will pay dividends whether or not any automated information system is the result.

Systems analysis should provide answers to a series of questions regarding the proposed new system. What are the weaknesses of the present system? What are its strengths? Why is a new system needed? What specific kinds of information should the system generate? When does this information need to be available? Who will use it? In what ways will it be used? Where does the needed data originate? Answering questions such as these is the basic task of systems analysis.

Note the question that is *not* included here: "How will the new system provide the requisite information?" This is the basic task of the design phase of the project. The details of how information requirements are to be met should not constrain a systems project too early. Rather, requirements should be stated and ways should be found to meet these requirements. More problems in health information systems have resulted from inadequate analysis and lack of specification of system requirements than from shortage of available information technology.

Systems analysis is the process of collecting, organizing, and evaluating data about IS requirements and the environment in which the system will operate. Figure 8.3 shows the steps to be carried out in the conduct of an information systems analysis.

1. Study existing systems. If the proposed information system is to replace an existing one, regardless of whether information is obtained manually or through machine processing, then the first step of systems analysis should be a complete study of existing procedures, their strengths and weaknesses. The information obtained serves as a basis for the establishment of realistic requirements for the proposed new information system.

2. Define end-user requirements. Future business needs and end-user requirements should be defined in detail. The project team may find that major reengineering of existing work processes is required rather than simple refinement of current procedures.

3. Identify alternatives. The project team should look for cost-effective alternatives in deciding how far to go in attempting to meet all user-defined requirements for the proposed system. Reynolds (1995, 376) suggests that system requirements be divided into three categories: high, medium, and low priority. He recommends that at least three alternative approaches be considered:

a. the "do-everything alternative," which meets or exceeds all user requirements regardless of priority assigned to them;

Figure 8.3 Information Systems Analysis

---

1. Study existing systems.
2. Define end-user requirements.
3. Identify alternatives.
4. Evaluate alternatives.
5. Prepare report.
6. Obtain management review and approval.

---

b. the "lots of features alternative," which includes all high-priority requirements, most medium-priority requirements, and many low-priority requirements; and

c. the "low-cost alternative," which meets most high-priority requirements, a few medium-priority requirements, and almost none of the low-priority items.

4. Evaluate alternatives. The choice among these alternatives will be dependent on the priority assigned to the proposed information system in meeting business objectives tempered by the resources available for system acquisition and implementation. The alternative of doing nothing should always be considered. If the project team fails to identify high-priority requirements and benefits from the new system, it may be appropriate to invest scarce resources in other areas of the organization where the payoffs would be higher.

5. Prepare the systems analysis report. Careful documentation of the systems analysis is essential, both for management review and to serve as the basis for preparation of system design specifications. The report should include:

a. the purpose and scope of the project, the user departments involved, and procedures followed in the study;

b. the objectives to be served by the information system being considered; and

c. the major findings of the study including strengths and weaknesses of the present system, user requirements for the proposed new system, and justification for proceeding to the next step, if this is the recommendation.

6. Obtain management review and approval. The systems analysis report should be reviewed by executive management as well as middle-level management from all user departments involved in the proposed new system. Signatures of approval should be obtained before proceeding to the next step.

Systems Analysis Tools

A number of tools have been developed to assist in the process of systems analysis. (See Figure 8.4.) This section includes a brief description of some of these tools.

1. Data collection tools. Data on system requirements are collected through a variety of mechanisms. Key personnel in the operating departments involved in the information system should be interviewed as one means of documenting present procedures and obtaining input on new system characteristics that are desirable. Interviews should be carefully planned, and a structured interview guide should be prepared in advance

Figure 8.4 Tools of Systems Analysis

Data Collection
1. Interviews
2. Questionnaires
3. Observation
   a. Work Sampling
   b. Continuous Monitoring
Data Organization
1. Summary Tables and Statistics
2. Interview Summaries
3. Flowcharts
4. Narrative Reports to Accompany Data Tables and Flowcharts
Data Analysis
1. Workload
2. Output Utilization
3. Input and Data Collection
4. Coding Systems
5. Database Analysis
6. Procedures and Information Flow
7. Cost Analysis

to facilitate the interview and to be sure that key points are covered. An example of an interview guide to be used in obtaining information from the director of the clinical laboratory in an integrated delivery system is shown in Figure 8.5. Following a structured format, data are obtained on departmental organization, staffing, workload, facilities, current procedures, information flows, problems, and unmet information requirements.

Data can also be obtained through the use of questionnaires. Time and resources permitting, however, a face-to-face interview is preferable because it permits elaboration and dialogue not possible with a questionnaire. Questionnaires can be particularly useful in obtaining a representative sample of data from a larger group—for example, patient opinions on an existing service or proposed new procedure.

Interviews and questionnaire development require special skills that are developed through education and experience. Systems analysts should be trained in these techniques and be familiar with the extensive literature available on this subject.

In questionnaire development, decisions must be made between the use of open-ended and closed-ended questions. Responses to open-ended questions provide more freedom to the respondents, but they may provide answers that are not relevant to the intent of the question. Open-ended questions require interpretation by the analyst and coding before

Figure 8.5   Interview Guide: Director of Clinical Laboratory

Background Information
1. Describe goals and objectives of laboratory. Is a copy of the goals statement available?
2. How is the laboratory organized? Is a chart available?
3. What are current staffing levels (numbers of personnel by job category and levels of training)? Are position descriptions available?
4. What are current lab workloads? What is the volume of work by type of tests? What is the percentage of stat orders? Is a statistical summary available?
5. What kinds of equipment and other specialized facilities are used? Are there any urgent needs for new equipment at present?
6. Describe relationships with other units of the health system: (a) frequent interaction (e.g., daily); and (b) less frequent interaction.

Departmental Procedures
1. How are specimens obtained from patients?
2. How are stat orders handled?
3. What degree of automation is used in testing?
4. How are test results transmitted back to the patient's chart?
5. How are charges transmitted to the business office?
6. What kinds of quality control procedures are used?
7. Is a procedures manual available?

Information Flows
1. What reports are generated in the lab?
2. What other kinds of information are produced? telephone communications? verbal reports?
3. What kind of input information do you receive from other departments? Are sample forms available?
4. What kind of data-coding systems are used? Are code lists available?
5. What master files do you maintain in the lab?

Assessment and Problems
1. What are your major problems in lab operations? What are some of your less serious problems?
2. Are there any specific problems in information flow?
3. What are the major gaps and inefficiencies in your lab information system? Are error rates too high? Are input forms or reports consistently late?
4. How could a new or revised information system serve you better? What would you like to see in such a system?
5. Are there other comments or suggestions?

the results can be analyzed. Closed-ended questions, on the other hand, facilitate uniformity and ease of analysis. However, too much structuring can potentially result in omission of issues that might be considered important by those completing the questionnaire (See Figure 8.6 for suggested guidelines to be followed in developing questionnaires.) This is only a brief introduction to the important topic of survey research and collecting information through interviews and questionnaires. Readers

Figure 8.6 Guidelines for Questionnaire Development

1. Respondents must be competent to answer the questions included on the survey instrument.
2. Questions should be relevant to the topics under study.
3. Each question should deal with only one issue.
4. Questions should be clear and unambiguous.
5. Questions should be kept as short as possible.
6. Response categories to closed-ended questions should be exhaustive and mutually exclusive.
7. Negative questions and biased items or terms should be avoided.
8. The questionnaire format should be spread out and uncluttered.
9. The order of questions is important and can affect the answer given.
10. A questionnaire should include a concise introduction explaining its purpose and should contain clear instructions for completion.

Source: Babbie 1986.

interested in more detail should consult specialized reference material on this subject.

In addition to using interviews and questionnaires, those involved on the project team, particularly the project leader and other members of the technical staff, should observe operations in the departments to be involved in the information system. Observation will supplement information obtained through interviews and often will point up the need for system characteristics that did not surface during conversations with user personnel. Of particular importance, systems analysts should pay close attention to environmental factors while observing departmental operations. Physical facilities, leadership styles of supervisors, degree of formality or informality in departmental procedures, and other elements of the day-to-day working environment can have a tremendous impact on how a system will function in a given organization.

Observation may be continuous over a fixed period of time, or work sampling techniques may be employed. Work sampling is based on statistical sampling theory. It is more efficient than 100 percent continuous observation of work processes.

> Work measurement . . . involves the measurement of tasks or component parts of a job. The number of times each task is performed is tabulated and a time standard for the job is determined. This is later converted to human labor requirements, once all activities are applied to a time standard and the total time required to perform the job is calculated. ("Guide to Effective Health Care Management Engineering," HIMSS 1995, 11)

Notes should be taken throughout the data collection process, and other written documentation should be obtained, including sample reports, completed forms, procedural manuals, and organizational charts.

2. Tools for data organization. The collected data should be analyzed according to standard formats, and summary tables should be prepared. In addition to tabular and graphic organization of data, interview reports and observations of department operations should be written up in concise narrative format.

One of the most useful tools in systems analysis is the flowchart. Flowcharts provide a concise, logical, and standardized mechanism for depicting and analyzing current information flows. They help to pinpoint errors, inconsistencies, and inefficiencies in information flows and are very helpful in estimating the effects of changes on current operations. Flowcharts illustrate relationships among various organizational functions as far as information interchange is concerned. This is a critical element of information system analysis, since the identification of interfaces among functions is most important when attempting to achieve systems integration.

Figure 8.7 is an example of a system flowchart produced as part of a systems analysis of the clinical laboratory of a 273-bed general medical and surgical facility. The flowchart indicates the process followed in ordering lab tests, obtaining specimens, conducting the tests, and reporting results. The flow of information throughout this process is shown in a concise and logical format through the flowchart.

Several problems were identified as a result of the analysis. These included breakdowns in communication between ward and lab personnel, lost charges for tests performed, problems with the pneumatic tube system used to transmit information, and the need for more preadmission testing. With the aid of the flowchart and other tools of systems analysis, immediate solutions to each of these problems could be recommended to management. In addition, the flowcharts and other analyses served as the basis for an automated information-processing system in the laboratory.

Note that process flowcharts usually follow a top-down format and the shape of the boxes are indicative of a particular type of activity. For example, note in Figure 8.7 that rectangular boxes are used to identify individual processing steps and diamond-shaped boxes indicate decision or switching points in which alternative paths are followed depending on the results of the decision being made. Flowcharting software is available and is commonly used by systems analysts to simplify and speed the construction of process flowcharts, often as part of a broader information engineering methodology. (Reynolds 1995, 297–302)

Figure 8.7 System Flowchart—Ordering Tests, Obtaining Specimens, and Testing and Reporting

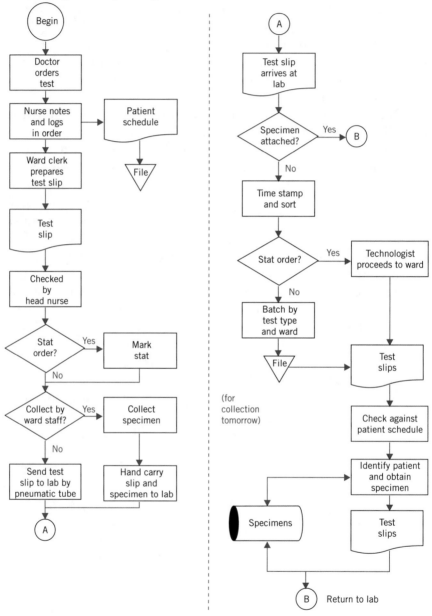

Continued

Figure 8.7 Continued

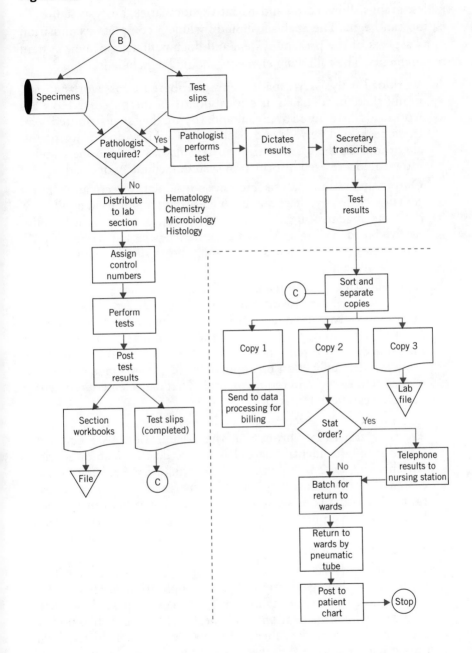

3. Analysis tools. After data have been collected and organized into tables, graphs, flowcharts, and narrative summaries, analysis and evaluation can begin. The analysis should include a complete examination of all aspects of the present system and documentation of new system requirements. The following elements should be included:

a. Workload analysis. Are loads evenly distributed across workstations, or are there bottlenecks at critical points in the process? How are workloads distributed over time and why are they so distributed? Are there peak load periods and slack periods? How does information aid or impede the work of the departments involved in the system? How could a revised information system facilitate workload?

b. Output utilization analysis. How are output data screens and reports actually used? Are there some which really are not used at all? Are the costs of generating a particular system output worth the benefits received from having it? What are the deficiencies in current output? What new or revised data screens and reports should be included in the new system?

c. Input and data collection analysis. What are the current problems in data collection? Are forms efficiently designed? Are data unnecessarily copied from document to document, increasing the possibility of errors in transcription? What are the error rates on data entry? Are the same data captured repetitively by various organizational units? How can data collection be improved? What new kinds of data are needed to meet system requirements? What data elements currently collected can be eliminated?

d. Code analysis. What codes and coding systems are presently used? Are they consistent throughout the organization? Are codes designed simply to identify data elements or do they also categorize? Are checking systems built into coding structures? Are codes flexibly designed and expandable to handle an increased volume of transactions? Are codes consistent with those used by other organizations for comparative purposes? Are the codes consistent with external reporting needs? What kinds of coding systems are needed in order that the new information system may be designed?

e. Database analysis. Are data elements duplicated in databases throughout the organization? Is such duplication necessary? Can needed information be obtained easily from existing databases maintained by other organizations in the health system? Are files updated according to a periodic schedule? Have files become cluttered with out-of-date material? Are the files properly indexed and accessible for retrieval of needed information? What data are being retained needlessly? How can files be improved? What new databases are needed for the new system?

f. Procedures and information flow analysis. How efficient are current operating procedures? What improvements are needed? Does information flow smoothly and on a timely basis? How can information flow be handled more expeditiously so that information truly supports operations and management decisions?

g. Cost analysis. What are the current costs of processing information in the area under study? Are these costs reasonable? Higher than expected? The cost analysis should be a complete study of all costs incurred in collecting, storing, processing, retrieving, and utilizing information under procedures presently employed. Cost data gathered at this phase of a system project provide important benchmark information for later comparison with costs of the proposed new system.

CASE Tools

The systems analysis process itself has been aided by automation. Computer-aided systems engineering (CASE) is a technology that provides a set of software tools for use in the process of systems analysis, design, and implementation. There are two major categories of CASE tools—upper and lower CASE. Lee (1996) describes them as follows:

> Upper CASE tools assist systems analysts in defining and graphically modelling the current information system and in describing and graphically modelling the systems users' requirements for the new information system. . . .
>
> Lower CASE tools are designed either to help programmers test and debug their program code or to automatically generate program code from the analysis and design specifications. (Lee 1996, 3–4)

There are a large number and variety of CASE products on the market. They are designed to increase productivity in the system analysis process, provide a vehicle for communication between analysts and users on the project team, provide a set of standards for the design requirements, and simplify system documentation.

Limitations of CASE tools include high cost, a steep learning curve associated with their use, and a failure of some tools to meet user expectations often due to vendors who overstate the capabilities of their products. (Lee 1996)

Process Reengineering

Many health services organizations have used information technology as a tool for automating existing processes. Currently, increased emphasis is being placed on reengineering processes rather than simply mechanizing existing procedures. Project teams involved in systems analysis of healthcare information systems are well-advised to follow principles of process reengineering rather than simply looking for ways to automate existing activities in the organization.

Michael Hammer (1990) defines reengineering as basic analysis and redesign of everything associated with a business process to achieve dramatic performance improvement. Management must take advantage of the power of information systems to revamp the way things are done.

> Everything is challenged: work flow, job definitions, management procedures, control processes, organizational structures, and even corporate values and culture. . . . Every company operates according to a great many rules—most of them undocumented, many of them decades old, and some of them no longer valid. Reengineering requires finding and vigorously challenging the rules blocking major business process changes. (Reynolds 1995, 11)

Benefits of Systems Analysis

There are many benefits from systems analysis, whether or not a new information system is developed. Systems analysis requires careful self-examination of current procedures. Any such analysis, properly performed, will result in procedural changes and methods improvement which in themselves should be worth the cost of the analysis. Systems analysis will also result in the development of standards for both procedure and performance. In most health services organizations, such standards are needed badly in order to improve management control and accountability of operations. The analysis also provides documentation of existing procedures and information flow, which many organizations do not compile in a systematic manner. Finally, systems analysis permits decisions about information systems to be based upon objective data and careful examination of requirements rather than intuition. As such, it provides a strong foundation upon which a new information system can rest.

Systems analysis is a critical first step in the process that should not be bypassed or cut short even when predesigned applications software will be used for implementation of the new system.

Analysts developing an automated appointment scheduling system for the Harvard Community Health Plan noted: "The first and most important step in the process was to define the needs of the users in detail." (Osteraas and Kelliher 1990) Eight sets of functional requirements were defined in detail including (1) provider scheduling, (2) appointment structure, (3) inquiry into the scheduling database, (4) appointment booking, (5) reporting, (6) required interfaces with other systems, (7) backup, and (8) security.

This chapter presents a limited description of the processes and tools of systems analysis. The reader interested in more detail is directed to one of the references on this subject included in the Additional Readings at the end of the chapter.

Selection of a Design Approach

Functional system requirements determined through systems analysis are used by the project team in selecting an approach to systems design. (See Figure 8.1.) Alternative approaches include:

1. use of predesigned (packaged) systems;
2. in-house design;
3. use of contractual services; and
4. combinations of the above.

Most health services organizations will choose to use a predesigned or packaged software system if one is available which meets organizational needs as specified in the statement of functional requirements. Use of a predesigned software system will eliminate most of the costs of the in-house design effort, particularly if no modifications of the standardized system are required. However, in some situations, the packaged system must be modified to meet specific institutional needs and organizational idiosyncrasies. Before making a decision to employ a predesigned system, the project team should carefully review the costs and benefits of this approach. Savings in computer programming costs will be offset to some degree by the purchase price or lease cost of the packaged system plus the additional costs required to modify it, if any.

The second design approach involves in-house development of a new information system tailored to the organization's specific requirements. The system is designed in detail and computer programs are written using functional requirements as specified during the systems analysis phase of the project.

Some health services organizations carry out detailed design and development of information systems through contractual services. For large systems, this may involve a competitive bidding process in response to an RFP developed by the organization after a systems analysis and statement of functional requirements have been completed.

Many healthcare organizations are turning to the use of outside contractors for software development, arguing that they will not have to develop the expensive technical expertise required and, consequently, their overall costs will be lower. Whenever outside services are used, health services organizations should protect themselves by (1) developing clearly stated and detailed specifications for the work; and (2) developing a written contract with performance requirements enumerated so that both parties have identical expectations for the results of the systems work or software package to be developed.

Chapter 9 presents detailed information on converting functional requirements into design specifications and evaluating, selecting, and contracting for packaged software and contractor services.

Conclusion: How Well Are We Doing?

There is a very limited amount of research on how well health services organizations use accepted principles of systems analysis in the development of information systems for their organizations.

In a recent study, Wong, Sellaro, and Monaco (1995) conducted a survey of U.S. hospitals to determine practices followed in the development of information systems. Responses were received from 216 hospitals. Some of the findings from the survey include the following:

1. 91 percent of the respondents identified information needs through interviews, questionnaires, current system documentation reviews, and observation.
2. 82 percent surveyed user feelings about the new or updated system.
3. 68 percent developed a cost-benefit analysis for the new or updated system.
4. 64 percent evaluated the advantages and disadvantages of using in-house developed software versus purchasing commercial software packages.
5. 11 percent used CASE tools for analysis and design.
6. 85 percent prepared a report to management that recommended whether or not to proceed with development of the new or updated system. (Wong, Sellaro, and Monaco 1995, 61–63)

The results of this survey seem to indicate that most hospitals follow the basic steps in the IS development life cycle. However, the results also indicate that improvements are needed in user involvement, cost-benefit analysis, evaluation of in-house programming versus use of software packages, and use of modern technology, such as CASE.

Summary

The life cycle for development of an information system in healthcare organizations includes seven steps: (1) systems analysis of functional requirements; (2) selection of a design approach; (3) system design; (4) system acquisition or construction; (5) implementation; (6) operation and maintenance; and (7) system evaluation and improvement.

Applications development projects should be carried out by a project team, headed by a senior systems analyst and including representatives of relevant user departments, the medical staff, and management. If an outside contractor is to be employed for systems development work, the same form of project organization should be a requirement of the contract.

Systems analysis is the process of collecting, organizing, and analyzing data about IS requirements *prior* to decisions being made about system design and implementation.

Data about system requirements are obtained through interviews, questionnaires, observation of operations, and review of written documentation. Data analysis includes: workload analysis, report utilization, input and data collection, code analysis, database analysis, procedures and information flows, and estimates of present system costs. Computer-aided systems engineering (CASE) provides a set of software tools for use in systems analysis and design.

Systems analysis provides the benefits of self-examination, improvement of operations, and development of standards. Of greater importance, systems analysis provides a strong foundation on which to build automated information systems.

In selecting an approach to system design, the project team can choose among the following alternatives: (1) purchase of predesigned "packaged" software from commercial vendors; (2) in-house design and programming; (3) employment of contractors for design and programming; and (4) a combination of these approaches. Most healthcare organizations are using commercial software for the majority of their applications because of the wide array of products available and the lower cost of development.

Discussion Questions

8.1 What is the purpose of systems analysis in health organizations?

8.2 Give examples of the kinds of questions that systems analysis should address.

8.3 What kinds of data are collected in a systems analysis?

8.4 What are some of the specific analytical tools and techniques that can be employed once data are collected and organized?

8.5 What are CASE tools? How are they used?

8.6 What are some of the benefits to the organization from a well-conducted systems analysis? Should the analysis always lead to development of an automated information system?

8.7 What alternatives are possible in the selection of an approach to system design? Discuss the advantages and disadvantages of each alternative.

Problems

8.1 Draw up an organization chart and work plan for a systems analysis of the order entry and results reporting process for clinical laboratory testing in a university medical center.
8.2 Conduct a study of information flow of the patient registration process in a health maintenance organization. Develop a systems flowchart with accompanying narrative notes. Describe improvements that could be made in the present system as a result of your study.
8.3 Interview the CIO or IS director of a healthcare organization in your area. Discuss the extent to which commercial software is used in developing systems and the extent to which in-house programming is employed. Prepare a report of your interview.

References

Babbie, E. 1986. *The Practice of Social Research*, 4th Ed. Belmont, CA: Wadsworth Publishing Company.
Hammer, M. 1990. "Reengineering Work: Don't Automate, Obliterate." *Harvard Business Review* 90 (4): 104–12.
Healthcare Information and Management Systems Society (HIMSS). 1995. *Guide to Effective Health Care Management Engineering.* Chicago: The Society.
Lee, F. W. 1996. "Can Computer-Aided Systems Engineering Tools Enhance the Development of Health Care Information Systems? A Critical Analysis." *Topics in Health Information Management* 17 (1): 1–11.
Osteraas, L., and M. Kelliher. 1990. "Appointment Scheduling." In *Information Systems for Ambulatory Care*, edited by T. A. Matson and Mark D. McDougall. Chicago: American Hospital Association.
Reynolds, G. W. 1995. *Information Systems for Managers*, 3rd Ed. Minneapolis–St. Paul, MN: West Publishing Company.
Wong, B. K., C. L. Sellaro, and J. A. Monaco. 1995. "Information Systems Analysis Approach in Hospitals: A National Survey." *Health Care Supervisor* 13 (3): 58–64.

Additional Readings

Austin, C. J., and R. C. Howe. 1994. "Information Systems Management." In *The AUPHA Manual of Health Services Management*, edited by R. J. Taylor and S. B. Taylor. Gaithersburg, MD: Aspen Publishers.
Gore, M., and J. W. Stubbe. 1988. *Elements of Systems Analysis*, 4th Ed. Dubuque, IA: William C. Brown Publishers.
Hammer, M., and J. Champy. 1993. "Reengineering the Corporation: A Manifesto for Business Revolution." *Harper Business* 18: 65–68.

Hepworth, J. B., G. A. Vidgen, and E. Griffin. 1992. "Adopting an Information Management Approach to the Design and Implementation of Information Systems." *Health Services Management Research* 5 (2): 115–22.

Kerr, J. M. 1991. "The Information Engineering Paradigm." *Journal of Systems Management* 42 (4) Issue No. 358.

Martin, J. 1990. *Information Engineering, Book II—Design and Construction*. Englewood Cliffs, NJ: Prentice-Hall, Inc.

Martin, M. P. 1995. "The Case Against CASE." *Journal of Systems Management* 46: 54–57.

Orens, J. 1996. "Grasp Operational Processes before Selecting Systems." *Health Management Technology* (July): 26–28.

Senn, J. A. 1989. *Analysis and Design of Information Systems*, 2nd Ed. New York: McGraw-Hill, Inc.

Valenta, A., C. Dixon, J. Finn, and S. Beller. 1995. "Developing an Enterprise Wide Strategy for Managing Healthcare Informatics." *Healthcare Informatics* 12: 30–31.

Whitten, J. L., L. D. Bently, and V. M. Barlow. 1994. *Systems Analysis and Design Methodology*, 3rd Ed. Burr Ridge, IL: Richard D. Irwin.

Williams T. 1994. "New CASE Tools Aimed at Coordinating Complex Projects." *Computer Design* 33: 65–67.

9

SYSTEM DESIGN, EVALUATION, AND SELECTION

A
S DESCRIBED in Chapter 8, the first two steps in the life cycle of information systems (IS) development are systems analysis and selection of an approach to systems design. This chapter discusses steps 3 and 4 in the cycle—specification of system requirements (system design) and system acquisition or construction. (Refer to Figure 8.1 in Chapter 8.)

Introduction

Design of a health services information system should flow readily from a carefully executed systems analysis. As discussed in Chapter 8, there are

---

Concepts and Applications

Design of a health information system should follow the functional requirements determined through systems analysis. Healthcare executives must choose between in-house design and programming or purchase of a commercial system.

After completing this chapter, readers should be able to evaluate options for system design and acquisition and will be familiar with criteria used in evaluating commercial software packages.

This chapter additionally addresses the essential elements of **requests for proposal** and **requests for information,** as well as the role of **consultants.**

---

four major alternatives available in the selection of an approach to systems design: (1) use of predesigned (packaged) systems; (2) in-house design; (3) use of contractual services; and (4) a combination of these approaches.

Detailed design specification are required for systems that are to be developed by in-house staff or through employment of contractual services. Less detail is required when packaged software is to be used. However, the system development project team must still develop a set of essential requirements to be matched against the capabilities of the software packages being considered. These essential requirements may serve as the basis for a Request for Proposals (RFP) or Request for Information (RFI) from vendors.

This chapter discusses the process of developing detailed design specifications for in-house development as well as recommended procedures to follow in the evaluation, selection, and acquisition of commercial software.

System Design Specifications

System design is the process of converting IS requirements into a detailed set of specifications for a system. The project team organization described in Chapter 8 should be continued during the design phase of a project. However, emphasis will shift to the more technical tasks requiring the skills of trained systems analysts or management engineers. Additional technical personnel may be needed at this point in the project. System users should continue to serve as a sounding board for the technical design characteristics developed by the analysts working on the project.

For systems to be developed in-house, the results of the design phase should be a formal, detailed set of system specifications. The content of specifications for an in-house development effort is shown in Figure 9.1.

The first step in the process must be the definition of system objectives. What are the specific goals the health services organization expects to achieve through the design of the new information system? Objectives should be as specific as possible and should be measurable later, when the system is operational.

Output specifications should flow readily from a specific statement of system objectives. Reporting requirements will be specified by departmental representatives on the project team working with the systems analysts. Each data screen and report to be produced by the system should be specified in detail. The specific content and format should be specified, and sample displays should be drawn up by the systems analysts.

Input specifications are derived from system objectives and output formats. Specific input data requirements are derived from the content of output reports and from data retrieval specifications. For each set of

Figure 9.1 System Design Specifications

1. Statement of System Objectives
2. Output Specifications
   a. Data Screens
      • Purpose
      • Content
      • Format
   b. Printed Reports
      • Purpose
      • Content
      • Format
      • Distribution and reporting schedule
      • Estimated volume
3. Input Specifications
   a. Sources of data
   b. Forms
   c. Procedures for converting to machine readable form
   d. Coding systems
   e. Schedule and estimated volumes
4. Database Specifications
   a. Content and format
   b. Estimated volumes and file sizes
   c. Updating and purging schedules
   d. Security procedures
5. Procedures and Data Flow
   a. Flowcharts
   b. Narrative
   c. Computer program specifications (if in-house development is planned)
6. Cost-Benefit Estimates
   a. System development costs
   b. Operating costs
   c. Maintenance costs
7. Management Approvals (Signatures)

input data to be processed by the system, the source of the data must be specified and forms or other means of capturing the data must be designed. As a general rule, it is desirable to capture data as close to the original source as possible, and it is also wise to minimize transcription of data before entry into the computer for processing. Direct input of data through terminals or capture of data in a machine readable format, if possible, is highly desirable. Good forms design also is an important step in the capture and entry of data into the system.

Input specification also includes development of codes and coding systems. Codes should be simple and easy to use. They should be flexible and easy to expand as the volume of transactions increases.

The fourth major element of system specifications is database design. Each master file must be specified in detail, including content and format of the file structure, estimated volume of transactions, and average file size. The system design should also include a procedure and schedule for periodic updating and purging of files in the database. The latter is often neglected, and the resultant system must cope with cluttered files of outdated information. Database security procedures are another essential element of design specifications. Protection of the patient's right to privacy must be paramount in the construction of medical record files, and safeguards should be built into the initial design to ensure that files are accessible only to authorized employees.

Inputs, outputs, and databases are system elements that must be related to one another through the specification of procedures and data flow. Flowcharts, similar to those used in systems analysis, are the basic tools employed in specifying information flow in the new system. In addition, narrative descriptions and elaboration of procedures, revised policies, and new organizational structures should be detailed in this section of the specifications. Also included should be written specifications for computer programs to be developed by in-house staff.

The sixth step in the development of system specifications should be a thorough estimate of the costs and benefits of the proposed new system. Three kinds of costs should be estimated: system development costs, operating costs, and maintenance costs. Development costs include the remaining costs of design and implementation, including computer programming, training of personnel, procedures writing, system testing, conversion of data files, and other similar tasks. Operational costs include labor, materials, and a prorated share of computer time used for the new system. Maintenance costs are often overlooked. These are the personnel costs incurred in keeping qualified systems analysts and programmers available to make necessary changes in the system after it goes into operation and to evaluate it periodically for improvements.

These costs must be matched against the anticipated benefits of the system, both tangible benefits that can be translated into dollar savings for the organization and also intangible benefits that cannot be measured directly in financial terms but which are expected to improve the effectiveness of service delivery.

Once the cost-benefit analysis has been completed, system planners should again critically evaluate whether or not to proceed with implementation of the system. It is quite possible that a system that looked attractive after an initial systems analysis could be found to be prohibitively expensive or not feasible after a detailed design is completed. In such a situation, the project team and management personnel must be bold enough not to proceed with implementation. A decision to proceed because a major investment has been made in the design phase is foolish; unfortunately many health services organizations have implemented computer systems when the results of a design effort dictated against such action.

The final element of the specifications should be a formal section for management approvals. The specifications should be submitted for formal review to the manager of each department and service unit involved and also to administration. Meetings should be scheduled to elaborate on the specifications, answer questions about them, and discuss possible problems with the system design. Once necessary changes have been made, signatures of approval should be required.

Appendix A to this chapter is a case study describing an actual system design effort at an academic medical center.

Evaluation of Application Software

As discussed previously, most healthcare information systems are developed using predesigned commercial software. Before considering the use of any application software package, health services organizations should develop a statement of functional requirements. A detailed list of functions and features should be prepared with requirements categorized into two groups, those that are *mandatory* and those that are *desirable*. If the software is to be used on an existing computer configuration, then hardware and operating system software compatibility requirements should be stated. Most applications will need to be linked to other operational systems requiring the specification of necessary system interfaces. For example, a proposed new system for scheduling patient appointments in an ambulatory care center might require linkage to the medical records and patient accounting systems already in place. In this case, the clinic must decide whether to require the new system vendor to supply the interface, contract with the vendors of the existing systems to build interfaces, or do the work in-house.

For major software acquisitions that involve multiple applications, consideration should be given to a formal bidding procedure through use of an RFP or an RFI. Guidelines for the development and use of RFPs and RFIs are included later in this chapter.

Information on application software in the health services field can be obtained from a variety of sources. (See Figure 9.2.) Guidebooks and directories provide general information about software products and their use in health services organizations. (See, for example, Ankrapp and Di Lima 1996, and *Health Management Technology* Annual Market

Figure 9.2   Sources of Information on Vendors and Software

1. Directories and Guidebooks
2. Exhibits at Professional Association Meetings
3. Internet Home Pages on World Wide Web
4. Direct Contact with Other Users
5. Hardware- and Software-User Groups
6. Consulting Firms

Directory.) Vendors display their products at major professional meetings such as the annual meetings of the Healthcare Information and Management Systems Society (HIMSS), the American Medical Informatics Association (AMIA), the American Health Information Association (AHIMA), the American Hospital Association (AHA), and the Medical Group Management Association (MGMA), to name just a few.

Many software vendors maintain home pages on the Internet via the World Wide Web, and general information on their products can be obtained through Internet searches (see Chapter 16 for more information on Internet resources). Information can be obtained directly from other health services organizations or from user groups that have been formed to share information about experiences with particular hardware and software products. Consulting firms can provide information on available products, but care should be exercised in selecting a consultant to be sure the firm has no business ties to any particular vendors. Use of consulting services is discussed in more detail later in this chapter.

Figure 9.3 lists some of the most important factors to consider in evaluating packaged applications software for a healthcare facility.

Using the statement of functional requirements as a base for comparison, an analysis of how well each package under consideration meets organizational requirements is essential. If a given software package does not exactly match stated requirements, to what extent is the organization willing and able to adjust operations to meet the general specifications of the software?

Consideration should also be given to the experiences of others who have used a particular packaged software system. Careful checking is essential and should be carried out independently from the vendor. Ask the vendor to supply a list of organizations that have purchased the software and make direct contact with a selection of these facilities through telephone interviews or site visits.

Determination of compatibility of the proposed application package with existing hardware and software must be part of the evaluation process. If hardware modifications or a complete new configuration is required, what are the costs involved (purchase and maintenance)?

Figure 9.3 Packaged Software Evaluation Criteria

1. Congruence with organizational requirements
2. Level of satisfaction of other users
3. Compatibility with existing hardware and software
4. Ability to interface/integrate with other applications
5. Support available
   a. Training
   b. Documentation
   c. Maintenance
6. Costs
   a. Software lease or purchase
   b. Additional hardware (if any)
   c. Implementation
   d. Operational maintenance and upgrades
7. Financial stability of vendor

Consideration must also be given to building system interfaces to other applications. Will this be done in-house, or will the vendor be responsible for them? What are the costs involved? If the health services organization follows an industry standard for data such as HL7 (see Chapter 7), is the vendor's software package compatible with this standard?

Support services available from the vendor are very important. These should include education and training programs for users and technical personnel involved in operating the system. What training is provided and what are the costs? Software updates and maintenance are important factors to consider in evaluating application packages. Will the vendor provide periodic updates to incorporate changes suggested by users or those required by changing regulations? How often will updates be offered and what will they cost? If the health services organization wishes to provide its own maintenance and make modifications as necessary, will the vendor offer contractual permission to do so and provide the source code for use by in-house programmers? In such circumstances, good documentation of the computer programs is essential if changes are to be made by in-house programmers.

Cost analysis is an important element in software evaluation. Costs fall into three categories: (1) the purchase or lease cost of the software itself; (2) the cost to implement the software including hardware modification (if any), building of interfaces to other systems, and personnel training; and (3) costs of software maintenance and updates once the package is operational. All three cost elements must be carefully estimated in comparing vendor products. The software package with the lowest purchase cost may not have the lowest overall cost when these other elements are considered.

The financial stability of the vendor must be considered as well. The applications software industry is volatile with frequent changes in vendors due to mergers, acquisitions, and business failures. Carefully review the financial history of each company under consideration. How long have they been in business? Do the company's financial statements and ratings appear stable?

Use of Contractual Services (Outsourcing)

An alternative to in-house development or purchase of packaged systems is the use of contractual services for design and implementation of systems. These services can be purchased from several vendors specializing in systems analysis and programming. Contracts can range from purchase of services on an hourly basis to fixed-price contracts for a total turnkey effort, in which the entire process is handled on a contractual basis. The following steps should be taken when evaluating contract services:

1. Review carefully the prior experience of the contractor. Talk to several previous clients.
2. Investigate the financial stability of the contractor.
3. Review the credentials (experience and training) of the specific personnel to be assigned to your project. Insist that the contractor identify those individuals to be assigned to your project rather than presenting a general portfolio of credentials for all professionals in their firm.
4. Be sure that the contractor employs well-established principles of systems analysis and design in its work plans and procedures.
5. Carefully examine all cost estimates and be sure they are thoroughly prepared, complete, and comprehensive. For major projects, insist on fixed-price and fixed-time contracts.
6. If necessary, use a neutral, disinterested party (independent consultant) to assist in the technical evaluation of proposed services.
7. Design a formal review process to evaluate the work of the contractor and manage the contract closely.

A discussion of negotiations and contracting for major projects is included later in this chapter. Further discussion of outsourcing as an alternative to in-house staffing is covered in Chapter 10.

The Selection Process

Selection of a vendor to provide software, hardware, or other contract computer services is a critical step in the IS development process.

Depending on the size and complexity of the system involved, an informal or a formal, more structured, process may be followed.

1. RFI. For smaller system acquisitions, an informal process requiring limited documentation is most common. The process often includes development of an RFI, which is used to obtain general product information and to prescreen vendors and their capabilities. The RFI includes a general description of the product (hardware and/or software) that the healthcare organization seeks to acquire. Vendors are asked to respond with information about their products and how they would meet the general requirements stated in the RFI. Responses to the RFI are used to screen the vendor list and select a smaller number (2 to 5) from whom additional information will be obtained. Those selected will be invited to submit proposals for providing the product including price, delivery, and support services included. These proposals are evaluated through meetings with vendor representatives and comments from other clients.

2. RFP. The formal vendor selection process usually involves a selection team of users and analysts, requires more documentation, and includes a formal RFP. An RFI might also be used to prescreen vendors and limit the number to be included in the formal bidding process.

There is some debate about the degree of specification that should be included in an RFP. Some argue for minute specification of every detail for the proposed system in order to insure that the health services organization knows in advance exactly what it is buying. The counterargument calls for greater flexibility and latitude in the specifications so that vendors are free to propose a variety of approaches in meeting the functional requirements included in the RFP. The answer usually lies somewhere between these two extremes. Specifications should be reasonably focused to ensure that system objectives are met and to provide a common base for evaluating proposals. Some flexibility should be included, however, to permit creative approaches on the part of prospective bidders.

The RFP describes functional requirements and states guidelines for bidders to follow in their proposals. For a major system acquisition, the RFP should include:

1. an introduction to the organization in which the system will be used, including organization charts, operating statistics, number of personnel, and financial information;
2. statement of functional requirements, categorized as mandatory or desirable, and listed in priority order;
3. specification of content and format to be followed in proposals, including vendor profile, software and hardware descriptions, training plans, documentation to be provided, maintenance coverage, list

of other clients who have used similar products or services, cost schedule, and performance guarantees;

4. statement of criteria to be used in evaluating proposals;
5. requirements for on-site demonstrations and system testing;
6. requirements for the vendor's role in system implementation; and
7. general contractual requirements including warranties, performance bonds, payment schedule, and penalties for failure to meet time schedules specified in the contract.

In the introduction to the RFP, the vendor should find information on how the system is to be used and who will use it. The number of users and their geographic dispersal is extremely important in the increasing number of integrated healthcare delivery systems. The vendor should understand all functions expected of the system. Thus the introduction should contain a thorough outline of all computer-based transactions, organized by department or other units of the organization.

Statistics on normal and anticipated levels of activity (bed capacity, occupancy rate, admissions/discharges, outpatient service levels, number of records on file, number of personnel, and levels of activity by category in departments) are necessary to "size" the system needed. A description of the current computer configuration will help in orienting vendors to the operation and will provide detailed information on interface and conversion problems. The implementation schedule should be outlined.

If collaborative proposals (in which more than one vendor is responsible for the system) will not be accepted, a statement should be included stating that all hardware, software, and maintenance is to be supplied by a single vendor. It should be clear whether or not a turnkey system is required. If facilities management can be bid by either the system vendor or separately, a statement to that effect should be included.

It is prudent to stipulate that the successful vendor will be responsible for any interface problems between the system acquired and any existing installations, such as a data switch or local-area network (LAN). Where modems and communication lines are involved, there is a tendency for each party (installations at both ends and the communication facility, such as a telephone company) to assume the problem is in someone else's territory.

To avoid unexpected charges in conjunction with the proposal and bid process, a clear statement should be included disclaiming responsibility for expenses of the vendors for demonstrations or delivery of information. The name, address, and telephone number of the contact for proposals should appear in the introduction, together with rules designed to prevent problems with clarifications and exceptions. In the case of public-supported and nonprofit institutions, it may be necessary to state that no amounts identified as taxes can be paid as part of the purchase. The key elements of the proposal evaluation process may be summarized, with a reference to the details of evaluation.

General requirements for proposals should specify the format for the reply to the RFP. If all the vendors adhere to the reply format, it will be easier for the buyer to compare proposals. The description of the format for the reply should encourage vendors to supply all relevant information, but it should request that stated section headings, such as these given above, be used in the order listed. A table of contents and divider tabs may be requested. If multiple copies are required, then the number needed should be stated. Complete sets of brochures, descriptive information, operation manuals, and technical reports will aid in evaluating competing proposals. An offer to return certain materials, except in the case of the successful bidder, may be included.

The vendor profile is intended to ensure that the company is stable financially and is capable of providing the kind of long-term support needed for computer products. Examples of pertinent information are the most recent annual report and the company's Dun and Bradstreet rating. The vendor's quality-control program should be adequately described to satisfy the purchaser. Information about the life cycle, or history of availability, of the product offered can be useful. Within the context of the vendor's established practices regarding systems marketed, this information may assist the buyer in evaluating the level of maintenance support that will be sustained for a particular product over the period of use intended by the health services organization. If the system proposed has appeared on the market recently, attention will be focused on assurance of reliability of hardware and software.

The vendor should state what types of training will be necessary for the system, what training materials will be needed, and the minimum skill levels of the persons to be trained. It should be clear where training is to be conducted by the vendor, how long it will last, and what it will cost. In the discussion of training and orientation, the purchaser can elaborate on the number and categories of personnel to receive training. All procedures and categories of personnel should be included in order to obtain accurate training costs.

The purchaser may wish to have a system demonstration. Any demonstration should be of a system identical to the one proposed for purchase. The purchaser should select the demonstration site from a client list provided by the vendor. It is preferable that the vendor not be present during the demonstration in order to allow free exchange of information with personnel from the organization demonstrating the system. The fault tolerance of the system and conditions of transfer to backup systems in emergencies should be determined.

Criteria for evaluating responses to the RFP will vary depending on the nature of the system to be acquired. However, general criteria would include:

1. established record of performance of the software, system, or equipment the vendor is proposing;
2. extent of vendor support to be provided, including expertise, availability, and capacity for support;
3. reliability, maintainability, and quality control;
4. projected economic and noneconomic benefits;
5. adaptability and provisions for expansion;
6. costs of acquisition, implementation, and maintenance; and
7. number and scope of any conditions attached to the proposal.

Once the RFP has been finalized and evaluation criteria have been developed, the document then is submitted to selected vendors. As mentioned previously, initial vendor screening can be accomplished by reviewing the responses to a preliminary RFI. After the RFP has been distributed, the health services organization may wish to schedule a bidders' conference in order to answer questions about the RFP in a public forum with all vendors present and receiving the same information.

All vendors should be required to submit proposals by a common date specified in the RFP. After proposals are received, screening can begin. The screening process may involve vendor demonstrations. Proposals will be evaluated in reference to stated criteria with a small group of vendor finalists selected as a result of the evaluations. Careful reference checking of each finalist, including site visits to organizations where vendor products are installed, is an essential step in the final selection process. It may be desirable to conduct preliminary contract negotiations with the two top finalists in order to determine if there are any insurmountable contract problems before the final selection of a vendor is made. Once the finalist has been selected, contract negotiations can begin.

Alternatives to the RFP

There is considerable disagreement about the value of using formal RFPs for acquiring information systems in healthcare organizations. The process can become so involved that prospective bidders may be discouraged from responding. Healthcare organizations often need to move quickly in developing or modifying information systems in response to competition and changing requirements in the managed care environment.

Smaller information system selections will rely more on prototyping and gathering of information for quick decisions. Roper Care Alliance in Charleston, South Carolina, employs an abbreviated RFP process for system selection. Appendix B describes the Roper process and includes as an example the System Requirements Definition for a Physician's Practice Management Application.

Negotiation and Contracting

The health services organization should take the lead in contract negotiations. As stated, negotiations should proceed concurrently with the vendors of first and second choice for as long as possible. This provides leverage during the negotiations and offers an alternative if negotiations with the primary vendor break down completely.

Vendors may propose using their standard contract. This should be rejected out-of-hand since the standard contract will contain features favorable to and designed to protect the vendor. The health services organization should form a negotiating team and utilize legal counsel from the beginning of the process. Although internal legal counsel may be utilized, consideration should be given to retaining assistance from a law firm that specializes in computer software and hardware negotiations because of the complexities and nuances involved in these types of contracts.

The final contract should be designed to put the vendor at financial risk for failure to meet requirements as specified in the RFP. In general, the health services organization should insist on fixed-price and fixed-time conditions in the contract. The RFP should be made part of the contract by reference in the main document.

Important issues that should be addressed in the contract include the following:

1. Delivery dates. Financial penalties should be included for failure to deliver and install software and hardware on the dates specified in the contract.
2. Acceptance testing. The contract should spell out performance requirements and the nature of an on-site acceptance test(s) to verify that these requirements have been met.
3. Payment schedule. As a general rule, no payments should be made until the system has been installed and acceptance tests have been met.

Final payments should be scheduled to allow some period of time for the system to function satisfactorily in operational mode, perhaps six months after system conversion. Cancellation provisions, including penalties (if any), should be clearly stated.

4. Warranties and guarantees. Hardware warranty periods should be specified and reliability guarantees on software should be included. The contract should specify the response time for service calls and the maximum allowable time for correcting software errors. Penalties for failure to meet these response time requirements should be included.

5. Software ownership (source code). The contract should specify who owns the software included in the system acquisition. If the vendor retains proprietary rights to the software (as often is the case), then the contract should specify the conditions under which the health services organization may modify the software for its own purposes.

6. Interface responsibilities. If the system to be acquired must interface with existing information systems, the contract must clearly state who will be responsible for building the necessary interfaces: new system vendor, existing system vendors, or the healthcare organization's programming staff.

7. Maintenance and updates. The contract should specify the responsibilities of both parties for system maintenance. If periodic software updates or upgrades are part of the agreement, the time intervals for them and costs should be clearly stated.

8. Personnel training. Vendor responsibilities for training user personnel, if any, should be clearly specified in the contract.

9. Documentation. The contract should specify the level and types of system documentation to be provided, including technical manuals for hardware and software and user manuals specifying operating procedures to be followed.

10. Expiration date and cancellation provisions. The contract should state the period of time that it will remain in effect and should include provisions covering a request for cancellation by either party.

Negotiations with vendors should be carried out in a professional manner, and efforts should be made to obtain a final contract that is satisfactory to both parties. Most new IS acquisitions result in a long-term partnership with the vendor, and mutual respect and trust is important to the success of that relationship.

Role of Consultants

Healthcare organizations frequently use consultants to assist in the evaluation and selection of IS vendors. Consultants can provide the following services:

1. Facilitate the selection process. Consultants with special expertise in system evaluation and selection can help design an objective process to be followed. However, decisions must ultimately be made by appropriate management and technical personnel from the healthcare organization, and the role of the consultant should be limited to that of a facilitator.

2. Provide technical information. There are a large number of vendors providing information services to the health services industry. It is difficult for any one organization to keep current on the technology that is available. Consulting firms offer specialized information services to assist in the evaluation process.

3. Provide an outside perspective. An independent consultant can help provide objectivity and expertise to the process, unencumbered by organizational politics or other internal factors that may influence the decision process.

In selecting a consultant, it is important to avoid firms that may have a conflict of interest. Some consultants have joint venture agreements with software or hardware vendors that could influence the advice they provide. An independent consultant should have no ties to any particular product.

Always examine the credentials of the individual(s) to be assigned to your project. This is particularly important when working with large firms. Be sure that your agreement with the consultant contains a provision that those assigned to the project will not be pulled off and reassigned before the engagement is complete. Check with other healthcare organizations who have used the consulting firm you are considering before making a final decision. Reynolds (1995, 435) suggests exploring the following questions:

1. Do they follow a collaborative process?
2. Are they good listeners?
3. Are they enthusiastic?
4. Do they keep the client well informed?
5. Do they really know their field and stay current with it?

Summary

Design of a health information system should flow readily from the statement of functional requirements determined through systems analysis. Detailed design specifications are required for systems being developed in-house. Less detail is required when packaged software is used. However, essential requirements must be specified and matched against the capabilities of software packages being considered.

Detailed design specifications for in-house projects should include: (1) system objectives; (2) output specifications; (3) input specifications; (4) database specifications; (5) procedures and data flow; (6) cost-benefit estimates; and (7) management approvals.

Most health services organizations now use predesigned applications software and other vendor services in implementing information systems. Careful attention to software evaluation, system selection, and contract negotiations is essential.

Factors to consider in evaluating applications software include: (1) congruence with functional requirements; (2) level of satisfaction of other users; (3) ability to interface this software with other applications already in place; (4) support available, including training, documentation, and maintenance; (5) costs of software, system implementation, new releases, and maintenance; and (6) financial stability of the vendor.

In evaluating contract services, health services organizations should: (1) review the prior experience of the contractor; (2) investigate the company's financial stability; (3) review the credentials of personnel to be assigned to the project; (4) insure that well-established principles of systems analysis and design are followed; (5) carefully review costs; and (6) use a neutral consultant for technical assistance if necessary.

An RFP is often used in major system acquisitions. The RFP should specify functional requirements, content and format for proposals, criteria to be used in evaluating proposals, demonstration and system test requirements, and general contractual requirements. In less complex system acquisitions, an RFI sent to selected vendors may substitute for the more formal and costly RFP process.

Legal counsel should be employed in negotiating contracts. Special attention should be given in the contract to delivery dates, acceptance testing, payment schedule, warranties and guarantees, software ownership, interface responsibilities, maintenance and system updates, personnel training, and documentation.

Consultants can assist in the evaluation and selection process by serving as facilitators, providing technical information, and offering an outside perspective. Consultants should be chosen carefully to be sure they have the necessary expertise and have no conflict of interests through ties to particular information system vendors.

Discussion Questions

9.1 List the major elements that should be included in the design specifications for a computer application to be developed by in-house staff.

9.2 What are some of the sources of information for identifying health-care software packages?

9.3 Discuss some of the more important elements to consider in evaluating applications software packages.

9.4 Discuss the pros and cons of using an RFP in a system acquisition.

9.5 Describe the major elements that should be included in an RFP.

9.6 Why should legal counsel be used in negotiating contracts for major system acquisitions?

9.7 What are some of the major elements that should be included in a contract for information systems?

9.8 What role can consultants play in the evaluation and selection of systems?

Problems

9.1 Select five vendors who provide software for the healthcare industry. Using the Internet, determine as many as possible of the following:

a. headquarters address and telephone number;

b. names of the executive(s) in charge of marketing;

c. ownership status of the firm;

d. percent of gross sales due to healthcare software;

e. number of employees in the firm;

f. date the firm was established; and

g. profile of products (software packages) offered by the firm.

9.2 Select three software products that perform the same or comparable tasks. Compare these products with regard to user ratings of reliability, ease of use, documentation, and maintenance of the products by the vendor. On the basis of this information, specify which one you would recommend for acquisition.

9.3 Schedule a telephone conference with the CIO of a health services organization in your community. Obtain his or her opinion on the use of RFPs in selecting information systems for the organization.

References

Ankrapp, B., and S. N. Di Lima, eds. 1996. *Health Care Software Sourcebook*. Gaithersburg, MD: Aspen Publishers.

Health Management Technology. Annual Market Directory 1996. Atlanta, GA: Argus, Inc.

Reynolds, G. W. 1995. *Information Systems for Managers*, 3rd Ed. Minneapolis, MN: West Publishing Company.

Additional Readings

Braly, D. 1996. "System Purchases Support Vendors' Visions." *Health Management Technology* (February): 13–14.

DeLuca, J. M., and O. Doyle. 1991. *Health Care Information Systems: An Executive's Guide for Successful Management*. Chicago: American Hospital Publishing, Inc. (Note particularly Chapter 6, "Acquiring a Health Care Information System.")

Lorenzi, N. M., M. J. Ball, R. T. Riley, and J. V. Douglas. 1995. *Transforming Health Care Through Information*. New York: Springer-Verlag, Inc. (Note particularly Chapter 15, "Evaluating for Success.")

Mandell, S. F., J. R. Duke, and D. Taliaferro. 1989 "Advanced Multi-Attribute Scoring Technique (AMAST): A Model Scoring Methodology for the Request for Proposal (RFP)." *Journal of Medical Systems* 13 (3): 163–75.

Neal, T. 1993. "Evaluating and Selecting an Information System, Part 1." *American Journal of Hospital Pharmacy* 50 (January): 117–20.

———. 1993. "Evaluating and Selecting an Information System, Part 2. *American Journal of Hospital Pharmacy* 50 (February): 289–93.

Orens, J. 1996. "Grasp Operational Processes before Selecting Systems." *Health Management Technology* (July): 26–28.

Person, M. M. 1988. *The Smart Hospital: A Case Study in Hospital Computerization*. Durham, NC: Carolina Academic Press.

Tsay, B., and J. R. Stackhouse. 1991. "Developing a Management Information System for a Hospital: A Case Study on Vendor Selection." *Journal of Medical Systems* 15 (5–6): 345–58.

System Design Case Study

The following case study is an adaptation of an actual system design effort at an academic medical center. Several years earlier, the institution installed a clinical data repository, which is a longitudinal database of patient data, including laboratory and radiology results, discharge summaries, operative notes, and other miscellaneous patient reports. The data is fed into the clinical data repository using Health Level-7 (HL7) standards for message transmission from feeder systems through an interface gateway. As time progressed, both technical staff members and end-users of the system began to identify new potential uses for the data repository, as well as many other sources of data. The system design effort described is about the implementation of a subsystem to utilize the data repository in the Urgent Care/Trauma Center.

The director of the trauma center contacted system support staff to help him solve a problem with retrieval of patient information from reports transcribed outside medical center. The trauma center had earlier chosen to outsource the transcription of the physicians' notes dictated during the urgent care visit. This was accomplished through direct telephone dictation to the transcription company in another area of the country. The company then transcribed the dictation and digitally transmitted reports back to a printer in the trauma center within defined turnaround periods. Reports were then printed and placed on the patients' paper charts. While this process worked very well, the reports were not available

The authors wish to thank Mr. Mark Daniels, Manager of Patient Support Systems, at the Medical University of South Carolina for the preparation of this case study.

for review in the medical center's clinical data repository. It was felt that if this information could be available in the local repository, several clinical management problems could be solved.

1. System Objectives

- Provide clinicians access to Urgent Care/Trauma Center notes from the clinical data repository.
- Provide the ability for any authorized clinician to browse the urgent care record online.
- Assist in follow-up care with patients through quick access to records online.
- Assist in the monitoring and quality evaluation process of care delivery standards through online review of multiple episodes of urgent care.
- Improve the clinician's ability to obtain an in-depth history of a specific patient prior to arrival in the trauma center.
- Improve patient satisfaction through faster and better follow-up care by urgent care physicians.
- Improve relationships with referring and consulting physicians through online access of urgent care episodes.

2. Operational Specifications

- Available notes from the dictation system should be back-loaded to provide a historical database.
- Each urgent care episode should have an associated note so that historical visits and episodes can be reviewed by patient name or medical record number.
- Notes should be available on a real-time basis from the point of transmission by the transcription company back to the medical center.
- Notes should be able to be viewed simultaneously with other patient data housed in the clinical data repository, such as laboratory or radiology results for routine care audits.

3. Source System (Transcription System) Input Specifications

- The only input to the off-site transcription company's system is the physician's dictation. In order to correctly file the completed report against the correct patient, the physician must include the following items within the dictation (some items may be entered via phone keypad):

- physician number;
- patient number (medical record number);
- patient billing account number (this encounter); and
- patient name.

4. Source System Output Specifications

- The output from the transcription system consist of two files for each unique report. The first file is a print file. In addition to the text of the report, the "print file" contains all of the printer-specific formatting codes that are needed to print the file on the printer as desired. The second file is a plain ASCII representation of the print file. The plain ASCII file contains no printer-specific codes; it consist entirely of "printable" ASCII characters. The "plain ASCII" file is the file that is used by the interface being described and will be explained in more detail.

- At predetermined intervals, the transcription system gathers all of the reports that have been generated for a given site (print and ASCII files) and "batches" them together in a "zip" file. The transcription system then establishes an asynchronous connection (via modem) with a file server at the target site. The "zip" file is transmitted to the site and a batch job is run on the site's file server that will "unbatch or unzip" the file and place the "print" files in one directory and the "ASCII" files in another directory. A second batch job is then triggered that will print all of the files in the print directory on a local printer.

- At predetermined intervals, the communications manager of the interface gateway looks at the "ASCII" file directory on the site's transcription system file server. If files are found they are transferred to the interface gateway system for processing.

- The "plain ASCII" files that are output from the transcription system consist of two sections, a one line header record followed by the textual body of the report. The header record is pipe "|" delimited and contains all of the data necessary to file the report against the correct patient and account. An example of the header record follows with the definition of its elements.
123456|801993456|123X56ZZ9|JOHN|PAUL|JONES|MSD |MARCUS|J|WELBY|1431|199611221537

  - patient number (medical record number)
  - patient billing account number (this encounter)
  - filer number/accession number (unique for this report)

- patient first name
- patient middle name
- patient last name
- transcriptionist identifier (initials)
- responsible provider first name (dictated by)
- responsible provider middle initial (dictated by)
- responsible provider last name (dictated by)
- responsible provider number (doctor number)
- report creation date and time

5. Interface Gateway Input Specifications

- The primary input to the Interface Gateway is the set of "ASCII" files generated by the transcription system.
- Patient data is looked up in the clinical data repository and used to verify the information in the "ASCII" file prior to acceptance by the interface gateway.

6. Interface Gateway Output Specifications

- Under normal conditions, the only output from the interface gateway is the insertion of the report data into the clinical data repository (database server).
- If an error is found during the report acceptance process, a copy of the report will be e-mailed to a designated user in the Urgent Care/Trauma Department. No attempt will be made at this point to insert the data into the clinical data repository. These errors are limited to incorrect pairing of medical record number, account number, and patient name or their omission. The report will be investigated by the trauma department and corrections called into the transcription company where a revised report can be generated. This report flows through the same process as outlined above.

7. Output Data Screens

Figure 9.4 is a sample output screen of an emergency service note as viewed by clinicians in the Urgent Care/Trauma Department.

8. Procedures and Data Flow

- Figure 9.5 shows the general flow of information for entry and storage of information in the clinical data repository.

- Figure 9.6 illustrates the retrieval of clinical information in the Urgent Care/Trauma Department.

9. Anticipated Costs and Benefits

- A detailed cost-benefit analysis has not been performed, but expectations are that current time spent in retrieving and reviewing manual records will be cut by 50 percent.
- Expected costs for development of the interface (labor only) are $15,000.

Figure 9.4 Sample Output Screen—Emergency Service Note

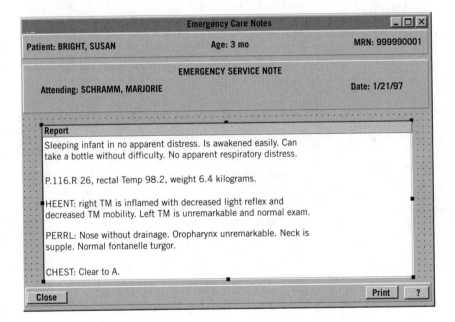

Figure 9.5 Flowchart—Entry and Storage of Information in the
Clinical Data Repository

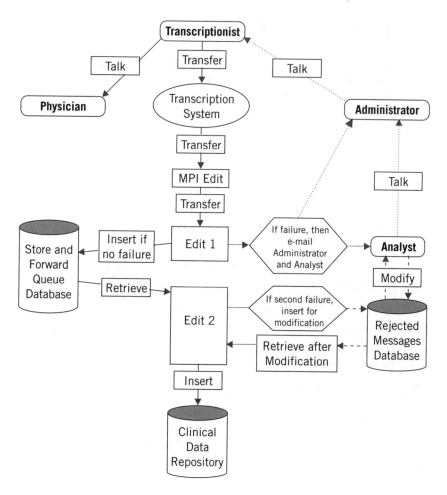

Figure 9.6 Flowchart—Retrieval of Clinical Information in the Urgent Care/Trauma Department

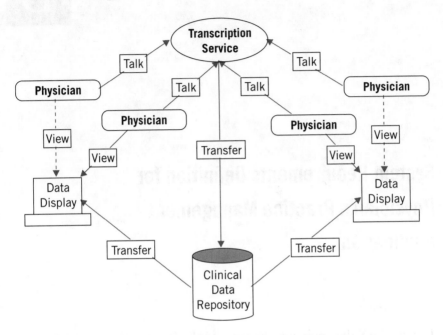

System Requirements Definition for Physician's Practice Management Application

The vendor will supply information on the following subjects:

1. Vendor Attributes

- Company profile, businesses involved
- Total years in business
- Years of this product support
- Number of employees by function (sales, technical support, development)
- Annual revenues, profits
- Research and development commitment, percent of revenue
- Number of installations for this product
- Demonstrated commitment to healthcare
- Demonstrated commitment to product, current and future
- Established comparable customer base, references supplied

The authors wish to thank Mr. Robert C. Johnson, Chief Information Officer, at Roper Care Alliance in Charleston, South Carolina for preparation of this System Requirements Definition.

2. Business Information

- Pricing:

  a. Software License(s)—Applications, Layered Software & Operating Systems, or Servers and Clients
  b. Installation
  c. Maintenance
  d. Hardware

- Corporate contract coordination with other vendors and contracts
- User groups, development partnership
- Site visits to Roper by other customers after installation
- Start-up resources, vendor/client

3. Technical Architecture/Environment

- "Best of fit," see separate scoring document attached
- Technical and industry standards confirmed
- Integration/interface capabilities, requirements
- Computer operations requirements for client and/or remote
- Single network protocol
- Uses existing "off-the-shelf" hardware/network equipment
- Flexible, modular components
- Custom modifications and screens
- Table maintenance, master files, codes
- Screen flow matched with user processes
- Inquiry and reporting
- Stated strategic direction and commitment
- Archive and retrieval/purge

4. Application System Software Functionality

- General

  a. Flexible, profile driven, user maintained
  b. Organizationwide operability
  c. Reporting, fast and easy, online
  d. Ability to expand and grow with company

- Application functionality

  a. Patient management and registration
  b. Resource scheduling, notices to patients, overrides, overbooking
  c. Patient instructions, walk-ins, no shows, tracking
  d. Charge posting
  e. Insurance processing, eligibility, and tracking
  f. Coding ICD-9, validation, cross edits to CPT-4 codes
  g. Data edits
  h. Referral tracking, incoming and outgoing
  i. Billing, single, sequential
  j. Payment posting, cash handling, electronic remittance, tracking
  k. A/R management and collections
  l. Management reporting
  m. Patient care and clinical data
  n. Medical records, links to hospital systems, orders, results
  o. Managed care and contract management
  p. Electronic submission
  q. Standard batch reports, custom
  r. Physician productivity and group practice

5. Product Stability and Support

- Application and hardware orders, installation and support
- User implementation methodology, requirements
- Training—who, where, when
- Documentation, hard/soft versions, how current
- Production support, toll-free help, logging and follow-up, hours
- Problem determination, reporting, follow-up/review procedure
- Problem escalation procedure
- Program corrections
- Routine, special maintenance
- Planned enhancements, how done, how frequent
- User-group participation, process
- Established plan for future product enhancements

Strategic Architecture (Best Fit) Scoring Scale:

Product Name: _____ Vendor Name: _____ Date: _____

System Architecture Requirement	Score (See below)
1. System is Three-tier client/server architecture (Presentation, Functionality servers, and Data)	
2. System is based on open architecture; hardware platform independent using RISC (Reduced Instruction Set Computing) DEC Alpha computers in UNIX operating system (i.e., Current hardware environment), engineered to take advantage of 64-bit Alpha architecture	
3. Client runs in Microsoft Windows environment (or Windows NT)	
4. Network protocol is industry standard TCP/IP (Transmission Control Protocol/Internet Protocol) and supports wide area topology	
5. System runs on relational database of user choice (Oracle, SQL Server, Sybase, Informix) and is directly accessible by user without proprietary intermediate connect program	
6. Code is industry standard (Visual Basic, C++, Open-M), not proprietary, and customer can support applications if vendor defaults	
7. Application settings, profiles, and functional parameters are user defined, managed with online screens	
8. System has built in "Hooks" to connect interfaces inbound and outbound to other foreign applications	
9. Applications are "Modular" and can be implemented in complex, mixed computer environment	
10. Application has integrated security by user identification	
11. Product is deployed in production in Integrated Healthcare System, similar to this company with proven success and positive references; designed for multicorporation, multi-entity, wide-area	
12. Functionality meets user requirements (defined in separate document)	
13. Application provides subsecond response time at any location	
14. Product is cost-effective	
15. Application is easy for users to operate with fully defined help functions online	
Total points:	
Total points divided by 15 for average score:	

Score: 1 = Unacceptable, does not meet requirements, not strategic
2 = Questionable, but meets some requirements; must negotiate tactical interim solution
3 = Meets most requirements with some modifications of product or procedure, requires impact study
4 = Acceptable, meets most requirements as delivered, identify specifics
5 = Meets all requirements

Comments: _____

MANAGING INFORMATION RESOURCES

CHAPTERS 8 AND 9 described the first four steps in the life cycle of information systems (IS) development: systems analysis, selection of a design approach, system design, and system acquisition or construction. This chapter describes the final three steps in the cycle: system implementation, operation and maintenance, and system evaluation and improvement. (Refer to Figure 8.1 in Chapter 8.) General issues in information resource management such as organization, staffing, and executive responsibilities are also discussed.

Concepts and Applications

After a system has been designed and selected, it must be implemented in the organization. Implementation includes procuring hardware and software, training personnel who will operate and use the system, and final testing prior to operation.

The reader will be able to discuss all facets of each phase of implementation, operation, and maintenance of a system.

Additionally, this chapter discusses the increasingly important role of the **chief information officer,** and analyzes the requirements for that position. Finally, **outsourcing** is discussed, along with its rationale, benefits, and pitfalls.

Managing System Implementation

Once a new or replacement information system has been selected, planning for implementation begins. System implementation may include acquisition of new hardware, computer programming, training, database preparation, system testing, and final documentation. (See Figure 10.1.) As with all phases of system development, implementation does not just happen; it must be carefully planned and managed.

1. Equipment acquisition. New equipment will be required for some system implementations. This task can range from complete installation of a general purpose computer or new computer network to the relatively simple addition of some workstations or terminals to an existing system. Whatever the magnitude of equipment requirements, equipment ordering and installation must be carefully planned. Sufficient lead time must be allowed to ensure delivery when needed. In some cases, renovations and site preparation will also be required, and good space planning must accompany all new equipment orders. (A detailed discussion of computer equipment is included in Chapter 3.)

2. Computer programming. For information systems being implemented by in-house staff, preparation of applications programs is part of the implementation process. However, most systems in healthcare organizations use applications software acquired from vendors, as described in Chapter 9. Nevertheless, some in-house programming may still be required for building interfaces to other applications or changing network configurations to accommodate the new software being installed. (See Chapter 4 for detailed information on computer programming and software.)

3. Training. An extremely important element of system implementation is training of personnel who will operate and use the new system. For systems designed and implemented in-house, training plans should be drawn up by the project team, and team members should take responsibility for coordinating and conducting the training sessions. For systems purchased from commercial firms, the company will usually include

Figure 10.1   Information System Implementation

1. Equipment Acquisition
2. Programming or Software Installation
3. Training
4. Database Preparation
5. System Testing
6. Final Documentation

initial training as part of the contract. These sessions should include general orientation for top management and more specific training for managers and first-line supervisors. Managers and supervisors, in turn, should take responsibility for training employees in their areas, and at the same time they will become more familiar with the new system. Training is critical when a system is installed. There has been considerable difficulty with many information systems in the first months of operation because user and operating personnel were not properly oriented and trained in advance.

For information systems procured from software houses, the vendor often will be required to provide some or all of the necessary user and operator training. As described in Chapter 9, the contract with the vendor should specify training responsibilities and costs. Some vendors have self-instructional, computer-based training packages available for use by clients. The health services organization should designate a training director who will plan and coordinate the training program and ensure that vendor responsibilities for training as specified in the software contract are carried out.

A well-designed and well-managed training program can help overcome employee anxiety and potential resistance to change and make the difference between a successful and unsuccessful system implementation.

4. Database preparation. Another task that is sometimes overlooked in implementation planning is database preparation or modification. Some health information systems will require that one or more organizational data files be converted from manual form to electronic storage in the computer. Other systems may require modifications to an existing electronic database prior to operation.

For example, an ambulatory care center installing an automated patient appointment and scheduling system must build a database that includes appointment times available for each physician and treatment facilities available for scheduling. The electronic database must be created prior to conversion to the automated system.

5. System testing. No health information system should be put into operation without complete system testing. This testing should be carefully planned and should cover all aspects of the new system in as realistic an environment as possible. Elements to be tested include system objectives, computer and network hardware, software, training of personnel who operate and use the system, accuracy of cost estimates, and adequacy of system documentation. (See Figure 10.2.)

The testing should be designed to determine whether specific goals and objectives for the information system have been met. Each objective

Figure 10.2   Elements of a System Test

1. System Objectives
2. Computer and Network Hardware
3. Computer Software
4. Personnel Training
5. Accuracy of Cost Estimates
6. Adequacy of System Documentation

should be measured against specific test criteria. The ability of the system to generate correct output data in a timely manner should also be tested.

A major element of the test is checking that data collection and input procedures are functioning properly. Is computer input generated with a minimum of errors? When errors do occur, does the system detect them and permit timely correction? Error and correction procedures are important elements of any information system. Most systems will handle routine transactions without difficulty, but those few exceptions that inevitably do occur often generate confusion and frustration unless good exception procedures are built into the system design. The adequacy of these procedures must be tested thoroughly.

The system test should also be designed to check the sufficiency of personnel training. Are procedures for gathering and reporting data understood and functional? Procedures manuals should be developed *before* the system test begins so that they are available to operating departments during the test period.

The test will check the adequacy of computer software and machine processes involved in the system. Problems are often uncovered when a program is operated under live conditions in conjunction with all the other system elements.

The system test should also aim at estimating as closely as possible the actual operating costs of the new system. If the costs appear to be much higher than the estimates contained in the system specifications, then management should carefully review the entire system and decide whether or not to proceed with full implementation. The system test should mark a critical decision to proceed or not to proceed with the implementation of an information system. Implementation in the face of evidence of significant cost overruns constitutes irresponsible management.

Finally, the system test should test the completeness of system documentation, including procedures manuals, documentation of computer programs, and machine operating manuals. Documentation is the key to good system maintenance, and it should be in order before the new system goes into live production.

Although every test element described above is important, the overriding purpose of a system test is to test the system as a whole. Will the various components function together in an orderly and systematic manner? To answer this question, the test should be as realistic as possible. Actual data from operations should be used if at all feasible. Although not always feasible, a parallel test may be the best way to simulate actual operation of the system. In parallel testing, the new information system operates along with the existing system and cross-checks for accuracy are conducted on a systematic basis. Parallel testing places considerable strain on day-to-day operations since two systems must be operated by the personnel involved. Temporary staffing often is required during this period, and it is recommended that the temporary staff be assigned to the old system so that permanent employees may gain experience using the new system procedures. Parallel testing requires careful advanced planning. Test plans should be approved by the department managers involved as well as central administration.

More than one system test may be required for complex applications. After the first test is completed, the system is modified, and the modified system is then retested. Conversion to full operation of the new system should not occur until all system tests have been completed satisfactorily and no further modifications are required.

6. Final documentation. The final aspect of system implementation is completion of all system documentation. Documentation should be a continuous process carried out during all phases of the system project. Just before production, the project team should do a final check to ensure that system documentation is adequate for effective maintenance of the new system.

System Operation and Maintenance

Information systems require both scheduled and unanticipated maintenance after they become operational. No matter how well a system is designed and regardless of how well it has been tested, there inevitably will be errors uncovered after the system goes into production. Systems analysts and programmers must be available to find such problems quickly and initiate immediate corrections.

In addition, alterations in the system will be required from time to time, since health services organizations are dynamic and subject to frequent changes in operating policies and procedures. These changes flow from a variety of sources: new programs initiated by the board of trustees; changes in the composition of the community served; expansion of facilities to meet increased demand; and ever-changing regulation by external agencies. Information systems must be sufficiently flexible so that these changes can be accommodated, and trained technical staff must be available to initiate them.

Adequate staffing is required if system maintenance is to be carried out properly. Although no general rule exists, it is not unreasonable to expect that approximately 25 percent of total technical staff time will need to be devoted to maintenance activities once several applications are operational. Failure to plan and provide for such staffing can result in many problems later. If staffing levels permit, it is also good practice to assign maintenance responsibilities to personnel not involved in the initial design and implementation of the system. The maintenance analyst or programmer should review all system and program documentation before accepting responsibility for the system, thus helping to ensure that maintenance can be carried out independently of the initial design team. This can be very important in a field where qualified technical personnel are in demand and turnover can occur rapidly.

If system maintenance is to be provided by outside contractors or software suppliers, contracts must be negotiated that guarantee timely response to requests for emergency maintenance and system updates.

In addition to providing quick-response maintenance, designers of health information systems must develop emergency backup procedures to be followed any time operational systems are down for any reason. These backup procedures should be carefully documented, and personnel must be well trained in their use so that they can be employed with a minimum amount of disruption to regular operations. Effective backup procedures are particularly critical for information systems that support direct patient care.

Continuous Quality Improvement

In addition to regular and emergency system maintenance, all operational information systems should be evaluated continuously in order to determine ways in which they can be improved to better serve organizational objectives. Total quality management (TQM) principles are being applied to improve performance and increase productivity within healthcare organizations. These same principles are applicable to the improvement of health information systems.

The guiding principles behind TQM are that all processes (clinical and administrative) can be improved and that the improvement must be continuous. The continuous improvement cycle includes measuring current performance, implementing actions to improve the process, verifying that the actual performance improvements have been realized, putting the new process into operation, and monitoring it continuously over time. (Austin and Boxerman 1995, 197–98)

Information system evaluations should include a formal review of at least the following four elements:

1. Functionality—the degree to which the system meets the organizational objectives for which it was designed (patient care, improved management, better decision making).

2. User Satisfaction—confirmation of the extent to which the system meets or exceeds expectations of personnel from the major user departments.

3. Costs and Benefits—analysis of the extent to which the system performs within cost estimates for it and documentation of benefits achieved.

4. Errors and Exceptions—analysis of system error rates to determine whether they are within tolerance levels as established in the design specifications for the system.

Periodic system reviews should be used as the basis for improvements to be made by maintenance personnel. Information system evaluation and total quality management are major responsibilities of information systems management.

Organizing for Information Management: Role of the Chief Information Officer

Determining the organizational locus for managing information resources in the healthcare organization is a key responsibility of the chief executive officer (CEO) and the governing board. Historically, many healthcare organizations have assigned this responsibility to the chief financial officer (CFO), reflecting the high priority assigned to fulfilling the need for accurate and timely financial information.

However, given the increasing importance assigned to clinical information systems and the use of information in strategic planning, many health services organizations have assigned the responsibility for information management and communications to the chief information officer (CIO).

Reporting directly to the CEO (or chief operating officer in some large organizations), the CIO serves two important functions: (1) assisting the executive team and governing board in using information effectively in support of strategic planning and management; and (2) providing management oversight and coordination of information processing and telecommunications systems throughout the organization.

In larger organizations, the CIO should be a full-time position. In smaller hospitals and clinics, these responsibilities may be assigned to another administrative officer. In either case, the CIO must possess a good understanding of the healthcare environment, be an experienced manager, and have sufficient understanding of information technology to insure that information systems are properly planned and implemented.

Healthcare CIOs have consistently listed the following as the three most important attributes needed for success in their job:

1. Leadership ability
2. Vision/imagination
3. Business acumen

Technical competence is *not* included as a top attribute with most CIOs, emphasizing their strategic role rather than their technical management role. (Morrissey 1996)

Diedling and Welfield state that the CIO should:

- be a leader of information utilization, not a controller of data and technology;
- focus on long-term strategy, not day-to-day operations;
- champion the development and constant monitoring of a strategic information plan, an intricate component of the corporate strategic plan; and
- participate as a full member of the executive team. (Diedling and Welfield 1995, 36)

To fulfill these roles competently, healthcare CIOs are highly educated. Fifty-seven percent of the CIOs responding to a 1996 survey held doctoral or master's degrees; 37 percent held bachelor's degrees. In addition, the scope of their responsibilities is increasing. Forty-six percent of the survey respondents have positions in the corporate office of a multifacility healthcare system. (HIMSS 1996, 43)

Staffing Requirements

The organizational structure for information systems development should be guided by the institution's strategic objectives and information systems plan (see Chapter 7). The size and complexity of tasks to be carried out by a central information systems department in a healthcare organization are affected by a number of factors including: (1) the degree of centralization or distribution of computer systems throughout the organization; (2) the extent to which systems are developed in-house or through use of packaged software; and (3) the extent to which tasks are *outsourced* to contractors.

A typical information systems organizational structure is shown in Figure 10.3. The IS department manager reports to the CIO along with the director of management engineering and the director of telecommunications.

The IS department is generally organized into three divisions. Professional staff in the systems development division are responsible for system design and implementation. The division is organized into three sections: programming, systems analysis, and system maintenance. The operations division includes three sections: network maintenance, data preparation and editing, and computer operations. The software evaluation and user support division is responsible for evaluation of software systems in the health applications area. This division also reviews and approves all hardware and software acquisitions proposed by user departments and provides technical support on software utilization. The user support staff often will operate a "help desk" that users can contact for hardware and software assistance.

An experienced technical manager, reporting to the CIO, should head the IS department. He or she must have up-to-date knowledge of the

Figure 10.3 Information Systems Organization

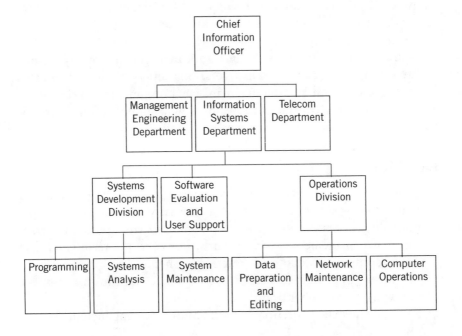

technical aspects of systems analysis, computer programming, hardware and software, networks, and telecommunications systems. The manager must be willing to spend the time and effort necessary to stay up-to-date with the latest technical knowledge in a rapidly changing field. In addition, the manager must be an experienced financial manager and must be skilled in interpersonal relations.

Three levels of personnel must be recruited in staffing an IS department: professional, technical, and clerical.

Professional staff include systems analysts and computer programmers. While it is possible to find talented persons who can fill both roles, care must be exercised in not equating the two. Systems analysis requires broad-based skills that computer programmers often do not possess. It is a highly creative process requiring someone with both technical knowledge of analytical and design techniques and also a broad organizational focus. Since most systems are complex and involve substantial man-machine interaction, the systems analyst must be able to deal effectively with people and must understand the way in which the organization functions in carrying out its mission. Programmers often have a more narrow orientation and are skilled in the technical tasks of software development and maintenance. Programming requirements are changing. As healthcare organizations move toward the implementation of client/server architecture (see Chapter 5), network programmers are replacing those who write and maintain large programs for mainframe computers. Staff retraining may be required for organizations who have employed large numbers of mainframe programmers.

Technician level personnel operate the computer and maintain the communications network. Skilled network managers are highly trained and are often in short supply. The operations supervisor must be both a skilled technician and an effective manager. Equipment maintenance is usually handled by a contract with vendors who supply periodic preventive maintenance and emergency repairs on call.

Outsourcing

Many healthcare organizations are considering outsourcing of some or all information systems functions as an alternative to in-house staffing. Traditionally, the term *outsourcing* has been associated with a contract for facilities management. More recently, however, the term is used in a broader context to denote contracting with the best qualified company to meet a specific information system objective. This may involve *multisourcing* to a number of different vendors.

Some of the major potential benefits of outsourcing include:

1. reduction of in-house staffing requirements;
2. smaller investment in capital equipment;
3. more flexibility in meeting changing requirements and adopting new technology;
4. reduction in the time required to implement new applications; and
5. more predictable cost structure, particularly if fixed-price contracting is employed.

Outsourcing is not without potential danger and risks. Some of these are:

1. too much dependence on vendors, with the possibility that a critical contractor might go bankrupt or change business direction;
2. high costs associated with vendor fees and profit structure; and
3. employment of contractors who do not understand the operation and culture of healthcare organizations.

Hensley (1997) describes some of the principles to follow in outsourcing in a list of "do's and don'ts." He emphasizes the importance of weighing the cultural fit with the vendor, suggests that outsourcing be part of a long-term strategy (not just a quick fix), and recommends good reference checking, in particular looking for staying power among vendors being considered. He states that healthcare organizations should not contract out the things they do best, should not become obsessed with short-term savings, and should not negotiate such favorable terms in a contract that a business partner is put out of business.

An increasing number of companies have entered the healthcare IS outsourcing market. The market exceeded $1 billion in 1994 and is expected to triple by the year 2000. (Morrissey 1995, 60) Twenty-nine percent of all healthcare organizations are outsourcing one or more services in the information technology area. (Hensley 1997, 40)

Executive Management Responsibilities

The basic thesis of this book is a simple one—information systems can be useful to management provided the process for planning, designing, installing, and operating such systems is itself well managed. The CEO and other senior managers of health services organizations must assume the responsibility for planning and controlling the development of effective information systems to serve their organizations. These tasks cannot be delegated to technical personnel if information processes are to be truly supportive of high-quality patient care and managerial decisions. Information is essential in today's competitive environment for strategic planning, cost and productivity management, continuous quality improvement, and program evaluation purposes.

Important executive management responsibilities that have been presented in Chapters 7 to 10 are summarized below.

1. Management must insist on a careful planning process that precedes all major decisions related to the installation of computer equipment or the design of complex information systems. A master plan for IS development should be created and updated at least once a year. This plan should be linked to the strategic plan of the healthcare organization and should guide all specific implementation decisions.

2. Management should employ a user-driven focus throughout the IS development process. Active involvement of personnel from all segments of the healthcare organization is essential. This participation should begin with a definition of information requirements that should always precede acquisition of hardware and software. It should continue through all phases of analysis, design, system evaluation and selection, and implementation.

3. Management must take the responsibility for recruiting competent personnel for the design and operation of information systems. Consideration should be given to recruitment of a CIO to serve as a member of the executive management team. When outsourcing is used, careful selection of vendors and contract negotiations with the assistance of legal counsel should precede the award of contracts for software, equipment, or services.

4. Intercommunication of data among systems is an absolute necessity in complex health services organizations, particularly those involving subsidiary units and central corporate management. Executives at the corporate level must establish policies and procedures to ensure integration of data files or interfacing among individual information systems for tracking patient flows, consolidating cost and financial data, monitoring quality of care, and evaluating individual products and services.

5. Management personnel at all levels have ethical obligations to maintain security of information systems and to protect the confidentiality of patient, personnel, and other sensitive information.

6. The design of individual systems should be carried out by an interdisciplinary project team. Systems analysts and computer programmers will take the lead on technical analysis and design activities. Representatives of departments to be involved in the system should help guide the specification of system requirements and evaluate the technical design plans of the analysts. Management should be involved in all major design projects to ensure congruence with organizational goals and objectives, and should insist on a user-driven system focus rather than a technology-driven focus.

7. Once a project team has been organized, careful systems analysis should precede any implementation decisions. Shortcuts in the systems analysis phase will inevitably lead to problems later on.

8. The preliminary design specifications for an information system should be in harmony with the master plan for IS development discussed in Step 1 above.

9. Detailed system specifications should always be required before any implementation activities take place. These specifications should be reviewed formally and approved by all user departments and by management before proceeding with the next steps in system development.

10. Throughout the analysis, design, and implementation phases of a systems project, management should require careful scheduling of all activities and should receive periodic progress reports as the project proceeds.

11. During the implementation phase, thorough training of all personnel to be involved in the new system should be carried out.

12. No information system should be put into operation without first carrying out a comprehensive system test. The testing should cover all phases of system operation, including computer programs and procedures, personnel training, user satisfaction, ability of the system to meet original objectives, and accuracy of the initial cost estimates.

13. Provision should always be made for adequate maintenance after an information system is operational. Maintenance provisions are essential to correct operational errors, to make system improvements, and to facilitate changes necessitated by changes in organizational needs.

14. Management must ensure that information systems are periodically audited and that all systems are formally evaluated once they are installed and operating normally.

In order to meet these responsibilities, a solid and mutually supportive relationship between the CEO and the CIO is essential. Stephen L. Ummel, President and CEO of Lutheran General Health System, Park Ridge, Illinois, states:

> Virtually all of our major growth in integration strategies is imminently linked to information technology and the leader thereof, namely our CIO. It's very important today that the CIO and the CEO form a new working partnership in order to co-sponsor the necessary investments, both financial and human, into information technology. (Bergman 1994, 36)

Stan Nelson, former CEO of Henry Ford Health System, Rochester Hills, Michigan, confirms the importance of this relationship: " . . . the role of the CIO has increased in importance to where it has become a critical component of the executive team." (Appleby 1997, 34)

Summary

Implementation of an information system includes ordering needed computer and telecommunications equipment, writing computer programs and/or procuring packaged software, orientation and training of management and operating personnel, database preparation, system testing, and final documentation.

System testing should include a complete check of system objectives, output screens and reports, input forms and procedures, error and correction procedures, computer programs and equipment operations, adequacy of system documentation, and accuracy of initial cost estimates. If the tests show that costs are much higher than estimated or that the system is not meeting its objectives, then the organization should not proceed with implementation.

Health information systems require both periodic and unscheduled maintenance after they are operational. Changing requirements in a dynamic healthcare environment will also necessitate system changes from time to time. Maintenance personnel should periodically evaluate the information system and make improvements based upon these evaluations.

Organizational placement of the IS department in a health services organization will be influenced by the priority assigned to various applications; the knowledge, attitudes, and style of the CEO; and the overall organizational structure of the institution. Many organizations have established the position of CIO to assist the executive team in using information for strategic management and for coordinating all information management and communication activities.

Competent technical personnel must be recruited to participate in the analysis, design, and implementation of information systems. A comprehensive IS department will include professional analysts and programmers as well as technicians for operation and maintenance of equipment.

An increasing number of healthcare organizations are turning to outsourcing some or all IS functions as an alternative to in-house staffing. In some cases, organizations are multisourcing different functions to a number of contractors. Potential benefits of outsourcing include reduced staffing requirements and smaller capital investments in hardware and software. Risks of outsourcing include too much dependence on contractors and potential high costs associated with vendor fees and profit structure.

The CEO and other senior managers must assume the responsibility for planning and controlling the development of effective information systems to serve their organizations. This cannot be delegated completely to technical personnel. Management must also ensure that careful planning precedes all decisions on acquisition of software and hardware and that well-established principles and procedures are followed in the analysis, design, and implementation of systems.

Discussion Questions

10.1 Why is careful planning of the implementation phase of an IS project important?

10.2 What kinds of training should be carried out before implementation of an information system in healthcare organizations? Who should be trained? Who should conduct the training?

10.3 What elements should be included in a system test?

10.4 What kinds of activities are involved in IS maintenance? Who should be responsible for operational systems maintenance?

10.5 Why is periodic evaluation and continuous quality improvement of health information systems important?

10.6 What factors should determine where an IS department is located in the overall organizational structure?

10.7 What kinds of skills should a CIO possess?

10.8 Discuss some of the potential benefits and dangers of outsourcing information system activities.

Problems

10.1 Prepare a system test plan for a patient scheduling information system for the outpatient clinics of a university medical center.

10.2 Assume that you are the CIO of a large general hospital. Write a policy statement for your hospital detailing how information systems maintenance will be carried out.

10.3 You are the CEO of a health services corporation consisting of a 500-bed tertiary care hospital, three smaller hospitals located in rural areas within 100 miles of the main facility, a long-term care facility, home health agency, outpatient surgery center, and several smaller units, some operated as joint ventures with other healthcare organizations. You are about to develop an organizational plan for development and management of information systems for the corporation. Prepare an outline of a presentation to your corporate board discussing the proposed organizational study and some of the major issues to be addressed.

10.4 Interview the CIO of a healthcare facility in your area to determine which information systems functions are outsourced and which are handled in-house and the rationale for each. Write a report summarizing the interview.

References

Appleby, C. 1997. "Interface (Or in Your Face)." *Hospitals & Health Networks* (February 5): 30–34.

Austin, C. J., and S. B. Boxerman, S.B. 1995. *Quantitative Analysis for Health Services Administration*. Chicago: AUPHA Press/Health Administration Press.

Bergman, R. 1994. "Health Care in a Wired World." *Hospitals & Health Networks* (August 20): 28–36.

Diedling, L., and J. Welfeld. 1995. "The Rise of the CIO." *Hospitals & Health Networks* (February 5): 34–38.

Healthcare Information and Management Systems Society (HIMSS). 1996. *1996 HIMSS Annual Compensation Survey*. Chicago: The Society.

Hensley, S. 1997. "Outsourcing Moves Into New Territory." *Modern Healthcare* (January 13): 39–43.

Morrissey, J. 1995. "CIOs Use Outsourcing to Revamp Systems." *Modern Healthcare* (July 24): 60–68.

Morrissey, J. 1996. "CIO Pay Averages $110,000 a Year." *Modern Healthcare* (March 4): 122–24.

Additional Readings

Austin, C. J., and R. C. Howe. 1994. "Information Systems Management." In *The AUPHA Manual of Health Services Management*, edited by R. J. Taylor and S. B. Taylor. Gaithersburg, MD: Aspen Publishers.

Brandt, M. D. 1994. "Making the Transition to CIO: Building Your Skills." *Journal of the American Health Information Management Association* 65 (4): 59–61.

Drazen, E., W. Reed, and J. Metzger. 1995. "The CIO of the Integrated Care Delivery System." *Healthcare Informatics.* 11 (6): 18.

Reynolds, G. W. 1995. *Information Systems for Managers*, 3rd Ed. Minneapolis, MN: West Publishing Company.

Sahney, V. K., ed. 1994. "Total Quality Management." Special Issue of *Healthcare Information Management* 8 (4).

PART

IV

Information Systems
Applications in Healthcare

11

PATIENT CARE APPLICATIONS

I N THIS FINAL section of the book, attention is focused on specific computer applications in healthcare delivery. This chapter will discuss *clinical* (or medical) applications, which involve the organized processing, storage, and retrieval of information to support patient care. *Administrative* applications, discussed in Chapter 12, are designed to assist in carrying out financial and administrative support activities such

Concepts and Applications

The ultimate goal of an information system is to provide information and feedback to users. A healthcare information system will provide timely, relevant information on a wide spectrum of clinical functions, including patient diagnosis, treatment planning, and performance measurement.

In addition, information systems allow for automated medical records, computerized order entry and results reporting, and clinical-decision support. Healthcare information systems also allow for remote-location patient care through the use of telemedicine.

After completing this chapter, readers will be able to identify the specific benefits of clinical applications for their organizations, discuss the potential role of clinical decision-support systems, and explain the role of information systems in ambulatory care.

as payroll, patient accounting, materials management, and office automation. *Strategic decision-support* applications, as presented in Chapter 13, provide information and analytical tools to support managerial decision making in health services organizations. *Managed care* applications, explained in Chapter 14, include HMO and PPO administration, marketing, contract management, and risk assessment and forecasting under capitation. The development of *enterprisewide networks and applications* within integrated delivery systems is described in Chapter 15. Finally, Chapter 16 discusses the rapid growth of healthcare applications on the Internet.

Introduction

Development of clinical information systems has become a top priority for healthcare organizations. Clinical systems provide direct support to the patient care process and establish data repositories that are essential for quality improvement and cost control programs.

Clinical information systems support diagnosis, treatment planning, and evaluation of medical outcomes across the continuum of care. They offer the potential for quality improvement and cost control by documenting that medically necessary procedures have been followed and that unnecessary tests and procedures have been avoided.

1. Quality of Care
   a. Treatment patterns for individual patients are planned and compared against regimens for a large number of similar patients in a clinical database.
   b. Risk is reduced through demonstration that medically necessary and historically mandated procedures have been followed.
2. Cost Control
   a. Clinical justification is required for tests and procedures that go beyond the patterns suggested by the clinical database.
   b. Generalized protocols are developed (nursing care, medical treatment, follow-up) that are both clinically effective and cost-efficient.

Recent surveys of healthcare executives confirm the importance that is being placed on development of clinical information systems. Respondents to the 1996 Healthcare Information and Management Systems Society (HIMSS)/Hewlett-Packard Leadership Survey listed the following as the three most important application priorities for their organizations:

1. implement a clinical data repository;
2. implement new clinical systems; and

3. implement an electronic medical record. (HIMSS/HP 1996, 1)

These results were confirmed in the 1997 *Modern Healthcare* survey of healthcare executives in which improved decision support for clinicians and improved patient care applications were listed as top priorities. (Morrissey 1997, 114)

The advent of managed care and development of comprehensive integrated delivery systems that provide care across a continuum of providers makes the development of clinical information systems essential.

> We are in a new age, in a world that focuses on the patient and his or her relationships (e.g., family, employer, insurer, provider) and on the multidisciplinary approaches to care across the continuum. This paradigm emphasizes prevention and care management for members of the community, not in a discrete episodic fashion, but across time truly, across lifetimes. Technology then becomes the enabler, the bond, that links communities together in the rapidly changing world of health care. (HIMSS 1996, 2)

The remainder of this chapter discusses specific patient care systems and their application across the continuum—ambulatory care, acute care, critical care, home care, rehabilitation, and long-term care.

Computer-Based Patient Records

The medical record is central to all patient care activities, serving several important functions. The medical record is a guide to, and continuous record of, treatment for active patients. For patients not currently receiving treatment, it serves as an archival record. Medical records also are working documents for medical audit, utilization review, quality improvement, and cost control. In many health services organizations, particularly teaching hospitals, the depository of medical records acts as a database for research studies.

Consequently, computerization of medical records is central to the development of clinical information systems in healthcare organizations. However, the development of a completely electronic medical record has been an elusive goal. "For 30 years, experts in the medical informatics community have been predicting paperless medical records systems. Although in reality, the movement toward electronic patient record systems progressed little during these past 30 years." (Waegemann 1996, 66)

A 1991 report by the Institute of Medicine (IOM), National Academy of Science, provided major impetus to efforts aimed at the development of electronic medical records. The IOM Committee on Improving the Patient Record called for "the prompt development and implementation of computer-based patient records (CPRs)" on a national basis in order to "improve the care of individual patients and populations and, concurrently, to reduce waste through continuous quality improvement." (Dick and Steen 1991, v) Key attributes of the CPR as defined by the IOM committee include the following:

1. The CPR includes a problem list that clearly delineates the patient's clinical problems and current status of each.
2. It encourages and supports the systematic measurement and recording of the patient's health status and functional levels.
3. It documents the clinical rationale for all diagnoses or conclusions.
4. It links to clinical records from various settings and time periods to provide a longitudinal record of events that have influenced a person's health.

The IOM report called for the development of computerized patient records by all healthcare organizations covering the spectrum from large medical centers to solo-practice physician offices. National standards for content of the CPR are under development by a "follow-on," nonprofit organization, the Computer-Based Patient Record Institute.

Although it is an ambitious goal, many healthcare organizations are moving forward with plans to develop and implement CPR systems. The current status of these efforts can be summarized as follows:

1. Many healthcare organizations have partially automated records that include items such as laboratory results, summaries of radiology procedures, current medications, and diagnostic and treatment summaries.
2. Integrated delivery systems are moving to develop master patient indexes that provide common patient identifiers for all patients in the system and facilitate electronic exchange of information among all providers in the network. (See Chapter 6.)
3. An increasing number of physician offices and group practices are installing practice management systems and ambulatory care records systems.
4. A small number of organizations, often university medical centers, are working on the development of complete electronic medical record systems, including the storage and retrieval of medical images as well as digital information.

Waegemann (1996, 69) discusses the major barriers to complete implementation of electronic patient records. These include: (1) legal issues (many states still have laws prohibiting paperless medical record systems); (2) the need for universal standards on record content and coding; (3) technological limitations (although modern multimedia approaches offer the promise of overcoming most of these limitations in the near future); and (4) the need to convince users of the importance of such systems. Overcoming user resistance, particularly among physicians, requires that systems be very user-friendly and make the caregiver's job easier—not more complicated.

The paragraphs that follow describe the efforts of three healthcare organizations in the development and implementation of computer-based patient record systems for their organizations.

City of Hope Medical Center is a major cancer research and treatment center located in Duarte, California. City of Hope has developed a patient data repository of electronic medical records serving users across its campus of 50 buildings. The first step was installation of a fiber-optic communications network with more than 40 file servers supporting approximately 1,000 users. The Medical Center selected the Oacis Healthcare Network and related clinical applications as the major software for the patient data repository. The repository collects data from ancillary systems using HL7 standard interfaces. After intitial development, the CPR contained clinical lab information, microbiology data, physician transcriptions, and encounter data on inpatient and outpatient visits with radiology and cardiology data soon to be added. (Edlin 1996)

Stuyvesant Polyclinic is an ambulatory care center located in an inner-city area of Manhattan, New York. The clinic, which serves a large number of HIV-positive patients, is affiliated with Cabrini Medical Center. Approximately 20,000 outpatient visits are logged each year. The clinic operates a CPR system linked to two sister clinics and the emergency department at Cabrini. The system provides physicians with a longitudinal record of clinical information including T-cell counts so important in treatment of HIV-positive patients. The result has been improved monitoring of patients' conditions and the ability to better analyze the clinical outcomes of interventions. (Hagland 1996)

Dr. Kim Charles Meyers is a physician in solo practice in Evanston, Illinois. Dr. Meyers installed a CPR system to serve his office staff of three (physician, nurse, and administrative staff member). The system utilizes HealthPoint ACS software operating on pentium processors at the network level and 486 laptops in the exam rooms. In evaluating the system, Dr. Meyers states: "I have greater access to information at the point of care, can provide more thorough care, and can practice medicine more efficiently." (Meyers 1997, 39)

A number of vendors are offering CPR products. The 1997 Annual Market Directory issue of *Health Management Technology* lists 132 companies that provide hardware, software, and/or consulting services related to CPRs. (*Health Management Technology* 1997; Directory Issue 1997)

Order Entry and Results Reporting

Clinical information systems, whether operated in a single healthcare organization (e.g., hospital, ambulatory care center, etc.) or across an integrated network of care, require software for efficient entry of orders for diagnostic tests and patient treatments and subsequent reporting of test results back to caregivers. Order entry and results reporting software systems are designed to meet this need. These systems provide computerized telecommunication of information throughout the various service areas of a health services organization. Physician orders are entered and transmitted to the appropriate clinical service units. Test results and treatment summaries are transmitted back for entry into patient charts, and records of charges for services provided are transmitted electronically to the appropriate business office for processing and entry into the accounting system.

When installing order entry systems, healthcare organizations must decide whether physicians will enter their own orders directly at computer terminals or whether clerical personnel will make the entries by transcribing physician paper notes. User-friendly operation is an essential element in the selection of order entry systems, particularly if physicians are to enter their own orders. Physicians and other caregivers will resist the use of systems that are time-consuming and difficult to understand. Well-planned user orientation and training programs are essential to the success of these systems. Based upon a comprehensive review of the literature, Sittig and Stead (1994, 108) conclude:

> Key ingredients for successful implementation [of physician order entry systems] include: the system must be fast and easy to use, the user interface must behave consistently in all situations, the institution must have broad and committed involvement and direction by clinicians *prior to* implementation, the top leadership of the organization must be committed to the project, and a group of problem solvers and users must meet regularly to work out procedural issues.

Shortliffe (1991, 3) believes that computer workstations will become a standard component of physician practice and will serve as "their windows on the world." He describes a scenario in which physicians have complete access to medical records (outpatient and inpatient) and use their workstations as a communications and practice support tool.

Tierney et al. (1993) describe a randomized controlled clinical trial of the use of microcomputer workstations for writing all inpatient orders in a major university medical center. Cost and time-motion studies were carried out. Results indicated that the use of workstations significantly lowered patient charges and hospital costs. However, the system required more physician time than use of paper charts, and the investigators call for additional research for ways to reduce time required by clinicians to operate these systems.

The 1997 Annual Market Directory issue of *Health Management Technology* lists 97 vendors who provide order entry/results reporting products (*Health Management Technology* 1997).

Clinical Services Applications

Given the complexity of the modern medical environment, many health-care organizations and integrated delivery systems operate separate clinical service information systems, particularly in areas such as pharmacy, clinical laboratory, and radiology. Advances in microcomputer technology and the availability of an extensive array of packaged software have facilitated the development of these decentralized departmental systems. As discussed in Chapters 5 and 7, corporatewide or institutionwide planning is essential when individual departmental systems are being installed in order to assure system integration and the ability to transmit data across organizational units both for medical and administrative purposes. This section presents an overview of some of the clinical service applications in common use in health services organizations.

1. Laboratory Information Systems. Laboratory information systems constitute one of the most common clinical computer applications in health services organizations. There are two phases to clinical laboratory systems: (1) automating the test processes themselves and (2) processing the laboratory data. Automation involves linking laboratory instruments directly to a computer. Signals from the test instruments are first converted to digital form (if not already digitized) for computer processing. For example, chemical autoanalyzers generate analog signals in which slide wire potentiometers are attached to continuous strip chart recorders. The same signals that drive the chart recorders are captured and converted to digital form. The computer then carries out calculations that would be made by the lab technician in a manual system. Computer calculations include determination of peak values and computation of the concentration of the unknown patient sample. The final results are then stored in a patient laboratory data file and test results are printed.

Laboratory data-processing systems can be used independently of, or in conjunction with, laboratory automation systems. A laboratory data-processing system would include recording of test requisitions, scheduling of specimen collection and test processing, recording of the results of completed tests, preparing test reports for immediate return to the nursing units or outpatient department, periodically preparing summary reports of all tests run for a given patient, preparing statistical reports for the laboratory, and record keeping for quality control and administrative control of laboratory operations.

Bar coding (see Chapter 3) is commonly used as an input vehicle for laboratory information systems. Willard and Shanholtzer (1995) describe the application of bar coding in the laboratory information system of the Minneapolis Veterans Administration Medical Center. Bar codes are used to identify individual lab specimens and on internal worksheets to link specimens back to the primary database. In addition, standard "bar-code scripts" are used for entering commonly occurring test results, thereby eliminating the need for keyboard entry of these results.

As integrated delivery systems become larger and more complex, healthcare organizations are increasingly looking for ways to decentralize clinical service functions. Jacobs and Laudin (1995) describe mechanisms for integration of information from satellite laboratories and point-of-care testing systems. The authors point out:

> Decentralized laboratory testing offers many advantages over the central laboratory as a mechanism for delivering rapid and accurate data. . . . However, these data must still be imported into a medical information system for overall coordination of medical care and follow up. (Jacobs and Laudin 1995, S34)

Although automation is most advanced in the clinical chemistry area, information systems are used extensively in other laboratory operations such as blood banks, microbiology, and virology.

Turnkey systems provided by vendors dominate the market for laboratory information systems. The 1997 Annual Market Directory issue of *Health Management Technology* lists ten categories of software products available for use in laboratory automation and information processing. Sixty-eight vendors are listed in the clinical laboratory information systems category alone (*Health Management Technology* 1997).

2. Pharmacy Information Systems. The pharmacy is one of the most informationally complex departments in the health services organization. Good records must be maintained in order to carefully control the ordering, stocking, and distribution of drugs and to avoid medication errors to the maximum extent possible. Accurate records are also important for billing.

The two basic approaches to the design of computer applications in the pharmacy include development of stand-alone pharmacy systems and integration of pharmacy activities with a larger institutional information system. Stand-alone pharmacy systems are available for control of dangerous drugs (particularly narcotics), drug ordering and inventory control, control of drug distribution to patients, storage and retrieval of drug information, the construction of patient drug profiles, the maintenance of the organization's formulary, and generation of charges for patient billing.

Pharmacy systems integrated into an enterprisewide information system will typically involve the entering of medication orders on computer terminals at nursing units and outpatient treatment centers. These orders are then communicated automatically to the pharmacy, where worksheets are generated, patient profiles are updated, and labels are prepared. Such systems often include automatic updating of the drug inventory and automatic generation of patient charges from the medication orders.

Computer systems are used to check prescriptions and monitor medications administered to patients. Current drug orders and prescriptions are checked against patient profiles to insure proper dosage, monitor contraindications, and protect against drug allergies and sensitivities.

The MENTOR clinical pharmacy system developed at Stanford University and the University of Maryland monitors drug therapies of hospitalized patients for possible adverse reactions.

> MENTOR determines the set of events of interest for any particular patient, based on the patient's current drug therapy, laboratory-test results, pending laboratory-test orders, and scheduled surgical procedures. . . . The system generates appropriate advisory messages to physicians and other health care professionals when it detects problems related to drug therapy. (Speedie and McKay 1990, 313)

A 1997 focus group survey of 19 pharmacists indicated that a majority plan to upgrade or replace existing pharmacy software systems. The major factors to be considered in selecting new systems include ease of use, the ability to integrate the pharmacy system with other information systems in the organization, and functions offered by the new software. (Wall 1997)

A wide array of software products is available. The 1997 Annual Market Directory issue of *Health Management Technology* lists products available in seven categories, including general pharmacy systems, archival, drug data services, inpatient, outpatient/retail, packaging/distribution, and pharmacy interface systems (*Health Management Technology* 1997).

3. Radiology Information Systems. Radiology systems fall into two general categories. Radiology data processing systems include recording test requisitions, scheduling procedures, recording and reporting test

results, reporting charges to the business office, and preparing management reports for the department. Medical imaging systems use computer technology for image processing and enhancement.

Image enhancement by computer has become an extremely important component of modern medical technology, particularly in the fields of radiology and nuclear medicine. Major diagnostic advancements have occurred as a result of the development of computerized image enhancement in computed tomography, gamma cameras, ultrasound scanners, digital subtraction angiography, and magnetic resonance imaging.

Computers are used extensively in the field of radiation treatment planning as well. Computerized treatment planning permits the preparation and evaluation of individual patient treatment plans utilizing complex mathematical models in conjunction with image enhancement of the treatment site. Given data about a patient and the location and size of a tumor, the computer determines the exact dosage to be applied at various treatment sites while minimizing the exposure to unaffected regions of the body.

Development of picture-archiving and communication systems (PACS) is an active area of development in clinical computing. PACS involve online storage and rapid retrieval of images transmitted over communications networks to user workstations that can display both digital information and images. Benefits of PACS include faster turnaround of images and reports, elimination of lost films, reliable retrieval of archived films, and reduced storage space requirements. (Drew 1997)

PACS are often used in conjunction with teleradiology communications systems to bring images from remote facilities to a central site for reading and interpretation. Teleradiology also provides the ability for physicians to call up images at workstations in remote locations, including their own homes. Use of teleradiology and medical imaging systems in conjunction with emerging telemedicine programs is discussed later in this chapter.

Beth Israel Health Care System in New York City initiated a major project in 1995 to move toward filmless radiology and state-of-the-art digital imaging throughout its network of care. Executives in the Beth Israel organization believe that teleradiology will play a key role in expansion of its network. "When Beth Israel offers affiliation to a community hospital, one of the incentives is the availability of subspecialty radiology services and the ability to connect immediately to a large, high-quality radiology department." (Stern 1995, 37)

Crabbe, Frank, and Nye (1994) report on the use of radiology information system data as a quality management tool. The system facilitates continual monitoring of work flow in the radiology department in order to improve report turnaround time and improve quality of reporting.

The 1997 Annual Market Directory issue of *Health Management Technology* lists a large number of radiology software systems in 12 different categories. Forty-one vendors of PACS products are included in the Directory. (*Health Management Technology* 1997)

4. Other service department systems. In addition to laboratory and pharmacy systems as described above, software is available for most other clinical departments and service areas of healthcare organizations. Systems are available to support clinical care and departmental management in physical therapy, pulmonary, emergency room, operating rooms, labor and delivery, and critical care units to mention only a few. For references on systems such as these, consult the Additional Readings included at the end of this chapter.

Ambulatory Care Information Systems

Increasingly, healthcare is being delivered outside the hospital in ambulatory care settings. The number of physicians in solo private practice is declining; consolidation of small practices into larger, multispecialty groups is increasing; and mergers of hospitals and clinics into integrated delivery systems has become commonplace. (Douglas 1994) As a result of these trends, increased emphasis is being placed on computer systems that support ambulatory care and assist physicians and dentists in their practices. The availability of powerful and inexpensive microcomputer and office practice software packages has brought this technology within the reach of small medical groups and solo practitioners (see Figure 11.1).

For larger clinics and group practices, typical computer applications include, but are not limited to:

1. patient scheduling and appointment systems;
2. electronic medical records and medical management systems;
3. patient and third-party billing;
4. managed care contract management; and
5. electronic communications with other providers in an integrated delivery system.

A typical practice management system for a solo or small group practice includes such functions as: (1) patient registration and scheduling; (2) billing and accounts receivable; and (3) limited medical records and document maintenance capabilities including transcription and word processing. Most of these systems would not be capable of connecting

Figure 11.1   Physician Office System

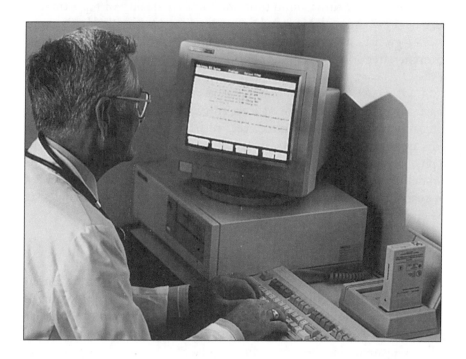

Courtesy of Hewlett-Packard Company.

to regional computer-based patient record systems because the practice systems do not contain complete medical records.

However, office practice computers can be linked to local hospitals in addition to serving the management needs of the practice. Many hospitals or integrated delivery systems have developed computer linkages to physician offices to enable clinicians to preadmit patients, order tests, and inquire into patient files for lab results, nursing notes, and other current clinical information. Healthcare organizations use such linkages as incentives to attract physicians to use their facilities in a highly competitive environment.

Mead, Powell, and Sevilla (1996) describe the development of an automated outpatient scheduling system at the University of Rochester Medical Center in Rochester, New York. The in-house developed system handles scheduling of some 400,000 annual outpatient visits and is linked to the Medical Center's patient registration and billing system, which contains more than 1.6 million patient records. Benefits reported include increased efficiency, reduction in no-shows, and improved patient tracking.

Dr. Steven Ornstein and colleagues at the Medical University of South Carolina in Charleston have implemented a computer-based preventive services system in the Family Practice Clinics of the University. Practice audits revealed that improvements occurred in several areas of preventive medicine including counselling, screening, and immunizations. The authors conclude:

> A CPR-based preventive services system coupled with an adaptable physician education program provides an ideal solution to improving the education about and delivery of preventive services. (Ornstein et al. 1995, 260)

Results from a 1995 survey of 580,000 physicians in the United States (BMI Medical Information 1995) indicated that more than 70 percent were using a computer. However clinical uses were limited and the most common applications included:

Access to clinical databases such as MEDLINE	18%
Maintenance of clinical records	7%
Continuing medical education	6%
Checking for drug interactions	2%

The 1997 Annual Market Directory issue of *Health Management Technology* lists 104 vendors providing ambulatory care/outpatient products and 70 vendors offering practice management systems (*Health Management Technology* 1997).

Nursing Information Systems

Information systems have become an essential component of nursing practice in most health services organizations. Computer systems have been developed to assist in patient care planning, critical care monitoring, and nursing unit management.

Protocol-based nursing care systems are available to assist in the planning and administration of patient care. Uniform standards of nursing care are programmed and stored in the computer's memory. When the nurse enters a specific care initiator code into the system, the computer responds with specific nursing orders and lists of interventions to be considered.

Vrooman (1996) describes the development and use of "care maps" by selected nursing units at Charleston Area Medical Center. The objectives of this pilot project were to improve the level of patient care being provided and reduce cost and length of stay in the process. Critical paths were developed for Medicare patients undergoing mastectomy treatment for breast cancer. The paths were developed jointly by a nursing team and general surgeon. Preliminary results indicated that patients' readiness for discharge improved as a result of use of the computerized care maps.

Financial analysis indicated a 40.7 percent increase in Medicare revenue and a reduction in average length of stay from 3.43 to 2.25 days.

As more and more patients receive care from large integrated delivery systems, continuity of care across the spectrum of providers in the system takes on increasing importance. Patterson et al. (1995) describe a study of nurse communication processes in a large medical center. A survey of 197 registered nurses in perioperative, intensive care, medical/surgical, outpatient, acute psychiatric, and long-term care units was carried out as part of a systems analysis for a nursing information system. The study suggests that "Nurse-to-nurse communication with database support can maintain patient momentum toward self-care, prevent rehospitalization for complications, and avoid risky medication errors." (Patterson et al. 1995, 28)

The development of point-of-care information processing through use of bedside terminals has been an important trend in nursing information systems. Drazen (1990) describes three types of point-of-care systems and software products: (1) dedicated products for general medical/surgical nursing care; (2) dedicated products for ICU or critical care; and (3) integrated hospital information systems that incorporate bedside data entry and retrieval. Bedside systems support entry of orders and care plans, retrieval of test results, and documentation of the nursing care (see Figure 11.2).

Potential advantages for point-of-care-systems include:

1. *Reduction in nursing service costs.* Recording patient data at the bedside can improve nursing efficiency by cutting down travel time to the nursing station and decreasing the amount of time spent recording patient data.

2. *Improved quality of care.* Since nurses are able to record and retrieve data at the bedside, they can spend more time with the patient and less at the nurse's station.

3. *More timely access and improved recording of information.* The patient record is updated at the bedside, and nurses do not tie up the chart when documenting their care. Current patient data can be viewed on the monitor at the bedside where physicians and nurses need it most. Since information is entered immediately as it is received, the patient record is more accurate.

4. *Cost reduction.* Bedside patient information systems can result in fewer lost charges since information is entered immediately on completion of a patient care activity. Length of stay could be reduced because every patient service will be delivered faster and better. The bedside terminal also permits more accurate logging of nursing activity, thereby producing more accurate data on nursing staff productivity and costs related to patient diagnosis.

Figure 11.2 Point-of-Care Terminal

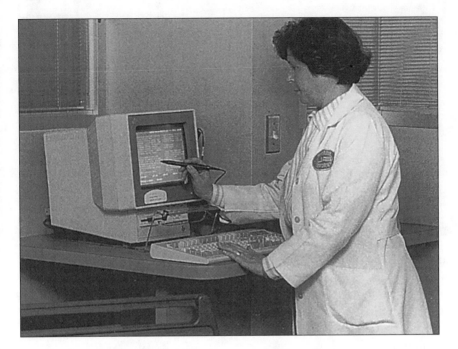

University of Alabama Hospital.

Hendrickson et al. (1995) studied the implementation of computerized bedside nursing information systems in 17 New Jersey hospitals. Four of the major findings of the study included:

1. The most positive comments from nurses related to improved quality and timeliness of documents produced by the system.

2. Staff in several of the hospitals reported that care had improved as a result of computer prompts. Nurses reported that patients believed that care was improved because the nurses spent more time in patient rooms.

3. Results were mixed with regard to the question of whether the computerized systems saved nurse's time; some reporting time savings and others indicating this had not happened.

4. Hospitals with the most timely implementation were those that purchased commercially available stand-alone nursing systems without the need for extensive interfaces to other information systems.

A wide variety of nursing information systems is available in the commercial software market. (See, for example, *Health Management Technology* 1997, 112–13.)

Clinical Decision-Support Systems

Clinical decision-support systems (CDSS) are computer-based information systems designed to assist physicians in diagnosis and treatment planning. CDSS fall into two categories: (1) passive systems that collect, organize, and communicate patient data to the physician (including data on the patient's medical history, physical examinations, and diagnostic tests performed); and (2) active decision-support systems that utilize medical data stored in the computer to suggest diagnoses and treatment protocols.

1. Passive CDSS. Passive systems use the computer to organize clinical data for interpretation and analysis by the physician. They make clinical information more readily available and useable but do not process the information for further analysis. The clinical information systems described earlier in this chapter (computer-based patient records, laboratory, pharmacy, radiology, and other clinical services applications) are examples of passive CDSS in that they capture clinical data and make it available to caregivers. These applications become more useful to clinicians for decision support when they are fully integrated and can provide complete medical information (both current data and historical information on the patient) through simple, user-friendly access from a computer workstation.

2. Active CDSS. Active CDSS employ the computer to provide direct assistance to the physician in diagnosis and treatment planning. They combine patient-specific data with generalized medical knowledge to reach a conclusion or make a recommendation to the caregiver.

Active CDSS generally fall into three categories: expert systems, systems that employ probabilistic algorithms, and reminder/alert systems. (Elson and Connelly 1995)

Expert systems contain three major components. A *general knowledge base* of medical information is obtained from a panel of experts in a given medical specialty. This knowledge base is matched against *patient-specific information* retrieved from the healthcare organization's clinical database. A *rule-based inference engine* generates conclusions for consideration by the physician. The system is dependent on the quality of the expert knowledge base and the "reasoning power" of the rules used by the inference engine.

Probabilistic algorithms use statistical information "on the prevalence of diseases in the domain of interest . . . as well as [information] on the specificity and sensitivity of symptoms and the findings associated with those diseases." (Elson and Connelly 1995, 370–71) These systems differ from expert systems in that they employ statistical probabilities rather than knowledge collected from expert human beings.

Clinical reminders and alerts are incorporated into clinical computer applications to alert the caregiver to potential medical conditions or other problems that should be given attention. Examples include pharmacy systems that alert the physician to potentially negative interactions between two drugs prescribed for the same patient and systems that suggest that certain drugs or treatments should not be employed when specific laboratory results contraindicate their use.

The Health Evaluation through Logical Processing (HELP) system developed at the University of Utah and Latter Day Saints Hospital provides an example of a CDSS that supports physicians in diagnosis and treatment planning. The system integrates general medical knowledge into other computer applications including a medical records system and a clinical laboratory system. HELP includes the following capabilities:

1. It can issues *alerts* to users prompting them to intervene when necessary in caring for patients.
2. It can *critique* new orders for patients.
3. It can offer *suggestions* for new orders and procedures.

The HELP database can also be used for retrospective studies of quality by assessing the medical decisions and treatments provided in the organization. (Haug et al. 1995)

Johnston et al. (1994) reviewed 28 controlled studies of the effects of CDSS on clinician performance and patient outcomes. Fifteen of the studies reported improved clinician performance through the use of CDSS. Three of ten studies that assessed patient outcomes reported significant improvements from the use of CDSS. The authors concluded: "Additional well-designed studies are needed to assess their effects and cost-effectiveness, especially on patient outcomes." (Johnston et al. 1994, 135)

In the future, physicians may be required for legal reasons to use computer-based systems as expert consultants. When CDSS become more widely available, the obligation to use them will become an integral component of the existing standard of care. A physician failing to consult the best available data could be held liable for failing to make an accurate diagnosis.

Expert knowledge bases increasingly will be used to support research into the clinical outcomes of alternative treatment modalities. Dr. Paul Ellwood predicts that outcomes management models will have profound impact on the future practice of medicine:

I expect that health care will be practiced epidemiologically, and that physicians will be absolutely dependent on outcomes data that allow them to determine how the patient fits into some larger cohort of similar patients, particularly in dealing with chronically ill patients. Outcomes data will be used in real time and will rely on artificial intelligence methods that permit the physician to enter various potential diagnostic or treatment strategies and then retrieve projections on how the patient is likely to respond to each. I anticipate a major paradigm shift as a result of the availability of this capability. (Elwood 1990, 17)

Computer-Assisted Medical Instrumentation

Computers have become an important component of many sophisticated pieces of medical equipment being utilized for instrument control, image enhancement, and processing of medical data in conjunction with a broad array of diagnostic and therapeutic protocols (see Figure 11.3).

Computer systems have been interfaced directly with patient-monitoring devices in critical care units of the hospital. Patient-monitoring systems employ the computer for continuous surveillance of a patient's vital signs and periodic display of physiological data for use by trained monitoring personnel. The first step in the process is acquiring data

Figure 11.3 Ventricular Angiography Workstation

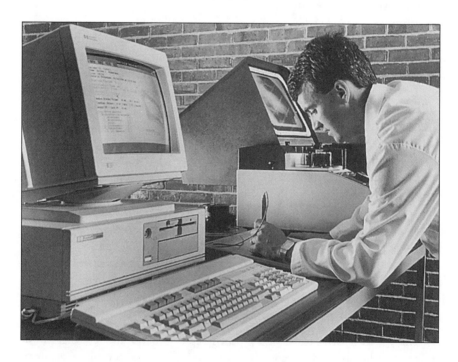

Courtesy of Hewlett-Packard Company.

from monitoring equipment attached to the patient and converting the data for computer processing and display. Data are then stored and made available for periodic display or display on demand. Computer programs enhance the measured data through structured analysis of clinical data in accordance with programmed decision rules. Trend data are also followed to monitor changes in patient vital signs over time. Patient-monitoring systems can operate at the individual patient bedside, at a central station designed to monitor a small number of intensive care beds, or at a remote location linked back to the critical care unit by telecommunication equipment. Many of these systems also have electronic linkages for transmission of clinical data to the centralized computer-based medical record.

Computer systems have also been designed for processing and interpreting data from various diagnostic devices. Much of the work in signal processing has been done in two areas: interpretation of electrocardiograms and analysis of electroencephalograms. Pulmonary function testing also makes extensive use of computerized results analysis with many of the devices containing built-in microprocessors. In addition to the devices mentioned above, virtually every piece of modern medical equipment used for diagnostic testing and treatment now contains a microprocessor that helps control, enhance, and interpret the results of the testing or treatment process.

Other Clinical Applications

1. Telemedicine. Telemedicine is the application of computer and communications technologies to support healthcare provided to patients at remote locations. Telemedicine often involves online communication between a family practice physician, nurse practitioner, or physician's assistant treating patients in a rural area with specialty physicians located at a distant medical center. Audio communications and video conferencing equipment are used in conjunction with online computer access to patient records. The systems often employ teleradiology for transmission of medical images for review by specialty physicians. "Clinically oriented specialties can capture and remotely display physical findings, transmit specialized data from tests such as electrocardiograms and carry out interactive examinations or interviews." (Perednia and Allen 1995, 483)

Telemedicine applications were still largely developmental in early 1997. Reimbursement and legal issues, rather than technological limitations, are the major barriers to more extensive use of telemedicine. Many health insurers will not pay for telemedicine services. As of early 1997, the federal Medicare and Medicaid programs administered by the Health

Care Financing Administration (HCFA) do not cover services delivered through telemedicine. However, HCFA has issued grants to several states to study telemedicine reimbursement issues in conjunction with the Medicaid program, and changes in policies may result from these studies. Licensing issues arise when services are provided across state lines. Can a specialist licensed in one state legally provide services to patients at locations in an adjacent state where he or she is not licensed? Patient confidentiality and data security issues also take on special importance in telemedicine applications.

Nelson, Stewart, and Schlachta (1997) conducted telephone interviews with 25 organizations involved in telemedicine applications. The type of consultations provided included radiology, cardiology, pathology, prenatal, and other medical/surgical specialties. Reimbursement mechanisms varied with several sites operating on grants and contracts and others using their own organizational funds for research purposes. Those interviewed were generally optimistic about the future of telemedicine. The authors concluded:

- Reimbursement will be less of a barrier in the future because of managed care and capitation.
- Use of telemedicine in primary care will enhance the quality of care as patients become more involved with physicians and specialists. (Nelson, Stewart, and Schlachta 1997, 16)

2. Long-Term Care. Requirements for information systems in long-term care are similar to those for other health services organizations. However, the long-term care industry has been slower to implement computer systems than have other components of the delivery system. This situation is changing as more and more care is being delivered in subacute and post-acute care facilities.

Leatham (1996) describes the development of an integrated long-term care information system in a 157-bed skilled nursing facility operated by the Group Health Cooperative of Puget Sound. Systems requirements include census management, resident care documentation and assessment, documentation of physician orders, menu-planning in the dietary department, and pharmacy applications.

As more long-term care facilities become components of larger integrated delivery systems, electronic sharing of clinical and administrative information with hospitals, clinics, ambulatory care facilities, and other system components will be essential. (See Chapter 15 for further discussion of integrated delivery systems.)

3. Home Health Care. Home health services have expanded rapidly in recent years as an alternative to more costly institutional care. A variety of

computer software packages have been developed to support the delivery of home care. (See *Health Management Technology* 1997, 96–97.)

Nurses in many home health agencies are using laptop computers and other remote access devices for on-site documentation of patient care. Calico (1996) describes an automated system for clinical documentation developed by Appalachian Regional Healthcare (ARH) of Lexington, Kentucky. ARH provides care across a large mountainous rural area with long distances between patient homes and ARH facilities. Home health nurses enter information directly at the treatment sites. The system reduces the amount of administrative work needed to document care allowing visiting nurses and home health aides to spend more time with patients.

4. Computer Applications in Clinical Research and Education. Information systems and medical databases are used extensively to support biomedical education and research. Computerized patient records serve as the basis for epidemiological studies of a variety of diseases and their potential linkages to social and environmental factors. In addition, computers are used to support medical, dental, nursing, and allied health education using such techniques as computer-aided instruction (CAI) and patient management simulation.

Computers are an integral component of most medical research projects. Effective project design requires close collaboration among clinicians, biostatisticians, and information systems specialists. Austin and Balas (1994, 28) describe the development of a structured knowledge base of clinical practice research results at the University of Missouri. The knowledge base will be used for a variety of purposes. "Results from a practice analysis can lead physicians to discuss the reasons for individual variations and examine their own practice patterns. . . . Health services researchers can . . . explore areas where quality descriptors require further development. . . ."

Hospitals, medical libraries, and many individual clinicians now utilize microcomputers to access references to the medical literature. The most widely used system is MEDLINE, developed at the National Library of Medicine. Articles from over 3,000 biomedical journals are indexed, stored in computer files, and available for searching and retrieval using standard medical subject headings and key word searches. The Internet is used extensively to retrieve clinical information from a wide variety of specialty databases. (See Chapter 16 for more detail on Internet applications.)

Computers are an important tool for the education of clinicians. Computer-based medical education is designed to involve the student actively in the learning process. Projects range from presentation of information to students at computer terminals to sophisticated simulations of clinical problems. Microcomputer-based simulation programs are used to teach clinical problem solving. Students are presented initial cues and additional information on request as they proceed through a diagnostic process. Final diagnosis, patient management, and follow-up plans selected by the students are entered and the system responds with a comparison to the "ideal" solution and a critique of the process followed.

Summary

Clinical information systems support diagnosis, treatment planning, and evaluation of medical outcomes across the continuum of care. The installation of clinical systems has increased as governing boards and healthcare executives recognize their importance for continuous improvement of patient care quality and for cost-control purposes.

Medical records are central to all patient care activities. However, the development of a completely electronic medical record remains an elusive goal. A 1991 report by the Institute of Medicine recommended the development of a national system of computer-based patient records (CPR). Many healthcare organizations are moving forward with plans to develop and implement CPR systems.

Order entry/results reporting systems provide computerized telecommunications of information throughout the various service areas of a health services organization. User-friendly design of these systems is essential since physicians and other clinicians will resist using them if they are difficult and time-consuming.

Clinical services applications support the various clinical service departments of a healthcare organization or integrated delivery system. Common clinical services applications include laboratory information systems, pharmacy systems, and radiology information systems. Picture-archiving and communication systems (PACS) provide online storage and retrieval of medical images transmitted to user workstations. Information systems also support clinical care and departmental management in areas such as physical therapy, pulmonary medicine, emergency room, operating rooms, labor and delivery, and critical care.

As more and more care is delivered in clinics and outpatient settings, development of ambulatory care information systems has accelerated. Typical functions include: (1) patient scheduling and appointments; (2) electronic medical records and medical management; (3) patient and third-party billing: (4) managed care contract management; and (5) electronic communication with other providers in a network of care.

Nursing information systems support patient care planning, critical care monitoring, and nursing unit management. Use of bedside terminals for nursing information systems has become common. Well-planned bedside systems have been shown to improve patient care quality and efficiency.

Clinical decision-support systems (CDSS) are computer-based systems designed to assist physicians in diagnosis and treatment planning. There are two types of CDSS. Passive CDSS systems organize clinical data for interpretation and analysis by the physician. Active CDSS combine patient-specific information with generalized medical knowledge to reach a conclusion or make a recommendation to the caregiver. The categories of active CDSS are expert systems, systems that employ statistical algorithms, and reminder/alert systems.

Computers have become an integral component of many pieces of medical equipment. They are used for instrument control, image enhancement, and medical data processing. Patient-monitoring systems employ the computer for continuous surveillance of a patient's vital signs and display of physiological data for use by trained monitoring personnel.

Telemedicine is the application of computer and communications technology to support patient care at remote locations. Primary care practitioners and patients in rural areas are linked to specialty physicians at distant medical centers through audio communications, videoconferencing, and online computer access. These systems often employ teleradiology for transmission of medical images.

As more care is delivered outside of the hospital, information systems have been developed to support long-term care and home health services. Long-term care systems support census management, residential care documentation, pharmacy, and other areas of operation in skilled nursing facilities. Home health nurses often use laptop computers or other remote access devices to document care at the location where it is provided.

Information systems are used extensively to support biomedical education and research. Automated databases of patient records support epidemiological studies of disease linkage to social and environmental factors. Computer-assisted instruction and patient management simulation programs support the education of physicians, dentists, nurses, and other allied health personnel. National databases of bibliographic information and other clinical knowledge can be accessed through personal computers located in hospitals, medical center libraries, and individual physician offices.

Discussion Questions

11.1 What are some of the potential benefits of the computer-based patient record (CPR)?

11.2 In your opinion, when will the fully electronic medical record be a reality? What are some the problems that must be overcome for this milestone to be reached?

11.3 Why is involvement of physicians important to successful implementation of clinical information systems? What are some ways to achieve this involvement?

11.4 What are clinical decision-support systems (CDSS)? What is the difference between a passive and an active CDSS? Discuss some specific applications.

11.5 What kinds of information systems have been developed in the clinical laboratory? Describe typical applications.

11.6 Discuss the application of computers in a hospital pharmacy.

11.7 Give examples of information systems being used in: (1) ambulatory care; (2) long-term care; and (3) home health care.

11.8 Discuss the application of computers and information systems to biomedical education and research.

11.9 What is telemedicine? How is it being used? What are some of the barriers to more extensive application of telemedicine?

Problems

11.1 Interview the chief information officer and medical director of a hospital or medical center in your area. Determine plans (if any) for development of a computer-based patient record (CPR) system for this organization. Write a report of your findings.

11.2 Conduct an Internet search and find software vendors who offer products in one or more of the categories listed below. Identify five vendors for each category and prepare a report for each.

1. Laboratory information systems.
2. Order entry systems.
3. Pharmacy systems.
4. Radiology information systems.
5. Ambulatory care information systems.
6. Home healthcare information systems.

In your report, include the name and address of each vendor, the number of years in business, the size of the vendor's business (e.g., total revenue, number of employees, etc.), and a profile of the software product(s) offered.

References

Austin, S. M., and E. A. Balas. 1994. "Advanced Information Support: Abstracting Evidence from Clinical Practice Research." *MGM Journal* (July–August): 24–28.

BMI Medical Information. 1995. *BMI Medec Physicians' Survey*. Arlington Heights, IL: BMI Medical Information.

Calico, F. 1996. "Home Health Moving Toward 'High Touch, High Tech'." *Health Management Technology* (October): 22–25.

Crabbe, J. P., C. L. Frank, and W. W. Nye. 1994. "Improving Report Turnaround Time: An Integrated Method Using Data from a Radiology Information System." *American Journal of Roetgenology* 163 (6): 1503–7.

Dick, R. S., and E. B. Steen, eds. 1991. *The Computer-Based Patient Record*. Washington, DC: National Academy Press.

Douglas, J. T. 1994. "Group Practice Computing: The Road to Managing Information." *MGM Journal* (July–August): 15–18, 42.

Drazen, E. 1990. "Bedside Computer System Overview." In *Bringing Computers to the Hospital Bedside*, edited by P. F. Abrami and J. E. Johnson. New York: Springer Publishing Company.

Drew, P. G. 1997. "Justifying PACS." *Health Management Technology*. (February): 84–88.

Edlin, M. 1996. "HOPENET Puts Center on Path for Year 2000." *Health Management Technology* (October): 13–16.

Elson, R. B., and D. P. Connelly. 1995. "Computerized Decision Support Systems in Primary Care." *Primary Care* 22 (2): 365–84.

Elwood, P. M. 1990. As quoted in "The Outcomes Management Model" by K. Kyes. *Decisions in Imaging Economics* 3 (Winter): 17.

Hagland, M. 1996. "Making Patient Records Meaningful to Patients." *Health Management Technology* (November): 16–20.

Haug, P. J., R. M. Gardner, K. E. Tate, R. S. Evans, T. D. East, G. Kuperman, T. A. Pryor, S. M. Huff, and H. R. Warner. 1995. "Decision SupportSystems in Medicine: Examples from the HELP System." *Computers and Biomedical Research* 27 (5): 396–418.

Healthcare Information and Management Systems Society (HIMSS). 1996. *Guide to Effective Health Care Clinical Systems*. Chicago: The Society.

Healthcare Information and Management Systems Society (HIMSS) and Hewlett-Packard Company. 1996. *Trends in Health Care Computing: Seventh Annual HIMSS/HP Leadership Survey*. Chicago, IL: The Society.

Health Management Technology. 1997. Annual Market Directory. Atlanta, GA: Argus, Inc.

Hendrickson, G., C. T. Kovner, J. R. Knickman, and S. A. Finkler. 1995. "Implementation of a Variety of Computerized Bedside Nursing Information Systems in 17 New Jersey Hospitals." *Computers in Nursing* 13 (3): 96–102.

Jacobs, E., and A. G. Laudin. 1995. "The Satellite Laboratory and Point-of-Care Testing." *American Journal of Clinical Pathology* 104 (4) Supplement 1: S33–S39.

Johnston, M. E., K. B. Langton, R. B. Haynes, and A. Mathieu. 1994. "Effects of Computer-based Clinical Decision Support Systems on Clinician Performance and Patient Outcome: A Critical Appraisal of Research." *Annals of Internal Medicine* 120 (2): 135–42.

Leatham, P. 1996. "Information Systems for Long Term Care." *HIMSS News*, 7 (10): 10–13.

Mead, A., D. J. Powell, and C. Sevilla. 1996. "Automated Outpatient Scheduling: A Step Toward the Integrated Delivery System." *Journal of the Healthcare Information and Management Systems Society* 10 (3): 11–21.

Meyers, K. C. 1997. "What Works." *Health Management Technology* (March): 39.

Morrissey, J. 1997. "Back to Basics, Survey: Execs. Refocusing on Technology Nuts and Bolts." *Modern Healthcare* (February 17): 112–26.

Nelson, R., P. L. Stewart, and L. M. Schlachta. 1997. "Outcomes of Telemedicine Services: Patient and Medicolegal Issues." *HIMSS News* (February): 14–16.

Ornstein, S. M., D. R. Garr, R. G. Jenkins, C. Musham, G. Harnadeh, and C. Lancaster. 1995. "Implementation and Evaluation of a Computer-based Preventive Services System." *Family Medicine* 27 (4): 260–66.

Patterson, P.K., R. Blehm, J. Foster, K. Fuglee, and J. Moore. 1995. "Nurse Information Needs for Efficient Care Continuity Across Patient Units." *Journal of Oregon Nurses Association* 25 (10): 28–36.

Perednia, D. A., and A. Allen. 1995. "Telemedicine Technology and Clinical Applications." *Journal of the American Medical Association* 2 (8): 483.

Shortliffe, E. H. 1991. "The Networked Physician: Practitioner of the Future." In *Healthcare Information Management Systems*, edited by M. J. Ball, J. V. Douglas, R. I. O'Desky, and J. W. Albright. New York: Springer-Verlag, Inc.

Sittig, D. F., and W. W. Stead. 1994. "Computer-based Physician Order Entry: The State of the Art." *Journal of the American Medical Informatics Association* 1 (2): 108–23.

Speedie, S. M., and A. B. McKay. 1990. "Pharmacy Systems." In *Medical Informatics: Computer Applications in Health Care*, edited by E. H. Shortliffe, et al. Reading: MA: Addison-Wesley Publishing Company, Inc.

Stern, S. M. 1995. "On the PACS Path." *Imaging Economics* (November–December): 37–38, 78–79.

Tierney, W. M., M. E. Miller, J. M. Overhage, and C. J. McDonald. 1993. "Physician Inpatient Order Writing on Microcomputer Workstations." *Journal of the American Medical Association* 269 (3): 379–83.

Vrooman, W. P. 1996. "Care Mapping: Measuring Clinical and Financial Outcomes." *Journal of the Healthcare Information and Management Systems Society* 10 (1): 31–36.

Waegemann, C. P. 1996. "When Will Complete Medical Record Systems Exist?" *Health Management Technology* (March): 66–69.

Wall, T. 1997. "Pharmacists Aren't Impressed with Old Systems; Majority Surveyed Plan Upgrades, Replacements." *Health Management Technology* (January): 36–38.

Willard, K. E., and C. J. Shanholtzer. 1995. "Innovative Applications of Bar Coding in a Clinical Microbiology Laboratory." *Archives of Pathology and Laboratory Medicine* 119: 706–12.

Additional Readings

Cannavo, M. J. 1996. "PACS Prices, Performance Showing Improvement." *Health Management Technology* (February): 22–24, 44.

Edelson, J. T. 1995. "Physician Use of Information Technology in Ambulatory Medicine: An Overview." *Journal of Ambulatory Care Management* 18 (3): 9–19.

Evans, R. S., and S. L. Pestotnik. 1994. "Applications of Medical Informatics in Antibiotic Therapy." *Advances in Experimental Medicine and Biology* 349: 87–96.

Fawcett, J., and E. L. Buhle. 1995. "Using the Internet for Data Collection." *Computers in Nursing* 13 (6): 273–79.

Fitzpatrick, K. 1994. "Computer-Enhanced Medical Decision Making." *Physician Assistant* 18 (10): 67, 70–72, 74–75.

Frank, M. S., and J. A. Johnson. 1994. "Computerized Tracking of Mammography

Patients: Value of a Radiology Information System Integrated with a Personal-Computer Data Base." *American Journal of Roetgenology* 163 (3): 705–8.

Friedman, B. A., and W. Mitchell. 1993. "Integrating Information from Decentralized Laboratory Testing Sites." *American Journal of Clinical Pathology* 99 (5): 637–42.

Gianni, R. N., E. Beasley, and D. Linson. 1996. "Online Documentation: Making It Work with POC Technology." *Health Management Technology* April: 46–50.

Gustafson, D. H. 1996. "Incentives to Promote Quality Improvement in Long-Term Care." *Quality Management in Health Care* 4 (3): 1–14.

Hagland, M. 1997. "Outpatient Clinics without the Paperwork." *Health Management Technology* (May): 14–19.

Hogg, W. E., and H. Crouch. 1993. "Incorporating the Family into a Computerized Office Registration System." *Family Medicine* 25 (2): 131–34.

Lazarus, S. S., ed. 1996. "Plugging In: Integrating Group Practice into Health Care Information Systems." *Journal of the Healthcare Information and Management Systems Society* 10 (3).

Markin, R. S. 1992. "Laboratory Automation Systems." *American Journal of Clinical Pathology* 98 (4) Supplement: S3–S10.

McMahon, L. F., A. M. Eward, A. M. Bernard, R. A. Hayward, J. E. Billi, J. S. Rosevear, and D. Southwell. 1994. "The Integrated Inpatient Management Model's Clinical Management Information System." *Hospital & Health Services Administration* 39 (1): 81–92.

Morrissey, J. 1997. "Telemedicine: A Fuzzy Picture." *Modern Healthcare* (April 7): 118–20.

Ornstein, S., and A. Bearden. 1994. "Patient Perspectives on Computer-Based Medical Records." *Journal of Family Practice* 38 (6): 606–10.

Pulliam, L., J. Valentine, J. Raymond, and D. Racine. 1992. "Implementation of a Computerized Information System in a Long-Term Care Facility." *Computers in Nursing* 10 (5): 201–7.

Reed, W. C., ed. 1996. "Integrating Home Health Care into Health Care Delivery." *Journal of the Healthcare Information and Management Systems Society* 10 (2).

Remmlinger, E., S. Ault, and L. Hanrahan. 1995. "Information Technology Implications of Case Management." *Journal of the Healthcare Information and Management Systems Society* 9 (1): 21–27.

Shabot, M. M. 1996. "Achieving Measurable CQI Results." *Journal of the Healthcare Information and Management Systems Society* 10 (1): 61–65.

Siwicki, B. 1996. "Artificial Intelligence." *Health Data Management* April: 47–53.

Tello, R., J. E. Potter, and T. C. Hill. 1994. "The Use of Personal Computers in Nuclear Medicine." *Seminars in Nuclear Medicine* 24 (1): 75–81.

Tierney, W. M., J. M. Overhage, C. J. McDonald, and F. D. Wolinsky. 1994. "Medical Students' and Housestaff's Opinions of Computerized Order-writing." *Academic Medicine* 69 (5): 386–89.

Warshawsky, S. S., J. S. Pliskin, J. Urkin, N. Cohen, A. Sharon, M. Binztok, and C. Z. Margolis. 1994. "Physician Use of a Computerized Medical Record System During the Patient Encounter: A Descriptive Study." *Computer Methods and Programs in Biomedicine* 43: 269–73.

Wynekoop, J. L., and J. A. Finan. 1994. "A Survey of Office Computing in Medical Practices." *M.D. Computing* 11 (2): 107–13.

ADMINISTRATIVE APPLICATIONS

Brian T. Malec

MOST HEALTH services organizations first use computer systems to support their administrative operations. This chapter discusses ways organizations can use these systems in their day-to-day operations. The application of computers and organized information systems for decision-support and strategic management is discussed in Chapter 13.

Concepts and Applications

Information systems are used to support administrative operations in healthcare organizations. Whether designed in-house or purchased from an outside vendor, an information system can assist in an organization's business decisions with data on finances, staff, materiel, and facilities management. An organization can also enhance its internal communications through the use of groupware and Intranet applications.

On completion of this chapter, the reader will be able to explain how an information system can provide information to better administer a healthcare organization, as well as list specific areas in the institution that can benefit from the system.

Introduction

In the past, healthcare organizations had three options for developing and installing administrative information systems: (1) design and program the software in-house; (2) participate in shared service arrangements; or (3) purchase predesigned or packaged software. Many larger hospitals and health services organizations installed medium- to large-scale general purpose computers, using them first for administrative systems. With the rapid advancement of mini- and microcomputer technology, many organizations, particularly smaller ones, have installed dedicated systems in the business office as a part of a distributed systems approach. (See Chapter 7.) These turnkey systems generally come with preprogrammed application packages for inpatient and outpatient accounting, accounts receivable, payroll accounting, general ledger and cost accounting, and accounts payable processing. Packaged software is available for human resources management, materials management, and other administrative operations. A few hospitals and nursing homes still participate in shared service arrangements offered by commercial vendors, organizational consortia, or nonprofit associations. Multihospital systems and managed care organizations may provide central computer services to their affiliates on a shared service basis.

The advent in the 1980s of prospective payment systems for Medicare reimbursement resulted in the need for highly sophisticated administrative and financial information systems. As a result, many healthcare organizations increasingly turned to software vendors for purchased systems. Administrative demands of the managed care environment of the 1990s have led healthcare organizations to purchase software solutions rather than develop them in-house. The "1997 Resource Guide" published by *Healthcare Informatics* lists hundreds of software vendors that provide a wide range of products for the healthcare industry. Table 12.1 lists selected administrative applications and the number of vendors who provide software in these areas.

Historically, the healthcare industry has lagged behind other industries in developing effective administrative information systems that support "business aims and shifting operations." (Ummel 1997, 12) The problems have resulted from a lack of sophistication in systems analysis, undercapitalization of the system development process, and management's failure to define information requirements adequately and oversee the implementation process. The situation has changed substantially in recent years, however. Heightened competition, increased regulation, and new payment mechanisms have caused healthcare managers to rely heavily on their computer systems to provide information essential to effective competition and, ultimately, survival.

Table 12.1 Estimated Number of Administrative Operations Software Vendors as of December 1996

Administrative Applications	Estimated Number of Vendors as of Dec. 1996
Financial-Related Subsystems	
Financial Systems	76
Financial Decision Support	115
Accounts Payable	99
Accounts Receivable	147
General Ledger	80
Admission/Discharge/Transfer	87
Human Resources (Personnel) Systems	48
Recruiting	21
Time/Attendance	44
Personnel Systems	19
Materials Management	57
Managed Care Related—General	83
Risk Management	93
Contract Management	100
Eligibility	93
Enrollment	82
Master Patient Index	119
Physician Practice Management	105
Scheduling Applications—General	37
Patient Scheduling	131
Resource/Facilities Scheduling	107
Staff Scheduling	93
Internet/Intranet-Related Applications	112

Source: "1997 Resource Guide," *Healthcare Informatics*, December 1996

The remainder of this chapter discusses specific administrative applications categorized as follows:

1. financial information systems;
2. human resources (personnel) information systems;
3. facility utilization and scheduling systems;
4. materials management systems;
5. facilities management systems; and
6. office automation, groupware, and Intranet systems.

Financial Information Systems

With increased competition and more governmental regulation, health services organizations must have timely and accurate financial information to monitor and guide operational performance. In the face of demands for accountability and cost containment (while still providing high-quality services), administrators are acutely aware of the importance of sound financial management in guiding operational performance. The purposes of a financial management program include: (1) providing management with quantitative data for making least-cost investment decisions; (2) developing operational financial subsystems that are effective and efficient; (3) providing management information for controlling and evaluating operations; (4) analyzing historical and current financial activity; and (5) projecting future financial needs. (Stair 1996, 313, and Berman, Weeks, and Kukla 1994, 5)

Financial information systems require input from transaction-processing systems (TPS), external sources, and strategic organizational plans. (See Figure 12.1.) Transaction-processing systems record the organization's routine activities, collecting information from other administrative subsystems including payroll, accounts payable, accounts receivable, general ledger, and inventory control. These transactions are the basis for many financial reports required by management. To support effective financial decisions, financial systems also need external information such as government statistics, inflation rates, and information about the marketplace. An organization's strategic plan should contain financial goals and objectives that help provide the framework for preparation of financial reports.

In summary, a fully integrated financial information system will bring related information together for planning, monitoring, and control. Individual financial subsystems include:

- payroll preparation and accounting, linked to a personnel data system;
- processing of accounts payable, linked to purchasing and inventory control systems;
- patient accounting, patient and third-party billing, and accounts receivable processing;
- cost accounting and cost allocation of nonrevenue-generating activities and general overhead expense;
- general ledger accounting;
- budgeting and budget control;
- internal and external auditing;
- financial forecasting;
- financial statement preparation; and
- financial reporting for operating supervisors, executive management, board members, external regulators, and third-party financing agencies.

Figure 12.1   Financial Information System

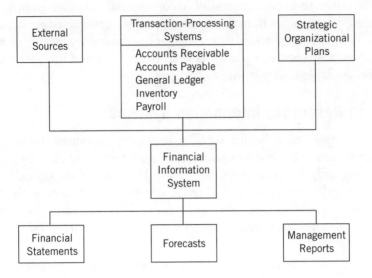

The development of a financial information system depends on the existence of a good accounting system. Sophisticated cost accounting is essential in today's environment. Berman, Weeks, and Kukla (1994, 10) define accounting as "the art of collecting, summarizing, analyzing, reporting, and interpreting, in monetary terms, information about the enterprise." An effective cost-accounting system enables the financial information system to generate accurate information on resources used to deliver services. In a managed care environment, both providers and managed care organizations (MCOs) need cost-accounting information to help negotiate capitation rates, monitor existing contracts, and evaluate the economic impact of managed care capitated contracts. (Toso and Farmer 1994, 1–12) Integrated financial reporting based upon a solid cost-accounting system provides information for product costing, analysis of labor productivity, inventory control, and examination of the productivity of capital.

Increasingly, payment for healthcare is based either on a fixed payment per case (such as diagnosis-related groups) or on a fixed payment per person per month (capitation payment systems). For effective management in this environment, a financial information system must have the capability to convert, or link, cost and net revenue information among multiple units of payment.

Dassenko (1997, 36) describes the implementation of a new integrated financial application that became necessary when the University of Wisconsin Hospitals and Clinics were separated legally from the State of Wisconsin and the University. A commercial software package was installed that includes human resources, payroll, general ledger, accounts payable, purchasing, materials management, and fixed-asset accounting. The system is reported to have reduced paperwork and improved information available to department managers.

Human Resources Information Systems

The employees of a health services organization constitute its most important resource. Most organizations spend 60 to 70 percent of their operating budgets on employee salaries and benefits. Thus a good human resources information system (HRIS) is very important to assist management in workforce planning and productivity analysis. The growing number of important functions that a human resources information system can perform, include:

- maintaining, updating, and retrieving information from the employee permanent record file;
- providing automatic position control linked to the budget;
- producing labor analysis reports for each cost center;
- producing reports for analyzing personnel problems, such as turnover and absenteeism;
- maintaining an inventory of special skills and certifications of employees;
- producing labor cost allocations with linkage to the payroll system;
- providing information on employee productivity and quality control (assuming that appropriate labor standards have been developed);
- providing an analysis of compensation and benefit packages compared to outside industry norms; producing salary surveys and benefit reports;
- helping management in labor relations negotiations and enforcement of labor contracts;
- providing access to training, skill development, and continuing education;
- providing assessment of staff needs and strategic HR planning;
- producing job applicant reviews and profiles; and
- providing scheduling and assignment reports to management.

An automated database of employee information used in conjunction with a human resources information system might include the following elements:

1. personal information such as name, address, Social Security number, birth date, marital status;

2. position information such as job title, department, employment date, date of last promotion, salary history;
3. benefits information such as medical insurance coverage, life and disability insurance coverage, pension plan data; and
4. miscellaneous information such as special skills, performance awards, disciplinary actions, physical limitations. (Austin, Johnson, and Palestrant 1994, 170)

The availability of computerized employee record files creates a security issue. Since protecting the employee's right to privacy is essential, organizations need to establish both software and hardware security systems and set policies for access, updating, and review of electronic personnel files. (See Chapter 7 for a discussion of data security policies.)

In addition to supporting operational work in the Human Resources Department, a well-designed HRIS will produce reports for management planning and control. (See Figure 12.2.) For example, HRIS management reports can be used to monitor:

1. turnover rates;
2. unfilled position vacancies;
3. attitudes of employees and physicians determined through satisfaction surveys;
4. proportion of position vacancies filled internally;
5. utilization of benefits and claims experience;
6. deficiencies identified in employee performance appraisals;
7. labor costs; and
8. employee productivity.

Human resources information systems support the analysis of workload data and help predict staffing needs. Staffing of the nursing service

Figure 12.2 Human Resources Information System

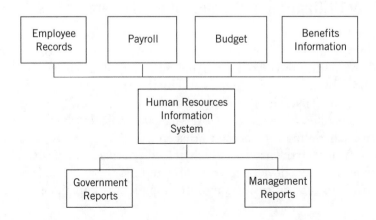

department, for example, is often one of the most difficult challenges in the recruitment and assignment of personnel. Patient care needs must be balanced with the availability and desires of nurses for individual work schedules. Nurse staffing and scheduling systems have ranged from simple manual systems listing rosters of staff members available for particular periods of time, to more complex decision-support systems assigning specific nurses to units for each shift.

Some larger hospitals and multiinstitutional health services organizations have developed automated databases to support recruitment of physicians. St. John's Regional Medical Center in Joplin, Missouri, implemented a physician recruiting database and software system. The system is used to identify staff needs, plan searches, and coordinate site visits of candidates for appointment to the medical staff. (Fanning 1992)

Computer systems are also available to maintain current records of physician credentials and practice privileges in the organization. These systems are very important for monitoring quality standards and for maintaining documentation required by accreditation surveyors.

Some healthcare organizations use HR software to review employee applications and resumes and match applicants' qualifications, experience, and education with current job openings. In the past, these reports would be performed manually, but today, HRIS software can perform the same task more efficiently. With computer-assisted job matching, an individual applies to an organization, rather then applying for a particular job, and the organization's HRIS matches the applicant with the best job opportunity.

A number of HRIS software packages are available. The "1997 Resource Guide" (see Table 12.1) lists 48 vendors that provide full human resources systems, 44 that provide time and attendance systems, and 21 that provide staff recruiting software.

Facility Utilization and Scheduling Systems

The need to contain costs in an era of rapid inflation and diminishing resources is an important reason for every health services organization to utilize facilities and resources to their fullest. Utilization review is mandated both by regulatory agencies and by insurance companies that provide payment for services rendered. Administrators are also charged with the responsibility of ensuring that services are available when needed, and effective scheduling is essential to this end.

In response to the need for efficient facility utilization, health services organizations have developed computerized monitoring and scheduling systems. Information systems monitor inpatient occupancy rates, clinic and emergency room activity, and utilization of individual service facilities, such as the operating suite. Patient scheduling systems are used for advance booking and scheduling of facilities, both for patient and physician convenience and for efficient allocation of resources, particularly staffing.

Advance bed booking and preadmissions systems are particularly useful in situations where most of the admissions are elective (e.g., a specialized surgical facility). Advance booking also provides time for necessary preadmission certification for Medicare patients and others covered by private insurance, which may require review and certification of the medical need for the admission. Preadmission information systems can be linked to individual physicians' offices as well. Computer programs can project the average length-of-stay for each elective admission once historical data (including diagnosis, surgical procedure, age, and sex of patient) have been accumulated. After admissions are scheduled and the data entered into the computer's master files, the system keeps track of projected occupancy levels for each day.

Admissions monitoring and scheduling improves staffing and work flow in healthcare organizations. It can reduce daily fluctuations in a hospital's census and improve employment of flexible staffing systems. If they are to survive, acute general hospitals must maintain an accurate accounting of bed census and occupancy. Census data helps compare projected income against projected budgets. Administrators can also track demands for specific services and adjust staffing and facilities as demand patterns change.

Reimbursement for hospital care increasingly is based on fixed payment (diagnosis-related or capitation). Consequently, software packages have been designed that schedule inpatient services automatically. These systems provide information and schedules specifying " . . . where and when a patient will be during his or her day in the hospital, such as when a patient is due in radiology for a scan, needs to undergo blood tests or must go to physical therapy." (Appleby 1991, 27) These systems require centralized scheduling rather than scheduling by individual departments. Benefits of centralized service scheduling include reduction in length-of-stay and resultant cost savings, particularly important considerations under fixed reimbursement systems.

Computer programs are also available for scheduling operating rooms in hospitals and ambulatory surgery centers. These systems are designed to improve operating room utilization, contain costs, facilitate planning, and aid in the scheduling of specific surgical procedures.

Outpatient clinic appointment and scheduling systems are common in organizations with a large volume of outpatient activity. (White 1996)

Scheduling systems must maintain continuous records of appointments made and appointment times available. They accumulate data on no-show rates, displaying variations by clinic, type of patient, time of day, and day of week. Such data are important for staff scheduling. Scheduling systems also provide automatic planning data, including lists of patients scheduled on the next day, for use in pulling clinic medical records.

Rapid growth in the formation of integrated delivery systems makes the development of enterprisewide scheduling systems important. These systems are designed to coordinate patient scheduling among providers in the network and be more responsive to user needs.

A large number of scheduling software packages are available to healthcare organizations. Table 12.1 indicates that in 1996, 131 vendors offered patient scheduling systems, 107 provided resource/facilities scheduling systems, and 93 offered staff scheduling systems.

Materials Management Systems

Computers assist health services organizations in more effective management of supplies and materials. These systems include computerized purchasing, electronic data interchange with suppliers, inventory control, use of bar-code devices for encoding supplies and materials, and computerized menu planning and food service management.

In a typical materials management system, requisitions for supplies and materials are entered into the computer and matched against budgetary authorization for financial control. Overdrafts on supply accounts are flagged and sent to the appropriate supervisor for follow-up action. Once requisitions are cleared, the computer generates purchase orders. As materials are received, receipt notices are entered into the computer and matched against an open order file. Many automated purchasing systems also include direct linkage to the accounts payable system if system integration has been planned. Some systems also provide the capability for automatic reordering of selected items. (See Figure 12.3.)

Purchase orders can be transmitted electronically to suppliers. Modern systems offered by many vendors allow healthcare organizations to obtain materials on a "just in time" basis, thus reducing the need to carry a large inventory. The savings that result can be significant.

In an era of managed care, the control of costs is essential. Many current software and hardware improvements focus on reducing costs of materials and supplies. Tim Darnell presents several examples of healthcare organizations that have used materials management strategies to reduce costs. (Darnell 1996, 15–19)

Figure 12.3 Materials Management System

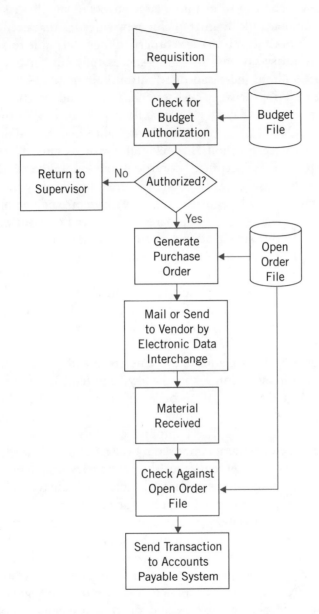

Peninsula Regional Medical Center in Salisbury, Maryland, has implemented a "point-of-use" strategy. Nurses on the floor can log onto the system to order supplies. The order automatically updates the medical record and adds a charge to the patient's account. (Darnell 1996, 16)

St. John's Health System in Springfield, Missouri, moved away from using off-site warehouses to maintain large stocks of supplies issued to departments on demand. By introducing new software that used hand-held data collectors and automatic reordering, they were able to achieve substantial inventory savings. St. John's successfully cut "inventory by a total of $15 million; increased distribution volume by $4.8 million; shortened its ordering/delivery cycle by 95 percent; and injected almost $4 million into the health center's capital flow." (Darnell 1996, 16)

The Summit Medical Center of Oakland, California, created through the merger of two organizations, had $2 million worth of inventory scattered in two facilities, department storerooms, and more then 60 locker locations. Not surprisingly, this resulted in great inefficiency including lack of control over both regular and nonstock items and the practice of reordering supplies "based upon perceived, instead of actual, need." (Darnell 1996, 19) By using handheld inventory control and ordering devices, and purchasing a materials management system (integrated with the admission/discharge/transfer and the financial system), Summit gained substantial savings. Inventory levels in its central storeroom fell from $450,000 to $208,000 in just four years. Inpatient surgery materials stored on-hand decreased from an average of $1,080,000 to $360,000 over the same four-year period. (Darnell 1996, 19)

Computerized menu planning systems store and analyze data on patients' minimum nutritional and dietary requirements, food items available and their costs, and decision rules on factors other than nutrition and food costs. This system helps plan nutritionally balanced and aesthetically pleasing meals. The computer presents a set of least-cost menus meeting the constraints imposed by the nutritional model.

Many suppliers who serve the healthcare industry utilize bar codes that conform to an industry standard, the Health Industry Bar Code Supplier Labeling Standard. (See Chapter 3 for a description of bar codes and bar-code scanners.) Material shipped to healthcare organizations will have the bar codes attached to each item. By scanning the bar code every time an item is used from inventory, organizations can monitor inventory turnover and determine appropriate reorder volumes. Understanding what supplies are used for each patient or diagnostic category helps an organization develop guidelines and other management tools for controlling costs. The ability to know instantly when an item is used from inventory, combined with the ability to transmit that information directly to suppliers, can greatly reduce inventory stocks and improve cash flow.

Facilities Management Systems

Computerized systems can help organizations plan, manage, and maintain physical facilities. Examples include preventive maintenance systems, energy management systems, and project scheduling and control systems (particularly useful in construction and remodeling projects).

Preventive maintenance monitoring systems help extend the life of equipment and facilities and reduce costly failures. Automated facility maintenance systems offer several potential benefits including:

- cost savings through reduced inventory of spare parts for equipment repair;
- reduced staffing of housekeeping and maintenance department personnel through improved scheduling; and
- improved risk management through better record keeping on equipment maintenance and reduction of safety hazards.

Energy conservation has become an important cost saving strategy for health services organization as it has for all major industries in the United States. Computer packages have been developed to assist in monitoring energy utilization. Actual utilization figures are compared against calculated requirements, and the computer model points at possibilities for reduced consumption.

Health services organizations are frequently involved in capital construction and major remodeling projects. Computer systems have been developed to aid in project management. One such system, Program Evaluation and Review Technique (PERT), assists in project scheduling and control. (Austin and Boxerman 1995, Chapter 8) System users first construct a network that shows: (1) all activities required to complete the project; (2) the relationships of these activities to one another (including those that can be carried out simultaneously and those that must follow a time sequence); and (3) time estimates for completing each activity. The computer responds with a schedule that shows the critical path for project completion. As activities are completed, actual completion times are entered back into the computer system, the program is rerun, and new schedules are prepared for the remaining work. This system is an excellent tool for dynamic scheduling and control of major projects. Good packaged software systems are available. For example, Microsoft Project Management software runs on a personal computer and provides excellent tools for monitoring and managing many projects at the same time (Microsoft 1996).

Office Automation Systems

Health service organizations use computers to carry out office functions such as word processing, electronic mail, project management, meeting scheduling, and maintenance of calendars for management personnel.

Office automation helps to coordinate and manage people and work flows, link organizational units and projects, and coordinate work in the organization across levels and functions. (Laudon and Laudon 1994, 515)

Managing documents can consume 40 percent or 50 percent of an office staff's time when all functions are considered: document creation, storage, and retrieval; desktop publishing; and converting documents to other forms. Use of systems for integrated word processing, scheduling, electronic filing of documents, and transmitting messages/documents can dramatically improve efficiency and reduce the costs of office operations.

Office systems can link parts of the organization together by scheduling individuals and groups using electronic calendars and electronic mail (e-mail). (Laudon and Laudon 1994, 515) E-mail systems link offices and/or individuals together, allowing word-processed documents to be forwarded to others or filed in computer storage for future reference.

A growing number of organizations are even expanding the concept of office automation to include groupware and office applications of Intranets.

Groupware is a broad term that refers to the specifically designed combination of software and hardware that enables managers to share information in an interactive networked environment. This software/hardware combination facilitates real-time interaction among members of the group in order to improve problem solving and project management. Groupware activities include e-mail, teleconferencing, interactive two-way compressed video conferencing, relational databases (used to search for data and information), document editing and management, group calendars, and scheduling.

The application of groupware to healthcare organizations is a part of a growing industry trend called computer-supported cooperative work (CSCW). CSCW enhances collaboration among members of administrative work groups or teams across geographic locations, levels, and functional relationships. (Darnton 1995) The goal of the CSCW movement is to change the way people work together. Organizations often move groupware applications that reside on the desktop computer into conference rooms, board rooms, or connecting video systems. This allows people to use their best computerized tools and applications no matter their location. Groupware applications run over existing organizational networks: local area, wide area, or Intranet. (See Chapter 5.)

Office operations are benefitting from Intranet technology. This technology helps organizations increase effectiveness of their business management systems. Organizations use Intranet technology to simplify internal communications and to navigate and search databases and other information sources. Intranets link employees together enabling easy communication, collaboration, and work flow.

Some Intranets include internal organizational documents such as office phone directories, newsletters, training material, policies and procedures manuals, and human resource information. They save on the costs of printing, duplicating, and distributing these documents. The Intranet can also be used to provide a source for current news from external sources indexed and delivered to employees on the internal Web system. The formation of discussion groups is another aspect of Intranets that organizations have found to increase productivity and engage employees in constructive problem-solving activities. (See Chapter 16 for a more detailed discussion of Intranet applications.)

Summary

Health services organizations use computers and information systems to support administrative operations, including financial management, human resources management, monitoring and scheduling of services and facilities, materials management, facilities management, and office automation.

Most health services organizations begin using electronic data processing by developing or purchasing financial information systems. Financial data are essential for making least-cost investment decisions, for providing quality services to patients, and for providing management information for planning, controlling, and evaluating operations. Within the healthcare field, financial software is available for payroll, accounts payable, patient charges, billing and accounts receivable, general ledger accounting, cost allocation, financial reporting, and budgeting and budget control. Various vendors have developed computer models to assist management in financial planning and forecasting.

Employees are the most important resource of health services organizations. Personnel or human resources data systems can assist in workforce planning and labor analysis. Human resources information systems maintain employee record files, provide position control, produce labor analysis reports, analyze personnel problems (e.g., turnover and absenteeism), maintain inventories of employee skills and certifications, produce labor cost allocations, and provide information on employee productivity.

Increasing pressure for cost containment makes it essential to use facilities efficiently. Computerized monitoring and scheduling systems help achieve this aim by allowing advance bed booking and preadmission of inpatients, preparation of bed census and occupancy reports, scheduling of service facilities such as operating suites, and scheduling of patients in outpatient clinics.

Computers are being used increasingly to manage materials and facilities. Administrative systems provide computerized purchasing, inventory control, menu planning and food service management, scheduling and monitoring of preventive maintenance, energy management, and construction project scheduling and work control.

Office automation has dramatically increased efficiency and reduced costs in the administration of health services. An integrated office automation system includes word processing, e-mail, electronic filing of documents, electronic calendaring, and scheduling of meetings. The Intranet gives employees the advantages of Web technology to increase productivity and reduce costs. Groupware, such as e-mail and teleconferencing, also influences worker effectiveness and improves the overall functioning of the administrative operations of healthcare organizations.

Discussion Questions

12.1 What are some of the more common administrative computer applications?

12.2 Why do most healthcare organizations usually enter the information systems field by first installing financial systems?

12.3 What are the principal purposes achieved by an effective financial management information system? Describe a typical set of health services financial applications.

12.4 How do Human Resources Information Systems contribute to effective personnel administration? What are the basic functions of an HRIS?

12.5 How can computers help management achieve more efficient utilization of facilities?

12.6 Briefly describe computer applications available for materials management.

12.7 Discuss office automation and its potential in the healthcare field.

12.8 How can Intranets be used to improve communications and office operations?

Problems

12.1 Contact a local healthcare organization and conduct a survey to determine what financial, human resources and facilities planning software applications are currently used. Determine vendor, product name, and date of implementation. Determine expectations for replacing or upgrading the applications.

12.2 The software market for administrative applications is constantly changing. Locate on the Internet four to five vendors for each of the administrative areas discussed in Problem 12.1. For each vendor: What information is contained on their home page? How long they have been in operation? How many clients do they have? Are they a single-product vendor or do they have a wide range of software applications? Find a recent article in a professional journal that describes use of one of these vendor's products. Compare and contrast the article with the information you found on the vendor's Web site.

References

Anonymous. 1996. "1997 Resource Guide," *Healthcare Informatics* December: 13 (12).

Anonymous. 1996. "Focus Survey: Enterprisewide Scheduling Systems Will Become more Responsive to Users' Needs." *Health Management Technology* (November): 40–42.

Appleby, C. R. 1991. "Traffic Systems in a Holding Pattern," *Healthweek* (November 18): 27.

Austin, C. J., and S. B. Boxerman. 1995. *Quantitative Analysis for Health Services Administration*. Chicago: AUPHA Press/Health Administration Press.

Austin, C. J., J. A. Johnson, and G. D. Palestrant. 1994. "Information Systems for Human Resources Management." In *Strategic Management of Human Resources in Health Services Organizations*, edited by M.D. Fottler, S. R. Hernandez, and C. L. Joiner. Albany, NY: Delmar Publishers.

Berman, H. J., L. E. Weeks, and S. Kukla. 1994. *The Financial Management of Hospitals*, 7th Ed. Chicago: Health Administration Press.

Darnell, T. 1996. "Materials Management Systems: All about Controlling Costs." *Health Management Technology* (December): 15–19.

Darnton, G. 1995. "Working Together: A Management Summary of CSCW." *Computing and Control Engineering Journal* 6 (1): 37.

Dassenko, D. 1997. "Restructuring and an Opportunity to Integrate Financial Applications." *Health Management Technology* (March): 36.

Fanning, R. J. 1992. "Physician Database Eases Staffing Headaches." *Healthcare Informatics* 9 (6): 46–48.

Laudon, K. C., and J. P. Laudon. 1994. *Management Information Systems: Organization and Technology*. New York: Macmillan Publishing Company.

Microsoft. 1996. "Microsoft Office 97 Whitepaper," Internet Homepage—http://www.microsoft.com/msoffice.

Stair, R. M. 1996. *Principles of Information Systems: A Managerial Approach*, 2nd Ed. New York: Boyd & Fraser Publishing Company.

Toso, M., and A. Farmer. 1994. "Using Cost Accounting Data to Develop Capitation Rates." *Topics in Health Care Financing* 21 (1): 1–12

Ummel, S. 1997. "Linking Information for Competitive Advantage." *Healthcare Executive* 12 (2): 12–15.

White, E. 1996. "Bringing Scheduling to the Enterprise." *Healthcare Informatics* 13 (7): 24, 26, 30.

Additional Readings

Bachus, K. 1994. "The New World of Groupware," *Windows Magazine* (March): 226–32.

Baker III, E., and S. A. Coltrin. 1993. "HR Managers Have Impact in Developing HRIS Course." *HR Magazine* (November): 90–96.

Borok, L. S. 1995. "The Use of Relational Databases in Health Care Information Systems." *Journal of Health Care Finance* 21 (4): 6.

Brennan, L. L., and A. H. Rubenstein. 1995. "Applications of Groupware in Organizational Learning." *Trends in Organizational Behavior* 2 (February): 38–49.

Coleman, D. 1995. *Groupware: Technology and Applications.* New York: Prentice Hall, Inc.

Dove, H. G., and T. Forthman. 1995. "Helping Financial Analysts Communicate Variance Analysis," *Healthcare Financial Management* 49 (4): 52–54.

Duffy, J. H. 1996. "Information Technology Needs for Integrated Delivery Systems." *Healthcare Financial Management* 50 (7): 30–31.

Ehreth, J. 1996. "The Implications for Information Systems Design of How Health Care Costs Are Determined." *Medical Care* 34 (March): 69–82.

Haughon, J. L., and L. J. Gibson. 1995. "Improving the Cost, Quality, and Access to Healthcare." *Medical Informatics* 34: 1558–61.

Hosking, J. E. 1995. "Containing Cost Through Effective Facilities Planning." *Healthcare Financial Management* 49 (4): 34.

McCormack, J. 1997. "The Paperless Business Office." *Health Data Management* 5 (6): 55–64.

Palley, M. A., and S. Cooger. 1995. "Health Care Information Systems and Formula Based Reimbursement." *Health Care Management Review* 20 (Spring): 74–84.

Russell, D. 1996. "Inventory Detectives Tap IT," *HealthcareInformatics* 13 (8): 25.

Worthey, J. A., and P. P. DiSalvo. 1995. *Managing Computers in Health Care: A Guide for Professionals*, 3rd Ed. Chicago: Health Administration Press.

Wynekoop, J. L. 1996. "Office Computer Systems in Healthcare: Use and Assessment," *Journal of End User Computing* 8 (1): 22–30.

13

STRATEGIC DECISION-SUPPORT APPLICATIONS

THE COMPUTER applications discussed in Chapter 11 are designed to support and enhance the delivery of care while those described in the previous chapter support routine, day-to-day administrative

Concepts and Applications

The executive decision-making process can be aided immeasurably with the right information, especially with such new business situations as capitation. Although information systems can be used in day-to-day management, healthcare leaders are increasingly using decision-support systems (DSSs) to make strategic decisions. DSSs are effective in that they can collect and collate requested data, display those data in an easy-to-understand format, and manipulate those data to yield different types of information. These systems provide information to analyze finances, do strategic planning, allocate resources, and oversee operations.

To function effectively, DSSs rely on a database of information. Like the DSSs themselves, information contained in a database can be developed either in-house or purchased from an outside source.

This chapter will enable readers to determine what long-term, strategic decisions can be made with assistance from a decision-support system, how to construct a DSS and its database of information, and how strategic plans can be made using a DSS.

operations. Although these systems provide many benefits to patients, nurses, physicians, ancillary personnel, and first-line managers, they have little direct impact on the functions of senior executives. In fact, most healthcare executives have historically viewed information systems (IS) as operational tools with no particular relevance to their senior management role.

One possible explanation for this perception of information systems is the tendency of senior executives to dismiss the role of data in the managerial decision-making process. Executives often view decision making as an art, based upon such qualitative features as experience, judgment, insight, astuteness, and political savvy. Certainly these are all important components of the decision-making process, but the increasing complexity created by managed care, patient demands, fixed revenues, and new approaches for delivering care creates a need for executives to employ more sophisticated decision-making techniques.

These decision-making techniques typically involve mathematical models and rely heavily on the availability of data. (See, for example, Austin and Boxerman 1995, Chapter 1.) While it is theoretically possible to create a custom computer-based solution each time a particular model and its data are defined, the availability of an existing information system to support the data retrieval, modeling, and reporting of results for executive questions as they arise is much preferred. Systems that perform these functions are known as decision-support systems (DSSs).

This chapter is designed to provide the executive with an understanding of these systems. Unlike the applications presented in previous chapters, whose users are a diverse group of clinicians, support staff, and departmental managers, the systems described in this chapter are designed for use by the executives themselves.

The Concept of Decision Support

Before specific applications of DSSs are presented, it is important to first understand the concept of decision support. "Broadly speaking, decision support can be defined as using an organization's data to aid in management decisions and efficient operations. The key, of course, is not just displaying the information, but also organizing it and using it intelligently." (Sempeles 1996, 28)

It is important to note that this definition of decision support makes no mention of computers. Decision support refers to an *approach* to problem solving that is based on the use of data. There are many strategies available for the actual *implementation* of this approach, ranging from a totally manual strategy to one that is totally automated. For example, consider the executive director of a multispecialty group practice faced with the decision of whether to sign a contract with a particular managed care plan. The contract provides for the group's physicians to be paid a fixed amount per month per patient to provide care to the plan's patient population.

The group's executive director could certainly make this decision based on intuition, the desire to generate additional revenue for the group, and/or a personal relationship established with the managed care plan. A better approach, however, would be to obtain appropriate *data*, including the time availability of the group's physicians; the demographics of the patients belonging to the managed care plan; the health services utilization patterns of these patients; and the costs incurred by the plan in providing various types of healthcare services. A *summarization* of this data provides a better understanding of the plan's patient population as well as the costs incurred by the group in providing care.

Using this understanding of the data, the executive director could then create a *model* that facilitates the computation of profitability as a function of variables such as payment mechanism, patient demographics, utilization patterns, method of delivering care, etc. By choosing reasonable values for these variables, the executive director can *examine* the expected consequences of signing the contract and thus come to an appropriate decision. In some cases the decision might involve choosing from among several alternative contract arrangements rather than the present simpler choice between accepting or rejecting a single contract. The steps followed by the Executive Director in deciding whether to sign the contract can be summarized in the flowchart shown in Figure 13.1.

Today's executives are typically faced with decisions that must be made within relatively short time frames and that require the analysis of large volumes of data. A manual approach to decision support is therefore impractical. Even with the use of spreadsheet or statistical software, the aggregation, management, analysis, and reporting of the data present a challenge to the timely completion of the decision-making process. Nor is it any longer viable for healthcare executives to continue their past practice of requesting that their Data Processing Departments generate special reports to provide the data needed for making pressing decisions. Frequently, the turnaround time for producing these custom reports has extended beyond the decision's deadline date.

Executives are thus becoming increasingly aware of their need for an information system with the following attributes:

1. Interaction with the system must occur with relative ease.
2. Executives themselves can retrieve the data they need.

Figure 13.1 Summary of Steps for Deciding Whether to Sign Contract

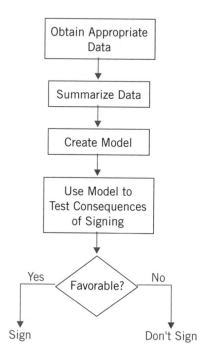

3. A summarization of the data that are retrieved can be displayed in a meaningful format.
4. Modeling capability built into the system allows alternative decisions to be evaluated.
5. The results of the analyses can be presented in a straightforward, easily understood report.

Figure 13.2 provides a summary of these desirable attributes.

An Overview of Decision-Support Systems

Historically, the concept of management DSSs began in response to the impending prospective payment system for Medicare patients and the related need for case-mix analysis. Beginning in the late 1970s and early 1980s, a parallel development in management decision modeling was initiated that combined industrial productivity systems engineering with units of hospital production (patient charges and procedures). These systems merged medical records data, patient billing data, utilization statistics, and human resources information to provide management with a basic decision-support model. (Raco, Shapleigh, and Cook 1989)

Figure 13.2   Desirable Attributes of a Decision-Support System

---

- Easy Interaction with the System
- Executives Can Retrieve Data Themselves
- Data Are Displayed in a Meaningful Format
- System Has Modeling Capability
- System Generates Clear Reports

Although today's decision-support systems have surpassed their predecessors in scope and direction, the integration of financial and clinical data into a single resource easily available to the decision maker remains one of their most important features. Today's decision-support technology "draws on operational and clinical information integrated from existing data sources, including provider billing or cost accounting systems, patient abstracting systems, hospital financial systems, and available external comparative databases." (Stearns and Mazie 1996) Executives can use this technology to examine specific performance indicators and analyze their organization along clinical, operational, and strategic lines.

A decision-support system, then, can be characterized in terms of the components that comprise the system as well as the functions that the system performs for the user. Each of these two perspectives is presented below, followed by a review of the characteristics of useful management information.

The Components of a DSS

An effective DSS must be more than a communication and data-processing system; it must contain modules that combine to produce the desirable attributes highlighted in Figure 13.2. A conceptual model of the components comprising such a DSS is shown in Figure 13.3, and each component is discussed briefly in the following paragraphs.

User Interface. The user interface allows the executive to communicate easily with the DSS. Whether communication with the system uses a menu format or free-text input, the key objective is to ensure that the input process is as simple and intuitive as possible. The same issues associated with accessing databases (see the discussion of data manipulation languages in Chapter 6) are also applicable to the design of the user interface for a DSS.

Model Manager. The system typically contains a model manager that is software designed to coordinate the creation, storage, and retrieval of the models that comprise the model library. Depending on the nature of

Figure 13.3 Conceptual Model of a Decision-Support System

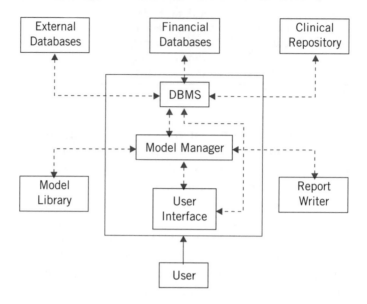

the request made by the user of the DSS, a linkage to the appropriate model would be made so that the desired analysis can be obtained.

Model Library. An important component of a DSS is its model library, which consists of an array of analytical capabilities, including statistical, graphical, financial, and "what-if" models.

- Statistical models support such functions as summarizing data, testing hypotheses, performing forecasting, and constructing control charts.

- Graphical models facilitate the construction of graphical displays of data in a variety of formats including scatter diagrams, pie charts, bar graphs, and multidimensional plots.

- Financial models provide the basis for performing break-even analysis, examining cash flows, and computing the internal rate of return associated with investments.

- "What-if" models allow users to determine how variations in one or more variables impact the value of an outcome of interest.

Depending on the type of decision being made, any of the models comprising the fields of operations research or management science might be utilized by the DSS. This use of modeling is in fact a major strength of decision-support systems.

Databases. Fundamental to the DSS is an array of databases, consisting of minimally of a clinical repository, financial databases, and external databases. These databases are typically relational, are designed for easy retrieval of needed data, and, as noted in Chapter 6, are separate from the organization's operational systems. Recall that this separation is designed to avoid having the DSS applications adversely impact the performance of the operational systems. Among the elements contained in these databases are: (1) units of service produced; (2) resources consumed in producing those services; (3) data for assessing the quality of services provided; and (4) indicators of the effectiveness of services provided in meeting perceived community health needs. Keeping the contents of the DSS databases current often requires a staff person with the designation of database manager.

Database Management System (DBMS). Access to the databases in the DSS is facilitated by the database management system (DBMS). For a specific decision-making problem, the DBMS retrieves the needed data and makes it available directly to the user and/or the model manager for use in a specific decision model. The components and operation of a DBMS have been discussed in Chapter 6.

Report Writer. Finally, the value of the DSS is enhanced by its report writer, which provides the user with a clear, easily understood report containing the decision problem solution. Depending on the application, this report might provide a comparison of several alternatives under consideration, the consequences of a particular decision, or a recommendation of an optimum action that should be taken.

A Categorization of the General Uses of a DSS

In addition to the components of the DSS, interest also focuses on the functions of the system. The DSS must be designed to perform well in the organizational environment in which it will operate. Alter (1976) has categorized decision-support systems in terms of what the users of the systems actually do with them; these categories include:

- systems in which the users retrieve isolated data items;
- systems used as a mechanism for ad hoc analysis of data files;
- systems that provide prespecified aggregations of data in the form of standard reports;
- systems that assist in estimating the consequences of proposed decisions;
- systems that propose decisions to management; and
- systems that make decisions according to predetermined decision algorithms.

Although proposed more than 20 years ago, Alter's categorization of these systems suggests an interesting paradigm for understanding the breadth of DSS capabilities. Figure 13.4 summarizes Alter's six categories and indicates for each category the type of contemporary DSS required. For example, the retrieval of isolated data items can be accomplished with any system having a database manager and direct query capabilities. Similarly, in order to perform ad hoc analyses of a single data file one can use any of the many available generic statistical packages. Tables based on prespecified aggregations of data comprised the standard reports that were the mainstay of managerial applications run on mainframe computers for many years. Today, colorful graphs and charts supplement tabular output in the executive information systems gaining increasing use. These systems are discussed in more detail later in this chapter.

The last three categories proposed by Alter define today's traditional applications of a DSS. To estimate the consequences of a proposed decision, the executive can use a DSS with a "what-if" modeling capability. The addition of optimization modeling to the system supports the search for optimal decisions that can then be offered as a proposed solution. Finally, unlike the uses described thus far where the DSS serves as a supplement to the decision maker, the last use involves systems that can actually make independent decisions. Such systems, often called expert systems, consist of a DSS that utilizes the science of artificial intelligence. More details of these systems are provided later in this chapter.

The Characteristics of Useful Management Information

The characteristics of useful management information were discussed in Chapter 2 and summarized in Figure 2.9. Because management

Figure 13.4 DSS Systems Corresponding to Alter's Categorization of Uses

Alter's Categorization of Use	Type of System
Retrieve Isolated Data Items	Simple Database Management System with Query Capability
Perform Ad Hoc Analysis of a Data File	Generic Statistical Package
Generate Aggregation of Data in a Standard Report	DSS with Report Generator; Executive Information System
Estimate Consequences of a Proposed Decision	DSS with "What-If" Modeling Capability
Propose Decisions to Management	DSS with Optimization Modeling Capability
Make Decisions According to Predetermined Algorithms	Expert System; DSS with Artificial Intelligence

information lies at the heart of DSSs, it is useful to once again summarize these characteristics. To be useful, management information must be:

- *information—not raw data*—intelligently processed in accordance with predesigned plans;
- *relevant* to the purposes for which it is to be used;
- *sensitive* enough to provide discrimination and meaningful comparisons for operating managers;
- *unbiased* so as not to meet self-fulfilling management prophecies;
- *comprehensive* so that all important elements of a system are visible to those charged with decision-making responsibility;
- *timely* so as to be available in advance of the time when decisions or actions are required;
- *action-oriented* in order to facilitate the decision process rather than just present passive facts about current operations;
- *uniform* so as to allow comparisons over time, both internally (against previous performance) and externally (against the experience of other institutions);
- *performance targeted* in order to allow comparison with predetermined goals and objectives; and
- *cost-effective* so that the anticipated benefits obtained from having the information available exceed the costs of collecting and processing that information.

Information Needs for Decision Support

The overviews of decision support and decision-support systems have emphasized the important role of information. The characteristics of useful management information were summarized in the previous section. Two logical questions naturally arise from these discussions: Where does the decision maker obtain the necessary information? What specific categories of information are needed? This section addresses these two questions.

Sources of Information for Decision Support

There are three basic sources for obtaining the information needed for decision support in healthcare settings: internal transaction processing systems; specially constructed databases; and external data sources.

Internal Transaction Processing Systems. A number of internal transaction processing systems are used in conjunction with the day-to-day delivery of healthcare. These have been described in the previous two chapters and are also discussed in the next chapter. In addition to serving an important operational function, these systems contain information that has a great deal of value on an aggregate basis. For example, the admitting system stores a number of important sociodemographic variables on each patient. When accumulated in a data repository, these data provide an excellent overview of the sociodemographics of the patients served by the healthcare organization.

Transaction processing systems also store valuable clinical information that indicates volumes of service provided, as well as the results of laboratory tests or radiologic procedures performed. It is important to bear in mind that these transaction systems were initially installed to facilitate communication of test orders and results as well as to support the billing function. Only recently have executives begun to realize the importance of aggregating clinical information for decision-support purposes. Therefore, special attention must be given to the process of ensuring this aggregation so that the information is not lost when the patient is discharged.

Specially Constructed Databases. There are a number of items of information about the healthcare organization that are needed for decision support but are not collected by the internal transaction processing systems. Examples include patient satisfaction data, waiting times associated with various patient flow processes, and times spent by nursing personnel in various categories of caregiving. A variety of data-gathering methodologies are required to obtain this needed information, including questionnaires and work sampling. The information gathered must then be stored in a database accessible to the decision-support system.

Similarly, many physicians and clinical departments, particularly in academic medical centers, will build and maintain dedicated databases. These systems store specific clinical information for a research study, maintain data to satisfy a physician's interest in various aspects of his or her practice, or support other uniquely defined departmental efforts, and are often a valuable source of information for a DSS.

External Data Sources. A number of decision-support applications will require information about the world outside of the healthcare organization. This information includes community demographic data, information on marketshare, age-specific national utilization data, information on physicians in the area, etc. Such information is available from a variety of sources, which are summarized in Figure 13.5.

The data obtained from sources such as those summarized in Figure 13.5 are essentially "raw data" that often require some degree of manipulation, or processing, in order to be useful for decision support. A number of vendors offer databases containing a variety of information that has already been aggregated and edited so that it is ready for use by healthcare organizations.

Figure 13.5   Some Sources of "External" Healthcare Data

- American Association of Health Plans
- American Hospital Association
- American Medical Association
- Bureau of Labor Statistics
- Census Bureau
- Center for Disease Control (Wonder System)
- Health Care Finance Administration
- Health Insurance Association of America
- National Center for Health Statistics
- State Hospital Association Data Sets

One example is the MEDSTAT Group, headquartered in Ann Arbor, Michigan. (Anonymous 1996, 14) This company offers a wide range of databases and software, including the "largest and richest private sector database of medical utilization and cost experience in the U.S. . . . ," a longitudinal hospital database that "links discharge abstracts, physician records, hospital facility reports and Medicare Cost Reports," and a database, of more than 600,000 respondents to a consumer survey, "used to project lifestyle-related health services demand."

Similarly, Sachs Group, a healthcare information firm based in Evanston, Illinois, also "specializes in turning data into useful information from which hospitals and health care systems can create strategies." (Anonymous 1995, 17) The company offers information to increase marketing effectiveness, including custom segmentation; local market research on 90,000 consumers in 33 major markets; and information for sizing a network, such as demand forecasting for inpatient, outpatient, and physician services.

Categories of Information Needed for Decision Support

There is a variety of decision-support information needs in the modern healthcare organization. These needs, which will be satisfied from a combination of the sources discussed above, can be categorized into the following groupings.

Information to Support Strategic Planning. The organization's strategic information needs are dictated by contextual variables such as size, competitive environment, and structure, and they are dependent on the organization's strategic orientation. Austin, Trimm, and Sobczak (1995) discuss several frameworks for understanding this relationship between strategic orientation and information requirements. One framework,

Porter's competitive analysis model, suggests three strategies that organizations employ to compete in the marketplace: cost leadership, differentiation, and niche-focused strategy. Healthcare organizations employing one of Porter's strategies will need to tailor their information systems accordingly. The strategies and associated information needs are tabulated in Figure 13.6.

All three strategies require continuous monitoring of marketshare. However, organizations following a cost-leadership strategy must continuously monitor costs of services and productivity in reference to competitors. Those employing differentiation (provision of products or services that are different from those of the competition) will need to monitor measures of patient satisfaction, quality, and changes in the demographic characteristics of the marketplace. Product-line management information will be essential for those organizations choosing to employ a niche-focused strategy.

Information to Support the Marketing Function. Austin, Trimm, and Sobczak (1995) describe how the Miles and Snow typology provides a conceptual basis for identifying information helpful in supporting marketing efforts. The application of this model is summarized in Figure 13.7. According to this framework, healthcare organizations can be classified into one of the following categories:

1. *Prospectors*—those that continuously and aggressively pursue new markets.

2. *Defenders*—those that try to be very good at what they do and follow a "stick to the knitting" approach to maintaining marketshare.

3. *Analyzers*—those that do not rush into new markets and services but continuously track and analyze trends, technology, and consumer demand.

Figure 13.6 Porter's Strategies for Competing in the Marketplace and Associated Information Needs

Strategy	Information Needs
Cost Leadership	• Marketshare • Cost of Services • Productivity Relative to Competitors
Differentiation	• Marketshare • Patient Satisfaction • Quality • Changes in Demographics Characteristics of the Marketplace
Niche-Focused	• Marketshare • Product-Line Management Information

Figure 13.7 Strategic Orientations to Marketing (Miles and Snow) and Associated Information Needs

Strategic Orientation	Information Needs
Prospectors	• Demographic Changes
	• Marketshare
	• Product-Line Performance
Defenders	• Productivity
	• Costs
	• Quality Factors
Analyzers	• Demographic Changes
	• Market Characteristics
	• Competitor Performance
Reactors	• Information Needs Vary, Depending on Perceived Threats and Opportunities

4. *Reactors*—those that are undirected and respond to forces after changes in the marketplace have occurred.

With regard to information needs, all of the strategic orientations require historical data on service utilization along with demographic projections to support forecasting demand for services. Also important is an understanding of the social and cultural determinants of service utilization along with demographic indicators to help predict how these factors may change. Prospectors must continuously monitor market-share, demographic changes, and product-line performance. Defenders will focus on productivity, costs, and quality factors. Analyzers need to track changes in demography, market characteristics, and competitor performance. The information needs of reactors will vary depending upon perceived threats and opportunities that arise.

Information to Assist in Resource Allocation. In order to remain competitive and survive under the cost pressures associated with managed care, healthcare executives must be very efficient in their allocation and utilization of resources. When healthcare organizations were compensated on a "cost-plus" basis, wasteful utilization of resources was a tolerable, if not optimal strategy. Today, however, providers typically receive a fixed payment, so that the wise allocation of resources is quite important. The availability of accurate and timely information to assist in the resource allocation process is a definite asset to the executive. Important items of information include cost estimates of personnel, materials, equipment, and other capital requirements for each program or major service line offered by the provider. In many cases, these data become the parameters in an optimization model, such as linear programming, which allows the executive to solve for the "optimal" mix of programs which should comprise the organization's product lines. (See, for example, Austin and Boxerman 1995, Chapter 5.)

Information to Support Enhancement of Productivity and Operating Efficiency. Once the "optimum mix" of programs and services to be offered by the healthcare organization has been identified, the pressures of managed care make it incumbent that each program comprising this mix be operated in a productive and efficient manner. A number of improvement techniques have been successfully used by healthcare organizations, including benchmarking (Mace 1995) and reengineering (Boland 1996). Common to these and other techniques for improving processes and systems is the important role of data in providing a basis for identifying the changes to be made and guiding the design and implementation of the new system. (Benson 1996)

Harrison (1995, 245) emphasizes the difference between *process* benchmarking, which seeks to understand "how processes work differently from one organization to the next," and *outcome* benchmarking whose focus is on a "comparison of metrics from one organization to another." The power of process benchmarking as a process improvement tool depends on the availability of data collected along process lines rather than the more traditional cost center orientation. Specific data needs are: cost data, defined as "operating cost per unit of throughput (e.g., cost per admission, cost per radiology procedure, etc.)"; process quality indicators, such as "waiting times in the Admitting office, denied claims due to inadequate data capture, subsequent transfers because of off-unit admissions . . ."; and cycle times or throughput times at the process and subprocess levels. (Harrison 1995, 248)

Hartless and Hager (1995) report similar data needs in their reengineering of patient care delivery of postpartum obstetric care. Phase I of the project, the planning phase, consisted of process definition, measurement, analysis, and design/redesign. Six categories of measurements were collected: process, including travel times, tasks completed, and task completion times; cost, measured in salary dollars per patient day and average hourly rate; quality measures, taken from their Quality Care Control Reports; staff satisfaction; patient satisfaction; and physician satisfaction. The satisfaction measures were based upon survey instruments.

Information to Support Outcomes Assessment. Health services organizations must evaluate their performance on a continuous basis, both to improve the quality of services delivered and to meet the scrutiny of a variety of external constituents, including regulatory agencies, managed care organizations, business coalitions, and patients. In fact Kachnowski (1997, 27) suggests that "The future success of the provider organization relies on a system that probably costs less than any other system in [the provider's] budget, and consists of about one-to-two percent of [the provider's] total IS expenditures: the outcomes system."

The literature tends to indicate general categories, rather than specific items, of information needed for outcomes assessment. Aller and Rosenstein (1996, 22) suggest that payors, researchers, managed care officials, providers, and patients each have different outcomes information interests. These are summarized in Figure 13.8. As a result, the authors suggest the need for systems capable "of measuring indicators that span the gamut of health care activities to reflect outcomes related to cost, utilization, quality and patient satisfaction."

The use of outcomes measurements appears to be shifting from a voluntary to a mandatory activity. In February 1997 the Joint Commission on Accreditation of Health Care Organizations (JCAHO) announced an initiative that "for the first time require[s] health care organizations to gather and submit data about the results of care." (Moore, Jr. 1997, 2) The program, known as "Oryx," initially applies to hospitals and nursing homes, requiring them to choose a performance measurement system by the end of 1997. "They must start submitting data on two clinical indicators of their choice, covering at least 20% of their patient population by the first quarter of 1999." (Moore, Jr. 1997, 2)

The extent to which accreditation would hinge on actual patient care was unclear as the program was being developed. What was clear, however, was the mandate that healthcare organizations must be using the data to drive their performance improvement, which of course implies that they must have systems in place to support the collection, storage, and retrieval of the needed data.

Approaches to Development of Decision-Support Systems

Once the healthcare executive has decided that decision-support capability is needed, a DSS must be developed and implemented. It is important to note that a DSS is software, so that the following four fundamental ways of obtaining any software capability apply to DSSs as well (Mallach 1994):

• Write the necessary programs from scratch in a suitable language.
• Use specialized tools, or "generators," designed for the task at hand.
• Customize a package.
• Purchase a turnkey package.

Figure 13.8 Categories of Outcomes Measurement Interests by Constituent Group

Constituent Group	Information Interests
Payors	• Overall Costs of Care • Information to Identify Cost-Effective Providers
Researchers	• Large Epidemiological Studies • Information to Assess Impact of Care on Health Status of Populations
Managed Care Officials	• Resource Consumption Assessments • Evaluation of Cost-Efficiencies of Care
Providers	• Evaluations of Impact of Care • Assessments of Quality of Care
Patients	• Functional Benefits Resulting from an Intervention • Perceptual Benefits Resulting from an Intervention

Adapted from Aller and Rosenstein 1996, 22

Early healthcare adopters of decision-support technology used third-generation programming languages (see Chapter 4) to write programs that extracted desired data from the files of their transaction systems. In many cases, the program had such a specialized focus that it was able to obtain only the data needed to answer a specific question. Subsequent management questions would require a new program. While in theory this approach would still work today, the time required to develop the software and make it operational creates unacceptable delays.

Fourth-generation development tools (see Chapter 4) do make the task of creating the DSS a bit easier. The system can be configured to meet the specific requirements defined by the healthcare organization, and when used in conjunction with a relational database (see Chapter 6) the resulting DSS can be quite efficient. But many, if not most, healthcare organizations recognize that their primary mission is to deliver health-care rather than create software. These organizations, therefore, tend to purchase rather than develop their software products.

Two alternatives are available to the healthcare executive seeking to purchase a DSS. One option is to obtain a customized package developed specifically for their needs. Most vendors offering these packages use a fourth-generation language to carry out the development effort. The advantage of customization is the opportunity to obtain a system with the specifically desired features. The disadvantage is the generally higher cost, although improved development tools and languages are enabling system developers to deliver customized DSSs at competitive prices.

Finally, the executive can choose one of the many turnkey packages available for use in the healthcare industry. A number of vendors offer turnkey decision-support systems for a wide range of applications. For example, the Annual Market Directory Issue of *Health Management Technology* (Anonymous 1997) contains ten categories of managerial financial decision-support systems. These categories, along with the number of vendors tabulated in each category, are shown in Figure 13.9. Some vendors offer products in several categories, others have only a single product, while others offer a decision-support component to one of their transaction systems.

Whether the DSS is developed in-house, custom-designed by a system developer, or purchased as a turnkey package, the system has no value without the availability of appropriate data. Early programs, developed in-house using a third-generation language, typically accessed the files that were part of the transaction processing systems. As was mentioned earlier, the data to support the DSS should not be stored as part of the organization's operational systems, but rather in a separate data repository, or *data warehouse*. Ladaga (1995, 26) indicates that a data warehouse "enables the collection and organization of disparate data sources, both internal and external, to an enterprise and provides users with a common, integrated subject-oriented view for decision-making. The data is time-variant and non-volatile, which means that updates occur in a scheduled manner."

When the DSS is developed in-house, the organization is free to choose the database format and structure. Turnkey systems, by contrast,

Figure 13.9 Number of Vendors Offering Decision-Support Systems by Category of System

Decision-Support System Category	Number of Vendors
Budgeting	62
Case-Mix Management	78
Contract Monitoring	88
Cost Accounting	56
End-User Reporting/Query	134
Executive Information Systems	105
Financial Modeling	63
Marketing/Marketing Analysis/Planning	64
Payor-Mix Status	68
Product-Line Management	69

Source: Adapted from "Product Breakouts," *Health Management Technology*, 1997 Annual Market Directory, February 1997

will come designed to operate with a database having a specific structure. In most cases it will be the responsibility of the healthcare organization to copy data from internal or external sources onto this database. This often is not an insignificant task. Furthermore, depending on how rapidly the source data change, daily, weekly, or monthly updates of this database must be made if the DSS is to remain a timely source of information for the decision maker. Healthcare executives planning for a new DSS must bear in mind that the system will require attention beyond its initial installation. Some larger health services organizations employ a database administrator in the IS department who has responsibility for maintenance and oversight of databases and database management systems.

Applications of Decision-Support Systems

Management databases and related decision-support systems have been applied to a variety of problems facing healthcare executives and their organizations. Benefits reported from the use of these systems include "improved access to and awareness of revenue performance . . . ," " . . . empowerment of end-users to generate their own reports . . . ," " . . . ability to maintain historical data . . . ," and the determination of "true costs and profit potential of various types of cases. . . ." (Evans 1997a, 37–38) Representative applications are reviewed in the following paragraphs.

Financial Modeling Applications

A California insurance company uses a simplified version of a DSS to manage fixed-income portfolios worth $370 million and to analyze 36 different types of fixed-income securities and derivatives for risk and return. (Sodhi 1996) Prior to implementing the DSS, the company accomplished these tasks with a spreadsheet, commercial software having a significant annual license fee, and manual methods. The new system was custom-developed by a management science PhD student using object-oriented programming, which facilitated the integration of mathematical models, database entities, and a user interface.

The DSS is used to perform a variety of tasks, including:

- making trades;
- analyzing individual securities and portfolios;
- performing "what-if" analyses to determine the effect of potential trades on portfolios;
- performing structured query language (SQL)–based ad hoc queries for accounting-related issues;

- generating a variety of reports for the corporate board; and
- generating monthly reports for the accounting department.

The portfolio manager has expressed extreme satisfaction with the system, indicating that the program "has and should continue to be an invaluable tool in increasing portfolio returns." (Sodhi 1996, 33)

A budgetary decision-support model, part of a financial management system implemented by a New Jersey academic medical center, "provides the foundation for evaluating needs of the nursing units while balancing allocation and deployment of resources." (Sengin and Dreisbach 1995, 33) The system uses a set of "key indicators" as the basis for its analyses: patient volume; occupancy rate; patient acuity; direct hours/patient day; paid hours/patient day; salary cost/patient day; and nonsalary cost/patient day.

Using both graphical as well as spreadsheet formats, the system generates a number of reports, including cost projections; staffing guidelines; budget breakdowns; overtime used; workload by unit; and holiday premium hours/dollars paid. The spreadsheets allow the nurse manager to update the report, experiment with different scenarios, and "obtain instantaneous data of how these changes affect her bottom line." (Sengin and Dreisbach 1995, 37) By assisting nursing management in "budgetary compliance and effective and efficient use of resources," the DSS is the foundation of the medical center's "success in maintaining the positive course of large and complex budgets while safeguarding high quality patient care for the community." (Sengin and Dreisbach 1995, 44)

Planning and Marketing Applications

Healthcare managers are now "catching up" with users in other industries in applying geographic information systems (GISs) and mapping software to a variety of planning and marketing studies. "The term 'geographic information system' is often used, appropriately, as an umbrella term for a system designed to process any type of information that traditionally would have been recorded on maps." (Mallach 1994, 428) By using a GIS and mapping software, healthcare executives and planners are able to gain a better understanding of their customers and potential customers as well as their competitors.

Evans (1997b) describes several applications of GIS and mapping software. A New York managed care organization uses this software to determine if its members are able to access physicians and other healthcare providers within a reasonable amount of time. Prior to having the software, the organization used tabular charts or a blank zip code map on which it manually filled in the information. Similarly, a large

Wisconsin insurer describes its mapping software as "a great tool for demonstrating how easy employee groups can access [their] provider groups." (Evans 1997b, 60) Finally, a New York–based home health care provider employs a mapping-based program to find the best routes for its drivers and professional field staff. The software helps the company assign new patients "to the appropriate nurse or aide in the correct sequence." (Evans 1997b, 60)

Forgionne (1991) describes the characteristics of a DSS for assistance in marketing prepaid medical plans. Several statistical models and a simulation model comprise the model base of the system. The system generates statistical reports and performance forecasts, including demographic information, consumer data, marketshare, predicted number of subscribers, and cost and revenue forecasts.

Resource Allocation Applications

Among the areas of application of decision-support systems to resource allocation processes in health services organizations are the following:

- labor planning, including analysis of staffing patterns, determination of optimal staffing levels, and projection of future staffing needs;
- supplies and facilities planning, including minimization of costs, consolidation of vendors/sources, and standardization of products/supplies; and
- equipment utilization control, including monitoring of equipment purchases, reviewing maintenance and lost charges, and determining future purchases.

McClean and Millard (1995) describe a decision-support tool that improves the efficiency of bed management and thus facilitates the more effective use of resources. Input to the system comes from data downloaded from the patient administrative system. A query-by-example function enables the decision maker to separate data into meaningful subgroups, and a "what-if" capability allows proposed changes to the system to be assessed prior to their implementation.

The design of a DSS for resource allocation in a clinical laboratory is discussed by van Merode et al. (1995). The system supports a variety of decisions, including how the laboratory should be divided into sections, how staff should be assigned to workstations, and how samples should be assigned to workstations for testing.

Applications for Improving Operations

With cost control an imperative to survival in an era of managed care, health services organizations are constantly looking for ways to improve the operation of the systems and processes within their organization. In many cases, the techniques that are available to accomplish these improvements use relatively straightforward models. The key is the presence of a DSS in which the data needed to apply the model are available, and a user-friendly interface enables managers with little technical background to use the system.

Mayo Clinic in Jacksonville, Florida, uses a DSS for their operating rooms that is "designed to help caregivers determine the total costs of inpatient and outpatient surgical cases while improving financial and clinical efficiency." (Siwicki 1995, 33) The system developer claims that while "Most information systems for operating rooms are designed solely for scheduling or anesthesia recordkeeping, . . . [this system] encompasses every aspect of the surgical process, from scheduling and anesthesia to interoperative procedures and recovery." (Siwicki 1995, 33) A variety of reports regarding costs, equipment and facility utilization, and volumes can be generated. But of particular importance is the ability to manipulate the data once they are stored in the relational database of the system.

The management engineering staff of a Tennessee hospital developed a graphical decision-support tool to help nursing managers answer daily staffing questions. (Graham 1995) By combining information from their hospital's patient classification system with the institution's usual staffing policies, a graphical display is generated that clearly shows whether a unit can economically justify the use of overtime, contract nurses, or nurses from other units. Implemented in a spreadsheet environment, the system enables a nursing coordinator to report the balanced hospital nursing hours, the approved overtime, and needed contract nursing hours.

In closing, one point bears repeating. While the systems described make data accessible and provide the modeling capability to allow alternatives to be evaluated, the final decision is made by the user. Systems that go beyond data aggregation and modeling are discussed in the next section.

Expert Systems

The DSS applications discussed thus far represent the administrative analog to the passive clinical decision-support systems introduced in Chapter 11. These systems are able to collect, organize, and communicate data to the user. This section of the text looks at a special type of administrative DSS, known as an *expert system*, which is the counterpart of the active clinical DSS, and is capable of reproducing "the reasoning process a human decision maker would go through in reaching a decision, diagnosing a problem, or suggesting a course of action." (Mallach 1994, 463)

Recall the three components of expert systems introduced in Chapter 11: a *knowledge base* (also known as a *rule base*), which contains the expertise of the system; a *database*, which the knowledge base is matched against; and an *inference engine*, which generates conclusions for consideration by the decision maker. Mallach (1994) suggests two additional components that might comprise the expert system: a *user interface* that facilitates interaction between the system and the user; and *workspace* where the system stores the facts about a situation. A possible conceptual model of an expert system comprised of these components is shown in Figure 13.10.

The field of expert systems is part of a larger discipline, known as artificial intelligence, that attempts to simulate human problem-solving techniques in a computer environment. Although artificial intelligence programs date back to the 1950s, applications in healthcare first appeared in the 1970s. These early applications, developed at academic medical centers, typically had a clinical orientation, and several representative applications were described in Chapter 11. But expert systems can be beneficial to managers as well, particularly for recurring, tactical, structured types of problems. Two representative applications are described below.

A Connecticut-based insurance company is making use of artificial intelligence to "find fraud and abuse in claims." (Siwicki 1996, 50) The system, which is capable of looking at vast amounts of data in a matter of minutes, identifies suspicious claims by looking for "subtle changes in behavior patterns" in a provider compared to his/her peer group. "By itself, a fraudulent claim might look normal. But when it's instantly compared with millions of other claims, . . . that normal-looking claim can be viewed in a new light." (Siwicki 1996, 50) Whereas considerable

Figure 13.10   Conceptual Model of an Expert System

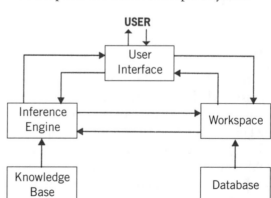

Source: Adapted from Mallach 1994, 461.

time was required to search for needed data when an allegation of fraud arose, the expert system has greatly reduced the time required to generate fraud and abuse reports and has made possible analyses of the behavior of providers.

Clerkin, Fos, and Petry (1995) discuss the use of an expert system for hospital bed assignment. The system is able to assign beds to a patient at the time of admission to the hospital or during the hospital stay. The assignment is based on a process of matching selected patient characteristics (sex, isolation status, acuity, special patient demands, etc.) with hospital bed characteristics (private vs. semiprivate; whether bed is clean, occupied, or dirty; floor/unit conditions; etc.). The goal is to optimize the match between the patient's needs and the hospital's bed characteristics.

Once the expert system has compared all of the information, a prioritized list of assignment options is presented to the hospital bed assigner, who then makes the assignment. "As such, the expert system serves as a decision consultant." (Clerkin, Fos, and Petry 1995, 390) The expert system then dynamically appends and updates the database to reflect the assignment.

While theoretically the assignment process could be carried out totally manually, the expert system offers several advantages:

- decreased information transfer and retrieval time;
- decreased probability of communication error;
- retained flexibility of a human expert system by providing the user with options; and
- formalized decision-making process with attempts to maximize the needs/availability match and minimize the workload fluctuation. (Clerkin, Fos, and Petry 1995, 398–99)

Adoption of decision-support technology by healthcare executives has proceeded somewhat slowly. This very likely parallels the historical reluctance of executives to use data and quantitative modeling as part of their decision-making process. However, executives are becoming increasingly aware of their need to monitor the key indicators or critical success factors that indicate the financial and operational "health" of their organization. Executives can monitor these indicators using printed reports, or they can access the information electronically using one of the information systems described in the next section.

Executive Information Systems

An executive information system (EIS) is "an information system which draws from multiple applications and multiple data sources, both internal and external to an organization, to provide executives and other decision makers with the necessary information to monitor and analyze the performance of the organization." (Hoven 1996, 49) Healthcare executives are typically interested in a variety of measures indicating their organization's financial performance, clinical outcomes, human resource utilization, access and continuity, and customer satisfaction. The EIS, a specialized database management system capable of query and data retrieval, graphic display, and report generation, can display values for all of these measures, or the executive might specify that only the values that have fallen "out of range" should be provided.

Executive information systems are only as good as the information that is loaded into them. Development of a system requires that the healthcare organization have accurate clinical and business information that can be quickly downloaded to a data warehouse where the information is consolidated into predefined formats and made accessible to the executive user. An Atlanta-based hospital, for example, reports that they "record about a million records every month, and data are updated monthly, although [they] may need to start updating more often." (Dotson 1995, 38) Similarly, Elliott (1996, 38) indicates that "Eighty percent of EIS success depends on how you structure your database. . . . The most important factor in a well-structured database is to visualize how multiple users want to receive the data and design it around their needs."

The extent to which the executive will utilize an EIS depends a great deal on its design. Senior managers who will use the system must therefore directly participate in its development. Milone (1995) suggests interviewing the executives to identify critical success factors that can then be translated into a system design. The system must provide relevant and desired information in a simple, user-friendly manner. By supporting high-quality graphics output, the EIS will allow executives to view their data in pictorial form, although many users still prefer tabular displays. The EIS can be built in-house (as indicated, for example, by a Detroit health system [Laureto-Ward 1996]), or acquired from one of the many vendors offering these systems. (See, for example, the listing of EIS vendors in the Annual Market Directory issue of *Health Management Technology* [Anonymous 1997].) (See also Chapter 8.)

A layered information format within the EIS facilitates probing for more detailed information about a particular measure. But an ongoing design issue is how deeply executives should be able to delve into their data. At some point, the executive will typically call on a functional specialist to obtain a detailed explanation of a value found to be "out of range." In fact one distinction that is often drawn between an EIS and the more general DSS is the greater depth of analytical probing and modeling that is supported by the DSS. Nevertheless, "managers are embracing the concept that more information is better. . . . 'They need access to all types of information, and are seeking to measure performances against standards which they've set.' Executives are seeking as many charts, graphs and reports as they can get their hands on—from all areas of operation." (Elliott 1996, 34)

A Final Thought

The development of DSSs requires an appropriate level of systems analysis and skilled system designers. Management's information needs and related information requirements must be fully understood and analyzed before an in-house system is designed or a packaged software system is purchased. It is the systems analyst's responsibility to pose appropriate questions, and the executive's responsibility to provide answers prior to any system design or implementation.

Performance failures are most likely to occur when the development process lies at either extreme of the design spectrum. An overly simplistic design results in a system able to merely collect and aggregate data rather than to serve as a DSS. Decision-support systems do not spring automatically from existing IS activities. Rather, they must be planned in advance according to a model or format specified by the managers who will use them. Information systems designed to produce periodic operating statistics for hospitals often simply aggregate data rather than breaking them down into meaningful categories, resulting in organizations that are "data rich and information poor."

At the other extreme, design teams often focus too much effort on developing overly sophisticated computing technology. These systems might have clever menus, sound effects, and "eye-catching" visuals, but have limited ability to interface with operational information systems and to provide the executive with needed information. In some cases the system developers feel it is necessary to include these "special features" in order to capture the executive's attention and interest.

These pitfalls can be minimized when the development process has the involvement and *sincere* interest of top management. Executives must look on the installation of a DSS in their organization as one of *their* strategic projects, rather than a necessary activity to be delegated to the IS staff.

Summary

Decision-support systems enable senior managers to adopt an approach to problem solving that is based on the use of data. These data serve as input to a model from which alternatives can be generated and a proposed solution can be identified. While this problem-solving approach could be implemented manually, a DSS has several favorable attributes including ease of interaction, ability to retrieve needed data, ability to appropriately summarize data, built-in modeling capability, and a report writer.

Decision-support systems can be characterized in terms of the components that comprise the system as well as the functions that the system performs. The six components of a DSS are: a user interface, which allows easy communication with the system; a model manager, which coordinates the creation, storage, and retrieval of the models used by the system; the model library, which contains statistical, graphical, financial, and "what-if" models; an array of databases consisting minimally of a clinical repository, financial databases, and external databases; a database management system, which retrieves the needed data; and a report writer, which generates clear, easily understood reports.

Decision-support systems can also be characterized in terms of the functions they perform: retrieve isolated data items; ad hoc analysis of data files; provide standard reports; assist in estimating the consequences of proposed decisions; propose decisions to management; and make decisions according to predetermined decision algorithms.

The information needed for decision support in healthcare settings can be obtained from three basic sources: internal transaction processing systems, which include a variety of financial, operational, and clinical measures; specially constructed databases, containing data obtained in special studies, attitudinal surveys, etc.; and external data sources, including demographic, marketshare, utilization, and physician data.

Management information needs in the modern health services organization include information to support strategic planning, the marketing function, resource allocation, enhancement of productivity and operating efficiency, and outcomes assessment. To be useful, the information must be relevant, sensitive, unbiased, comprehensive, timely, action-oriented, uniform, performance-targeted, and cost-effective. A management database should include information on (1) units of service produced, (2) resources consumed in producing those services, (3) the quality of services rendered, and (4) indicators of effectiveness in meeting perceived community health needs.

Like any software product, a DSS can be obtained in one of four ways. The first is to write the necessary programs from scratch in a suitable language. Second, specialized tools, or "generators," can be used to create the desired system. The third approach is to customize a package. And finally, a turnkey package can be purchased. Most healthcare executives choose one of the latter two options.

Whichever option is chosen for obtaining the system, the system has no value without the availability of appropriate data. The data to support the DSS should be stored in a separate data repository, or data warehouse. Keeping this repository current is often a full-time job performed by a database administrator.

Among the many applications of DSSs are: financial modeling, including analysis of investments and budgeting; planning and marketing, including geographic information systems, mapping, and simulation; resource application, including labor, supplies, and facilities planning; and operations improvement, including staffing and scheduling.

A system that goes beyond the data storage, retrieval, modeling, and reporting capabilities of a DSS is known as an *expert system*. This system attempts to simulate human problem-solving techniques in a computer environment. An expert system consists of a *knowledge base* containing the system expertise, a *database* that the knowledge base is matched against, an *inference engine* that generates suggested conclusions, a *user interface* that links the user to the system, and *workspace* which serves as a "scratch pad."

Executive information systems (EISs) are being used by an increasing number of health services organizations. These software products are sophisticated database management systems with data retrieval, graphics, and report generator capabilities. The EIS requires that the organization have accurate internal and external information available to download into the system. Executive information systems software products are available from several vendors or, occasionally, are developed in-house.

Information systems development in healthcare organizations has tended to focus primarily on applications that support day-to-day operations. Healthcare executives must begin to use information systems *strategically* for survival and growth into the next century. This requires that IS planning be guided by the strategic directions of the organization. The implementation of DSSs is one step in this reorientation.

Discussion Questions

13.1 Define the term decision support.
13.2 Discuss the factors that make having a DSS particularly important for today's healthcare executives.
13.3 Name and describe the six components that comprise a DSS.
13.4 What categories of information should be included in a management database?
13.5 According to Steven Alter, the uses to which decision-support systems are put fall into what six categories?
13.6 What are some of the characteristics of useful management information? How difficult do you believe it would be to build these characteristics into the design of a DSS?

13.7 Name and describe the sources of information for decision support.

13.8 Describe the three strategic orientations suggested by Michael Porter and the information needs associated with each of these orientations.

13.9 What is the relationship between information collected to assist resource allocation and optimization models like linear programming?

13.10 Explain the difference between process benchmarking and outcome benchmarking. What are the implications of this difference on information needs?

13.11 Briefly describe the information interests in outcomes measurements among the various healthcare constituent groups.

13.12 Name and describe alternative ways to develop a DSS.

13.13 Explain the importance of storing data for the DSS separate from the data for the transaction processing system.

13.14 Provide a brief overview of applications that have been made of DSSs in healthcare.

13.15 Name and describe the components of an expert system. How does an expert system differ from a traditional DSS?

13.16 What is an executive information system? Describe how it differs from a DSS.

13.17 Describe the importance of executive participation in the process of developing an executive information system.

13.18 Why do you think that an organization's strategic orientation is important to the development of its information systems?

Problems

13.1 Assume you are the chief executive officer of a health system consisting of a corporate office, a 600-bed teaching hospital, a 400-bed community general hospital, and a 325-bed community general hospital. You plan to appoint a special task force to develop a decision-support system for your health system. (a) What do you suggest should be the composition of this task force? (b) Develop an outline of the talk you will give at the opening meeting of this task force. Your focus should be the charge that you will give to this task force as they begin carrying out this project.

13.2 Conduct an audit of the DSS of a healthcare organization in your locale. Determine the extent to which good management information is available for the following:

a. financial modeling, including budgeting and investment analysis;

  b. marketing analysis, including overview of present patient population as well as a competitor analysis;

  c. productivity analysis;

  d. analysis of patient flow through a department, including waiting times and scheduling; and

  e. measurement of outcomes.

13.3 Use either the organization contacted in Problem 13.2 or another healthcare organization to determine whether their DSS was developed in-house or purchased. In particular, determine the issues that were considered as part of their decision. Finally, determine the support staff that is required to maintain their DSS, including the updating of their data repository.

13.4 Obtain information from vendors of three executive information system software packages. Compare and contrast the features of each of these packages. (The Internet serves as a good source for part of this information.)

References

Aller, K., and A. Rosenstein. 1996. "Outcomes Measurement: Collecting Data for Payors, Providers and Patients." *InfoCare* (September–October): 22–4.

Alter, S. L. 1976. "How Effective Managers Use Information Systems." *Harvard Business Review* 54 (November–December): 97–104.

Anonymous. 1995. "Sachs Group Data Helps Health Care Organizations Plan, Market, and Manage." *Health Care Strategic Management* 13 (9): 17.

Anonymous. 1996. "The MEDSTAT Group is a Market Leader in Healthcare Databases." *Health Care Strategic Management* 14 (2): 14.

Anonymous. 1997. "Product Breakouts—Decision—Support—Managerial—Financial." *Health Management Technology* 18 (3): 89–91.

Austin, C. J., and S. B. Boxerman. 1995. *Quantitative Analysis for Health Services Administration*. Chicago: AUPHA Press/Health Administration Press.

Austin, C. J., J. M. Trimm, and P. M. Sobczak. 1995. "Information Systems and Strategic Management." *Health Care Management Review* 20 (3): 26–33.

Benson, H. R. 1996. "Benchmarking in Healthcare: Evaluating Data and Transforming It into Action." *Radiology Management* 18 (1): 40–46.

Boland, P. 1996. "The Role of Reengineering in Health Care Delivery." *Managed Care Quarterly* 4 (4): 1–11.

Clerkin, D., P. J. Fos, and F. E. Petry. 1995. "A Decision Support System for Hospital Bed Assignment." *Hospital & Health Services Administration* 40 (3): 386–400.

Dotson, B. 1995. "For the Busy Healthcare Executive: Information Tools." *Healthcare Informatics* 12 (1): 36–38, 40.

Elliott, J. 1996. "Making the Executive Decision." *Healthcare Informatics* 13 (7): 33–34, 36, 38.

Evans, J. 1997a. "The Virtual Focus Group: Decision Support Systems." *Health Management Technology* 18 (6): 36–38, 52.

———. 1997b. "The Lay of the Land: GIS and Mapping Software." *Health Management Technology* 18 (5): 58, 60.

Forgionne, G. A. 1991. "Using Decision Support Systems to Market Prepaid Medical Plans." *Journal of Healthcare Marketing* 11 (4): 22–38.

Graham, M. V. 1995. "A Day-to-Day Decision Support Tool." *Nursing Management* 26 (3): 48I, 48L.

Harrison, M. 1995. "Process Benchmarking in Health Care." In *Proceedings of the 1995 Annual HIMSS Conference*. San Antonio, TX: Healthcare Information and Management Systems Society, Volume 3. 241–52.

Hartless, C., and J. A. Hager. 1995. "Data Driven Reengineering Results in Wellness Delivery Model for Obstetrics." In *Proceedings of the 1995 Annual HIMSS Conference*. San Antonio, TX: Healthcare Information and Management Systems Society, Volume 1. 309–21.

Hoven, J. van den. 1996. "Executive Support Systems and Decision Making." *Journal of Systems Management* 47 (2): 48–55.

Kachnowski, S. 1997. "Outcomes Management: A System Long Overdue." *Healthcare Informatics* 14 (1): 27–29, 32–33.

Ladaga, J. 1995. "Let Business Goals Drive Your Data Warehouse Effort." *Health Management Technology* 16 (11): 26, 28.

Laureto-Ward, R. A. 1996. "Searching for the Perfect EIS." *Healthcare Informatics* 13 (7): 74.

Mace, J. D. 1995. "Process Redesign: Making Your Film Library Work For You." *Radiology Management* 17 (4): 52–60.

Mallach, E. G. 1994. *Understanding Decision Support Systems and Expert Systems*. Burr Ridge, IL: Irwin.

McClean, S., and P. H. Millard. 1995. "A Decision Support System for Bed-Occupancy Management and Planning Hospitals." *IMA Journal of Mathematics Applied in Medicine and Biology* 12 (3–4): 249–57.

Milone, M. 1995. "Implementing an EIS, One Step At a Time." *Healthcare Informatics* 12 (1): 42, 44.

Moore, J. D. Jr. 1997. "JCAHO Tries Again. Agency Moves to Accredit Providers Based On Outcomes [news]." *Modern Healthcare* 26 (45): 2–3.

Raco, R., C. Shapleigh, and D. Cook. 1989. "Decision Support in the 1990s: The Future is Now." *Computers in Healthcare* 10 (12): 26–29.

Sempeles, S. 1996. "Decision Support: Simplifying the Information." *InfoCare* (September–October): 26–29.

Sengin, K. K., and A. M. Dreisbach. 1995. "Managing With Precision: A Budgetary Decision Support Model." *Journal of Nursing Administration* 25 (2): 33–44.

Siwicki, B. 1995. "Slicing Costs in the OR." *Health Data Management* 3 (9): 33–34.

———. 1996. "Artificial Intelligence." *Health Data Management* 4 (4): 46–48, 50–53.

Sodhi, M. 1996. "Development of a DSS for Fixed-Income Securities Using OOP." *Interfaces* 26 (2): 22–33.

Stearns, F. E., and J. Mazie. 1996. "Using PC-Based Decision-Support Technology to Improve Efficiency." *Healthcare Financial Management* 50 (11): 39–41.

Van Merode, G. G., A. Hasman, J. Derks, H. M. Goldschmidt, B. Schoenmaker, and M. Oosten. 1995. "Decision Support for Clinical Laboratory Capacity Planning." *International Journal of Bio-Medical Computing* 38 (1): 75–87.

Additional Readings

Bergman, R. 1994. "From the Top Down: EIS Works for Everybody." *Hospitals & Health Networks* 68 (18): 68.

Collins, L. W. 1994. "TQM Information Systems: An Elusive Goal." *Joint Commission Journal on Quality Improvement* 20 (11): 607–13.

Edwards, L. 1995. "Supporting Executive Decision-Making With EIS." *Healthcare Informatics* 12 (8): 58, 62.

Forgionne, G. A., and R. Kohli. 1996. "HMSS: A Management Support System for Concurrent Hospital Decision Making." *Decision Support Systems* 16 (3): 209–29.

Gilbreath, R. E., J. Schilp, and R. Pickton. 1996. "Toward an Outcomes Management Informational Processing Architecture." *Healthcare Information Management* 10 (1): 83–97.

Gove, D., D. Hewett, and A. Shahani. 1995. "Towards a Model for Hospital Case-Load Decision Support." *IMA Journal of Mathematics Applied in Medicine and Biology* 12 (3–4): 329–38.

Griffith, J. R. 1995. *The Well-Managed Health Care Organization*, 3d Ed. Chicago: AUPHA Press/Health Administration Press.

Griffith, J. R., V. K. Sahney, and R. A. Mohr. 1995. *Reengineering Health Care: Building on CQI*. Chicago: Health Administration Press.

Hampshire, D. A., and B. J. Rosborough. 1993. "The Evolution of Decision Support in a Managed Care Organization." *Topics in Health Care Financing* 20 (2): 26–37.

Hannah, K. J. "Transforming Information: Data Management Support of Health Care Reorganization." *Journal of the American Medical Informatics Association* 2 (3): 147–55.

Hoffman, T. 1997. "Maine Drives Medicaid Reform With Decision-Support System." *Computerworld* 31 (3): 67–68.

Hornig, D., and J. M. Vezina. 1997. "Knowledge-Based Decision Support: How to Deliver Solutions." In *Proceedings of the 1997 Annual HIMSS Conference*. San Diego, CA: Healthcare Information and Management Systems Society, Volume 4. 199–210.

Jacobs, S. M., and S. Pelfrey. 1995. "Decision Support Systems. Using Computers to Help Manage." *Journal of Nursing Administration* 25 (2): 46–51.

Kusters, R. J., and P. M. A. Groot. "Modeling Resource Availability in General Hospitals— Design and Implementation of a Decision Support Model." *European Journal of Operational Research* 88 (3): 428–45.

Laureto-Ward, R. A. 1995. "Looking for the Best EIS." *Healthcare Informatics* 12 (8): 58, 62.

Mattison, R. 1996. *Data Warehousing: Strategies, Technologies, and Techniques*. New York: McGraw-Hill, Inc.

Miles, R. E., and C. C. Snow. 1978. *Organizational Strategy, Structure, and Process*. New York: McGraw-Hill, Inc.

Porter, M. E. 1985. *Competitive Advantage*. New York: Free Press.

———. 1980. *Competitive Strategy: Techniques for Analyzing Industries and Competitors*. New York: Free Press.

Rafanelli, M., F. Ferri, R. Maceratini, and G. Sindoni. 1995. "An Object Oriented Decision Support System for the Planning of Health Resource Allocation." *Computer Methods and Programs in Biomedicine* 48 (1–2): 163–68.

Schneider, P. 1996. "Consult an Expert: Your Computer." *Healthcare Informatics* 13 (5): 37–38, 40, 42.

Shapin, P. G. 1994. "Washington Hospital Center's EIS Success." *Healthcare Informatics* 11 (6): 26, 28.

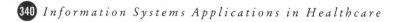

Shortell, S. M., E. M. Morrison, and B. Friedman. 1990. *Strategic Choices for America's Hospitals.* San Francisco: Jossey-Bass Publishers.

Stipek, C. E. 1995. "Grouping Systems Enhance Outcomes Analysis." *Topics in Health Information Management* 15 (4): 14–25.

Urden, L. D. 1996. "Development of a Nurse Executive Decision Support Database. A Model for Outcomes Evaluation." *Journal of Nursing Administration* 26 (10): 15–21.

Walker, L. 1994. "Unlocking the Information Vault." *InfoCare* (June): 14–16, 18, 20.

MANAGED CARE APPLICATIONS

Brian T. Malec

MANAGED CARE is an all-encompassing term describing the organizational arrangements by which health plans offer a comprehensive package of health services to members of a defined population for a set fee. The consumer/patient is given financial incentives to use physicians and facilities associated with the health plan.

Concepts and Applications

With the advent of managed care comes a host of new requirements for the healthcare executive. Decisions must be made about capitation, community health, and the cost and effectiveness of care. Similarly, healthcare patients, who are becoming more and more savvy about the care they purchase, can use healthcare information to make more informed decisions. An information system can collect and process healthcare data to assist in cost containment and quality assurance.

After reading this chapter, readers will also be able to discuss the implications of managed care for an organization's information systems. They will be able to list the users of healthcare information in the managed care environment and the type of information they need.

Enrollees' out-of-pocket costs are usually small and entail a copayment for delivery of service or the purchase of prescriptions. (See Chapter 1 and the Additional Readings at the end of this chapter for more detail on managed care.)

According to the 1996 Annual HIMSS/Hewlett-Packard Leadership Survey, "Managed care continues to be the dominant force in health care as organizations focus on the bottom line and control of costs." (HIMSS/HP 1996) Forty-nine percent of survey respondents believe that managed care is the single most important factor driving information technology in healthcare. Fifty-seven percent believe that managed care will have a positive influence on healthcare by either lowering costs or improving outcomes (both of which are information-intensive activities). However, 41 percent felt that managed care will have negative consequences for the delivery of healthcare to consumers. Respondents believe that knowledge of managed care, along with its implications for information systems and the management of those systems, will occupy a significant portion of a health administrator's day-to-day responsibility.

This chapter will discuss the application of information systems (IS) within the managed care environment, including: (1) information needs in the managed care marketplace; (2) users of information in the managed care environment; (3) the managed care software market; and (4) a brief case study of the IS needs of a Medicaid HMO.

Information Needs in the Managed Care Marketplace

Managed care plans have special needs for information systems that differ from those of fee for service systems. The healthcare market has responded to managed care in four ways: (1) the change in economic incentives; (2) the emphasis on wellness and prevention; (3) the shift to capitated payment; and (4) the need to demonstrate quality of outcomes. Information requirements resulting from these market responses are discussed.

Economic Incentives. The move to a managed care environment has resulted in many new economic incentives in the healthcare delivery system. These incentives to produce services in a way that balances the cost of production with the expected outcome are a departure from the past. Changing economic incentives have, in turn, resulted in a number of changes in the way services are provided, for example:

- delivery of care in the least costly environment (inpatient vs. outpatient vs. home based);
- use of generic rather than brand-name drugs;
- use of primary care physicians, "gatekeepers," and restricted access to specialists;

- use of clinical guidelines to ensure quality and reduce costs;
- more effective use of healthcare workers (multitasking);
- development of formal quality review programs; and
- financial incentives for patients to use physicians and providers within the plan for care rather than going outside of the plan.

Information systems take on great importance in this environment. For instance, providers, consumers, and purchasers of care need information to monitor the cost, quality, and utilization of services provided by the managed care plan.

Wellness and Health Promotion. Managed care plans emphasize wellness and health promotion in order to help reduce the costs of treating illness among enrollees. Conversely, the traditional healthcare system has historically been grounded in managing the delivery of services to sick or injured persons. It emphasized diagnosis and treatment of acute and chronic illnesses. But, under managed care, providers receive fixed payment for all covered persons; therefore they have an incentive to provide services to the "well" population in addition to treating those who are sick.

Managed care plans need information systems that enable them to continuously monitor the health status of the population being served. Epidemiological data on community health status can be obtained from public health agencies at the state and local level. Careful monitoring of service utilization by enrollees can help identify conditions that could have been prevented through wellness programs (health education, periodic checkups, screening, and immunization). Information systems to support epidemiological surveillance are essential in managed care. Managed care organizations (MCOs) are combining software that can analyze population-based information, such as census data and epidemiological information, with geographical information systems to evaluate and map the covered population. (DesHarnais, Marshall, and Dulski 1994)

Capitation. Capitation is a negotiated payment to a provider on a per member per month basis to provide care over a given time period. It places providers and insurers at risk should the cost of providing services exceed the available pool of resources. The provider must stay within the capitated rate or assume all or part of the financial risk for the additional cost of treatment. "Risk pools" are established based on capitated payments from members of the health plan. If money remains in the pool at the end of a contract period, then some or all of the remaining funds are paid to those who managed the risk. Under fee-for-service payment systems, the costs of production are passed through to insurers who pay usual and customary costs. In an "at-risk" contract, the provider has an incentive to reduce the use of resources and space in high-cost facilities and to use the least costly combination of labor to provide care.

Information systems that monitor costs and utilization of services are essential under capitation. They serve as the basis for negotiating rates to be paid under capitated contracts. In addition, they provide essential information to management for service planning and cost control.

Quality of Outcomes. Purchasers of healthcare (employers and public and private insurers) and consumers of care are demanding information on the quality of services provided by their health plans. Employers and health plan members demand information about the value of treatment received or information to "evaluate the effectiveness of treatments and compare results across settings." (Kibbe 1994) This focus on quality outcomes requires providers to design and implement information systems capable of reporting patient-care specific information on the quality of services rendered. "Increasingly, information about performance and outcomes of care delivery can be thought of as a product." (Kibbe 1994, 593)

"Report cards" on the costs and quality of healthcare have been developed by individual employers, industry coalitions, some large health maintenance organizations (HMOs), and accrediting organizations. (See Chapter 1.)

The National Committee on Quality Assurance (NCQA) is a non-profit, voluntary organization that accredits health maintenance organizations and other managed care plans. (Web site: http://www.ncqa.org) NCQA has developed the Health Plan Employer Data and Information Set (HEDIS) for use in accreditation of health plans and as a source of information for employers and consumers in making health plan choices. HEDIS currently measures HMO performance in eight majors areas:

1. effectiveness of care;
2. access to/availability of care;
3. satisfaction with the experience of care;
4. health plan stability;
5. use of services;
6. cost of care;
7. informed healthcare choices; and
8. health plan descriptive information. (Penner 1997, 254–56)

Within these eight categories, specific HEDIS measures include such items as consumer satisfaction, member disenrollment, immunization rates for children and adolescents, physicians under capitation, and length-of-stay in hospitals. To participate in the HEDIS rating system, HMOs must agree to be reviewed by NCQA. (DesHarnais, Marshall, and

Dulski 1994) At present, 87.2 percent of HMOs report either HEDIS or similar data to employers and the public. (McCormack 1997, 48) While the distribution of information is limited and the review is voluntary, the measurement does provide information that is useful for comparison.

The marketplace for quality information as a "product" is growing and new instruments will be developed to help employers, patients/consumers, and regulatory agencies make more informed decisions.

Users of Managed Care Information

Four groups generate, consume, interpret, or modify the information present in a managed care environment: (1) purchasers who pay health plan premiums; (2) consumers of services; (3) service providers (physicians, hospitals, and other health services organizations); and (4) managed care plans (HMOs, preferred provider organizations [PPOs], and exclusive provider arrangements [EPAs] developed by integrated delivery systems). These users expect to have the information they need to make decisions in a timely, cost-effective manner and at the location where they need it. This section reviews the information needs and related decision models of each group.

Purchasers

Employers are a primary purchaser of managed care products as part of their health insurance programs for employees. In addition, the federal government is a major purchaser of HMO products for Medicare recipients, and many state governments are contracting with HMOs for the Medicaid population. These purchasers need information to help evaluate the benefit package of each managed care plan, the costs and quality of services provided, and the service utilization patterns of their employees or recipients. To do this, they need information such as:

- comparison of the costs and benefits among alternate health plans;
- demographics of the covered population;
- utilization history and claims experience of the covered population; and
- report cards on plan performance (e.g., HEDIS scores).

There is growing demand being placed on providers from individual employers, as well as business and community coalitions, for information about the quality and utilization of health services. These purchaser groups are demanding accountability. They want to know how much care was consumed, from whom, and for what. This information helps the employer develop business strategies for reducing premium costs and selecting among health plans. Some businesses also use the information to develop employee education, wellness, and health promotion activities.

Consumers

Consumers who are considering enrolling in an HMO, PPO, or other type of health plan need information to decide among the competing alternatives. Whether the employer pays the entire premium or part of it, the consumer needs information to answer questions such as:

- What alternate enrollment choices are available?
- What is the cost of each alternative?
- How does the range of benefits differ among plans (limitations, copayments, deductibles)?
- What is the quality of the provider pool?
- Where is the nearest provider located?

HEDIS reports are helpful to consumers by providing some comparative information. The marketplace is also addressing the information needs of consumers by way of the Internet and various Web sites. Chapter 16 describes in greater detail how this emerging technology can support consumer as well as employer needs for information concerning managed care organizations.

Providers of Health Services

Healthcare providers need information to stay competitive in a managed care environment. Physicians and healthcare organizations with managed care contracts have information needs that differ from those of employers and consumers. Some larger health services organizations operate their own HMO or PPO plans and have information requirements similar to managed care plans as described in the next section.

Clinical and administrative information systems used by providers have been discussed in Chapters 11 and 12. These transaction processing systems produce much of the information needed by individual providers to respond to the demands of managed care. In this section, the focus is on those unique information applications needed under managed care. Figure 14.1 lists critical functions performed by providers in a managed care contract environment and the IS applications related to these functions.

Financial Monitoring. All healthcare organizations, whether operating under managed care or not, must have information systems that provide basic financial information. Within the managed care environment, the need for a cost-accounting system becomes critical because so much of what management has to do depends on the availability of accurate cost

Figure 14.1 Provider Functions and Associated Information Requirements

Provider Functions	Examples of Applications
Financial Monitoring	• Balance Sheets • Income Statements • Financial Statements • General Accounting • Cost Accounting • Premium Billing and Accounts Receivable
Management of Capitated Contracts	• Provider Profiles and Contracted Fee Schedules • Historical Data and Utilization of Services • Membership Reports by Age, Gender, Benefits Plan • Capitation Reconciliation and Verification Reports • Delivery of Services Reports: Utilization Rates, Charges per Service per Member per Month • Physician Profiling—Hospital Admission Patterns • Summaries of Hospital Admissions: Length-of-Stay, Hospital Days and Cost by Category, Physician Speciality, and Facility (Herrie and Pollock 1995)
Strategic Planning and Decision Making	• Forecasting Models • Contracting Models for Negotiation and Management • Budgeting Models • Utilization Management • Development of Clinical Pathways, Guidelines, and Other Physician Monitoring Devices • Member Demographics • Geographic Information Systems (Mapping) • Capitation Tracking and Modeling • Marketing Support (Posner 1996)
Patient/Member Services	• Health Promotion and Education • Access to Information About Services/Providers
Management of Multiple Lines of Business	• Multiple Managed Care Contracts • Government Accounts (Medicare, Medicaid, etc.) • Individual Coverage • Group Billing, Benefits Management, Eligibility • Management Service Organization (MSO)

information. An ideal cost-accounting system provides cost information by type of service, diagnostic category, physician and medical specialty, facility location, and managed care contract. (Hampshire and Rosborough 1996) Information generated by the cost-accounting system aids in contract negotiations, monitoring of existing contracts, and capitation rate setting.

Management of Capitated Contracts. Capitation contracts place the provider at risk and must be carefully managed. Special subsystems have been developed to help providers with electronic claims processing, enrollee profiles, details on health plans and their benefits, provider profiles, treatment authorizations, and other components. Managed care has generated the need for detailed information on the quality of services provided and the populations served under capitated contracts.

Strategic Planning and Decision Making. Chapter 13 examined decision-support systems for healthcare organizations. The need for such systems increases under managed care. Budgeting and forecasting models, development of care maps, and other management decision-support systems are essential Providers are also using geographic information systems (GISs) to map patient and facility location data to plan for better coverage of the capitated populations that they serve. (Franzblau 1994)

Patient/Member Services. With the increased presence of managed care in most marketplaces, providers are using information systems to communicate with patients and provide information on programs and services offered including health education and promotion. Chapter 16 will discuss Internet applications that support health education programs.

Management of Multiple Lines of Business. Providers often have contracts with multiple managed care organizations. Information systems that separate out unique aspects of each individual line of business are essential. Keeping lines of business clearly focused and separated helps the organization maximize its total profitability.

Managed Care Organizations

The information systems needed by HMOs, PPOs, EPAs, and other managed care organizations include those administrative systems discussed in Chapter 12. Managed care organizations are businesses that must have financial, human resources, facility scheduling, and other applications that support the effective management of the organizations. However, MCOs also need specialized applications to support their core managed care functions. Because MCO services span a wide portion of the continuum of care, management software also spans a considerable range of possible applications. John McCormack (1997, 45) points out that many HMOs are finding vendors to provide satisfactory solutions to core applications such as management of enrollment, referrals and treatment authorization, and processing of claims. However, these same

HMOs are then building in-house applications to meet specific needs such as tracking various market indicators to determine how the competition is doing.

Figure 14.2 presents both core MCO functions and other specialized functions supported by information systems. (Kissinger and Borchardt 1996)

Financial Monitoring. Managed care organizations are similar to provider organizations in the need for basic financial information on the operations of the business functions of the health plan. MCOs use financial information to monitor existing contracts with providers, aide in new contract negotiations, and set capitation rates.

Preparation of Standard Analytical Reports and Decision Models. An example of a Standard Analytical Report necessary for effective management of an MCO is "utilization management statistics." A utilization report might contain such information as: patient encounters, claims, referrals, use of ancillary services, and trend data. This series of reports is useful for negotiating future managed care contracts; deciding capitation rates; computing physician and other provider productivity measures; and helping with outcome research. (Posner 1996) Managed care information systems also are important in tracking referral patterns, out-of-network utilization, and provider profiles. The reports and decision models listed in Figure 14.2 help MCOs manage the relationship between input resources, the flow of consumers through the system, and the standards of productivity for the organization and its providers.

Actuarial and epidemiologic information systems are essential tools for MCOs. Health plans must track trends in health status and disease incidence among their members. Some organizations do not have the internal expertise to do the necessary analysis and therefore contract with consultants to provide actuarial reports on the covered populations.

Clinical pathways, or care maps, are becoming a standard mechanism for monitoring business practices and evaluating clinical outcomes. A care map is an optimum, standardized clinical care plan designed to provide care for a typical patient for a specific procedure or condition. (Meyer and Feingold 1995) When combined with other systems, a care map can help estimate the expected cost for each episode of care for a particular procedure. (Posner 1996) For example, epidemiological analysis of the covered population might result in an estimate that 0.2 percent of that population potentially could need a particular procedure within the next year (i.e., repair of a broken leg). Based on that analysis and the application of a care map, MCOs can allocate resources for an economically efficient and clinically effective treatment.

Figure 14.2 Managed Care Organization Functions and Associated Information Requirements

Core Functions	Examples of Applications
Financial Monitoring	• Balance Sheets • Income Statements • Financial Statements • General Accounting • Cost Accounting • Premium Billing and Accounts Receivable • Payment Tracking for Contracts, Subcontracts
Preparation of Standard Analytical Reports and Decision Models	• Performance Statistics • Utilization Management • Provider Reporting: Inpatient and Outpatient • Referral Patterns • Inpatient and Outpatient Out-of-Network Utilization • Case-Mix Analysis • Provider Profiling • Actuarial Analysis
Management Control and Reporting	• Membership Analysis • Eligibility/Verifications Tracking • Utilization Rates by Groups, Age, Gender • Quality Indicators • Financial Reporting • Regulatory Reporting • Budgeting Models • Forecasting Models • Contract Modeling and Projections
Claims Payment and Prospective/Capitation Payment Processing	• Capitation Payments • Claims Payment, Network and Out-of-Network • Claims Adjudication • Encounter Statistics • Claims Grouping by Episodes of Care
Management of Multiple Lines of Business	• Government Accounts (Medicare, Medicaid, etc.) • Individual Coverage • Group Billing, Benefits Management, Eligibility
Marketing and Sales Support	• Enrollment and Disenrollment Trends • Geographic Distribution of Members and Providers • Contract Negotiation and Management • Rate Management/Actuarial Services

Continued

Figure 14.2 Continued

Core Functions	Examples of Applications
	• Account Management and Analysis • Forecasting Models • Provider Databases and Credentials
Profitability	• Per Member Per Month Costs and Premiums • Medical Loss Ratios
Member/Customer Services	• Customer Service Inquiry • Internet Access to MCO • Member Health/Wellness Education and Promotion • Epidemiological Analysis
Employer Information Needs	• HEDIS Reporting • Outcomes Measurement • Employer Group Enrollment Tracking and Reporting • Utilization History and Claims Experience of Covered Population

Management Control and Reporting. In addition to standard financial reports, forecasts, and decision models, MCO managers need information on membership characteristics, utilization of services, and various quality measures.

Claims Payment and Prospective/Capitation Payment Processing. Claims payment and processing is a specialized function of a managed care organization. MCOs must have information systems that process claims and make payments to providers who are members of the health plan network as well as to out-of-network providers if authorized by point-of-service options available to members. Out-of-network claims will normally be reimbursed at a lower rate with the enrollee paying increased copayments.

Management of Multiple Lines of Business. MCOs are complex businesses that have contracts with numerous employers, governments agencies, and individual members. Information systems that monitor the performance of each individual line of business are essential.

Marketing and Sales Support. Information systems are needed to support the marketing and sales functions of MCOs. Marketing information systems will monitor trends in enrollment and disenrollment of members, the geographic distribution of covered populations, locations of providers and facilities, and general demographic characteristics of plan members and the community at large. Geographic information systems are useful tools for graphic analysis and modeling of demographic and marketshare information. (Environmental Systems Research Institute 1996)

Profitability. MCOs must monitor financial indicators that are commonplace in the insurance industry. Medical loss ratios (benefits paid divided by premiums received) are important indicators of the profitability of health plans. The smaller the benefits paid out, the larger the difference will be between expenses and revenue, resulting in a smaller "loss" ratio. The difference between revenue and expenses covers the administrative and marketing costs of the health plan and is also used to pay stockholder dividends in for-profit MCOs.

Member/Customer Services. A customer focus and service orientation is critical for success in managed care organizations. One tool is an information system used to communicate with the membership. Automated systems can provide information about hours and locations of operations, new services available, wellness programs, and healthier lifestyles. They can also answer common questions concerning benefits. Many MCOs are developing home pages on the Internet to provide information to current and prospective members. (See Chapter 16.)

Employer Information Needs. As discussed, the employer is an important consumer of managed care information. Through HEDIS reporting and analysis of utilization data, employers can design benefit packages that meet the needs of their employees and reduce the company's premium costs. Employers are demanding accountability from the health plans with whom they have contracts. Managed care organizations must be prepared to provide information on costs, quality, and utilization of services when requested by employers and other purchasers of care.

In summary, managed care organizations (MCOs) have all the basic needs for administrative information systems plus the special functional requirements discussed. The difference between an application of an information system in a managed care environment and other more traditional method of healthcare delivery is often a matter of degree. The special requirements of managed care plans and provider organizations who offer managed care products include information systems for the negotiation, monitoring, and management of capitated contracts; quality control; marketing and enrollment services; and customer support.

The Managed Care Software Market

The vendor market for managed care software applications is volatile and expanding rapidly. Figure 14.3 gives examples of the types of software

Figure 14.3   Healthcare Software Vendors

Representative Company	Number of Installations as of 1996	Target Market for Software	Examples of Modules and/ or Applications
Vendor A	3	IPAs PPOs HMOs	Enrollment/Eligibility and Benefits Encounter, Referral and Claims Tracking Tracks Practice Patterns of Primary Care Physicians Claims Adjudication Account Processing (Provider Reimbursement)
Vendor B	50+	IPAs HMOs	Provider Profiles Benefit Summary and Coverage Enrollee Profiles Specialist and Hospital Treatment Authorization Capitation Payment to Providers Risk-Sharing Arrangements
Vendor C	15	small-to-medium HMOs, PPOs, and PHOs	Enrollment and Eligibility Premium Billing Utilization Management Capitation and Fee-for-Service Reimbursement Ad Hoc Reporting
Vendor D	3	IPAs	Payor and Provider Contracts Claims Processing Central Data Repository User-Defined Reports
Vendor E	39	PHOs MSOs HMOs IPAs	Membership Eligibility Capitation and Provider Risk Management Utilization Management Reinsurance Management Check Processing Electronic Data Interchange Claims Status and Submission Authorization and Referral Processing Provider Reimbursement

products available in 1996. Because of the pace of software product changes and the volatility of the market, no company names are provided. The examples are abstracted and condensed from vendor literature, other printed sources, and various Web sites.

The vendor market has many small companies, each with speciality products. In the future it is expected that the market will consolidate with fewer and larger vendors who offer a full range of products and services. The healthcare manager can either use a strategy to select vendors carefully who will survive the test of time in the marketplace or be prepared to adapt quickly to new systems and vendors as the market changes.

Volatility in the managed care software market reflects the rapid change occurring in the healthcare delivery system. These changes create a challenging environment for management, including:

- the political and economic uncertainty of the healthcare market;
- the unstable nature and short life cycle of some vendor products;
- the high cost of conversion from older information systems; and
- the lack of management understanding and experience in using technology to enhance decision making in a managed care environment.

Case Study: L.A. Care

Across the United States, Medicaid and Medicare HMOs are being established in the hope of controlling the growth in state and federal government expenditures for populations covered by these programs. In California, the Medicaid program (called Med-Cal) has begun the process of moving all Medicaid recipients to a managed care plan. In the Los Angeles area, the state has authorized two managed care health plans for Medicaid recipients. One is a commercial for-profit health plan and the other is a local initiative nonprofit health plan. When fully operational, the local initiative plan (called L.A. Care) will cover more than 700,000 members, will have 3,000 primary care providers and 10,000 contracting physicians, and will result in 4 million outpatient visits and 210,000 inpatient days annually. (Massey 1997) L.A. Care is a "health plan for health plans" because the actual delivery of services will be carried out and administered through seven plan partners. The plan partners are existing MCOs that contract with L.A. Care to provide services to a specified number of Med-Cal recipients. The plan partners include Blue Cross of California, Care 1st Health Plan, Maxicare, Tower Health, United Health Plan, Kaiser Foundation Health Plan, and Los Angeles County Community Health Plan.

As a start-up organization, L.A. Care had to create an information system from the beginning. Calvin Massey, the chief information officer of L.A. Care, was charged with developing a high-level systems architecture, defining the business processes, and developing an RFP for managed care, financial, and other administrative systems. L.A. Care selected packaged software for general ledger, financial, and human resources systems. The managed care functions required a software system capable of a wide variety of activities including:

- sorting monthly tapes of current enrollees from the State of California by plan partners and doctors;
- reconciling enrollee income and payout to partners via contracts; and
- monitoring the demographic characteristics of enrollees in order to match them to the appropriate service providers.

L.A. Care chose a national vendor of managed healthcare information systems, CSC Healthcare Systems to be the principal software provider. Selected CSC applications used by L.A. Care include membership and enrollment monitoring; provider profiling; reporting on capitation, network penetration, and profitablility; and preparation of HEDIS reports.

Future plans call for a budget forecasting system capable of integrating enrollment data coordinated with the managed care system for continuous updates and management control. A geographic information system (GIS) is also planned to help manage the delivery of services by the plan partners and to support the matching of Medi-Cal recipients with service locations.

Summary

Managed care organizations have emerged in the current decade as a significant market force. These organizations, and the various constituencies associated with them, will continue to demand and need a wide range of information systems. The twin forces of cost containment and quality improvement challenge MCO organizations. The economic, quality, and marketing incentives of managed care drive the end-users of information to engage in decision-making activities that require integrated and flexible information systems.

There are four distinct groups that either generate, consume, interpret, or modify the information that is needed in a managed care environment. They are (1) purchasers who pay the premium; (2) consumers of healthcare services; (3) providers of services (physicians and health services organizations); and (4) the health plan or managed care organization.

Purchasers (employers and public or private insurers) require information about utilization of services by the covered population, availability of wellness programs and incentives for healthy lifestyles, ratings of quality such as HEDIS measures, and the satisfaction of consumers with the health plans. Consumers seek information on the costs and quality of alternative health plans and the ease of access to services. Providers of health services must respond to demands from health plans for cost and quality information. Providers need a range of information products that support capitated payment systems, normal business operations, quality improvement, clinical and management decision support, provider profiles, and demographic information on the covered populations. In addition to general administrative and clinical systems, managed care plans need advanced information systems to support a variety of special needs including systems for capitation management, tracking of utilization and referral patterns, actuarial analysis of financial risk, marketing, and membership and enrollment services.

The volatile nature of the managed care software market challenges administrators to select products that will be stable for more than just a few years.

Discussion Questions

14.1 How have financial incentives changed under managed care? What is the impact of these changes on information system requirements?

14.2 Who are the primary users of managed care information systems?

14.3 What kinds of information do consumers and employers need to make selections among health plans? How do the information needs of these two groups differ?

14.4 What is HEDIS? How is it used in evaluating managed care plans?

14.5 What are the similarities and differences between the information system needs of individual providers and managed care plans?

14.6 What is the overall impact of managed care on the demand for health information systems?

Problems

14.1 Survey a local managed care organization using the basic information systems functions found in Figure 14.2. Determine which of the basic functions: (1) are currently in use by the MCO; (2) are not in use at this time, but will be in the future; (3) will never be implemented; or (4) are additional information systems applications that were not included in Figure 14.2.

14.2 Survey local healthcare providers to find out what software vendors they are using to support managed care activities. Explore the World Wide Web (WWW) to find these software vendors and develop a brief report on the types of products they offer.

References

DesHarnais, S., B. Marshall, and J. Dulski. 1994. "Information Management in the Age of Managed Competition." *Journal of Quality Improvement* 20 (November): 631–38.

Environmental Systems Research Institute. 1996. "Geographic Information Systems (GIS) Solutions for Healthcare," unpublished material by ESRI. Internet Home-page—http://www.esri.com [Retrieved: March 1997].

Franzblau, D. 1994. "Hospitals Using Mapping Data to Plan Network Coverage." *Health Care Strategic Management*, 12 (July): 14–15.

Hampshire, D., and B. Rosborough. 1996. "The Evolution of Decision Support in Managed Care Organizations." *Topics in Health Care Financing* 20 (2): 26–37.

Healthcare Information and Management Systems Society and Hewlett-Packard Company (HIMSS/HP). 1996. *Seventh Annual Leadership Survey: Trends in Health Care Computing*, Chicago: The Society.

Herrie, G., and W. Pollock. 1995. "Multi-speciality Medical Groups: Adapting to Capitation." *Journal of Health Care Finance* 21 (3): 37–43.

Kibbe, D. 1994. "Designing Quality Into Health Care Information Systems." *Journal of Quality Improvement* 20 (November): 591–94.

Kissinger, K., and S. Borchardt, eds. 1996. *Information Technology for Integrated Health Systems, Positioning for the Future*. New York: John Wiley and Sons.

Massey, C. 1997. "Local Initiative Health Authority of Los Angeles County." Unpublished presentation at Southern California Chapter of HIMSS, May.

McCormack, J. 1997. "HMO Automation Strategies." *Health Data Management* April: 44–50.

Meyer, J. W., and M. Feingold. 1995. "Integrating Financial Modeling and Patient Care Reengineering." *Healthcare Financial Management* 49 (2): 33–40.

Penner, M. J. 1997. *Capitation in California: A Study of Physician Organizations Managing Risk*, 254–56. Chicago, Health Administration Press.

Posner, B. L. 1996. "The Development of an Integrated Decision Support System for Provider Risk Contracting." Unpublished master's thesis, Health Administration Program, California State University, Northridge.

Additional Readings

Anonymous. 1994. "Managed Care Software: The Next Generation." *Nursing Management* 25 (March): 28–29.

Anonymous. 1997. "Managed Care Systems: New Capabilities for Growing Markets." *Health Management Technology*, April: 62–67.

Austin, C. J., and P. M. Sobczak. 1993. "Information Technology and Managed Care." *Hospital Topics* 71 (3): 33–37

Bernard, A., R. Hayward, J. Anderson, J. Rosevear, and L. McMahon. 1995. "The Integrated Management Model, Lessons for Managed Care." *Medical Care* 33 (July 1): 663–75.

Brennan, C. 1995. "Managed Care and Health Information Networks." *Journal of Health Care Finance* 21 (Summer): 1–5.

Ciotti, V., and F. Zodda. 1996. "Selecting Managed Care Information Systems." *Healthcare Financial Management*, 50 (June): 35–40.

Coddington, D. C., J. Pollard. 1995. "Information Systems and Integrated Healthcare: An Essential Partnership." *Health Management Technology* 16 (July): 38–40.

Conrad, D., T. Wickizer, M. Maynard, J. Klastorin, D. Lessler, A. Ross, S. Naomi, S. Sullivan, J. Alexander, and K. Travis. 1996. "Managing Care, Incentives, and Information: An Exploratory Look Inside the 'Black Box' of Hospital Efficiency." *HSR:Health Services Research* 31 (3): 235–59.

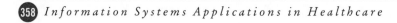

Davidson, H. L. 1996. "Contracting for Medicaid Managed Care. *"Healthcare Financial Management* 50 (11): 45.

Fox, S. J . 1996. "Medicaid Capitation and Information Management." In *The Capitation Sourcebook*, 235–55. Rockville, MD: Aspen Publishers.

Hard, R. 1992. "Well-Managed Information Vital to Effective Managed Care Contracting." *Hospitals* 66 (11): 50.

Keene, R. D., and F. F. Naus. 1994. *Negotiating Managed Care Contracts*, New York: McGraw-Hill, Inc.

Masters, G. M., and S. T. Valentine. 1995. *Health Care Capitation and Risk Contracting Manual.* New York: Thompson Publishing Group.

O'Connor, K. 1995. "Information Management for Managed Care." *Medical Group Management Journal* 42 (November–December): 52–56, 75.

Ribka, J. P. 1996. "Strategic Planning for Managed Care Information Systems." *Health Management Technology* (November): 30, 34, 55.

Shortell, S., R. Gillies, and D. Anderson. 1994. "The New World of Managed Care: Creating Organized Delivery Systems." *Health Affairs* 37 (Winter): 46–64.

Welge, W. 1992. "Managed Care is Limited by Information Systems." *Topics in Health Care Financing* 19 (Winter): 23–32.

Wright, C. M. 1993. "Information Technology Boosts Managed Care's Bottom Line." *Computers in Healthcare* 14 (7): 19.

HEALTH INFORMATION NETWORKS

Karen A. Wager

C HANGES IN the healthcare environment, including the growth of managed care and the expansion of integrated delivery systems (as discussed in Chapter 1), place new demands upon healthcare organizations and providers to establish information infrastructures that provide timely, accurate, and complete patient information across the continuum of care. Many integrated delivery systems in existence today are grappling with how to provide a true coordinated continuum of services to a defined population in a cost-effective manner. Although

Concepts and Applications

The rise of integrated delivery systems has required healthcare executives to access a steady stream of clinical and financial information. A health information network can provide executives with such information, but must be properly implemented to do so. Institutions wishing to construct a network must plan for it effectively, and must take into account several organizational factors when developing a strategy for implementation.

On completion of this chapter, readers will be able to describe an effective plan for implementing a healthcare information network, as well as discuss the issues that affect that plan.

there is a great deal of uncertainty about how to provide coordinated services, one thing is certain—integrated delivery systems are becoming the dominant model in healthcare. Despite the fact that estimates vary considerably, many experts expect that the U.S. healthcare market eventually will include 200 to 500 integrated delivery systems. (Bazzoli 1996) Results of a recent survey of leaders in healthcare computing affirm that the expansion of integrated delivery systems is indeed widespread; 60 percent reported that their healthcare organizations were part of or were in the process of forming an integrated delivery system, with another 11 percent planning to become part of such a system within the next year. (HIMSS/HP 1997)

For integrated delivery systems to be successful in managing care effectively across a continuum of services and organizations, studies have shown they will need strong governance and leadership, accessible primary care networks, greater physician alignment and involvement, sufficient capital, *and* responsive information systems. (Conrad and Shortell 1996; Shortell et al. 1993) In fact, one of the most comprehensive longitudinal studies to date on integrated delivery systems, conducted by researchers at the Center for Health Services and Policy Research at Northwestern University, found that information systems were central to an integrated delivery system's success. Two models that have emerged from their work and are used to illustrate their view of integrated delivery services have information systems as the hub holding the entities together at both the enterprise (Shortell, Gillies, and Anderson 1994) and community level (Shortell, Gillies, and Devers 1995). See Figures 15.1 and 15.2.

Based on these models, it is clear that healthcare leaders will need to assume a critical role in implementing information technologies that link the components of an integrated delivery system and support the unique clinical, financial, and administrative information needs of the delivery system. In particular, health information networks (HINs) or information infrastructures will need to be established in order to provide a true continuum of care. Likewise, HINs will need to evolve from the present enterprise level to the local community level and eventually to the national or international level if the goals of integrated delivery systems are to be fully realized. Creating these networks requires that healthcare leaders systematically plan for and address the complex issues associated with electronic exchange of information across organizational boundaries.

This chapter provides an overview of some of the critical issues that must be addressed in developing and implementing an HIN, whether it be an enterprise network or community network. This chapter begins

Figure 15.1 Model of Integrated Service Delivery

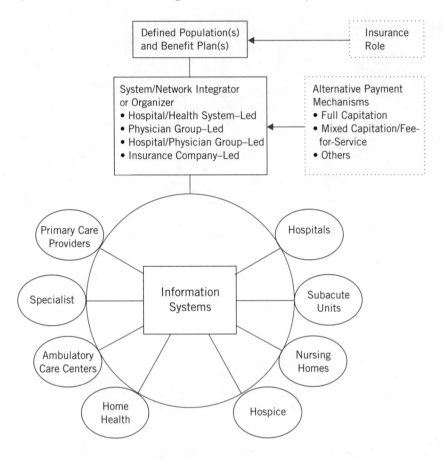

Source: Shortell et al. Copyright 1994. The People-to-People Health Foundation, Inc., Project Hope, http://www.projhope.org/HA/.

by introducing and defining the various terms used to describe the healthcare industry's movement toward a national HIN infrastructure. Two different models are presented to illustrate the different levels of HINs in the healthcare marketplace. Although the chapter focuses on the issues that should be addressed in planning for the development and implementation of enterprisewide HINs, also included is a brief discussion on community health information networks (CHINs) and some of the barriers to widespread implementation of such systems. Much attention has been given to CHINs in recent years. It is critical to examine some of the organizational, political, behavioral, technical,

Figure 15.2 The Community Health Care Management System

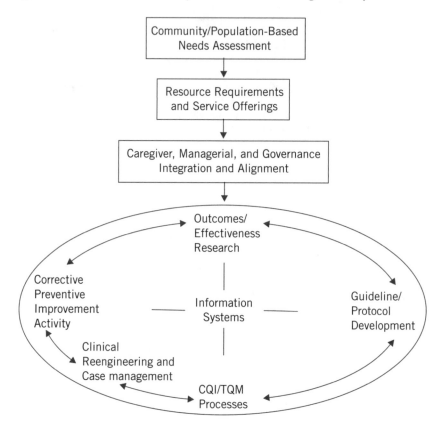

Source: Shortell et al. 1995. Copyright 1995. Blackwell Publishers.

and financial factors that have led to the success and failure of CHIN-initiatives to date, if we are to learn from the experiences of others and move forward in building an information infrastructure of healthcare for the new millennium.

Definition and Evolution of Health Information Networks

The plethora of terms used to describe HIN-related initiatives can be overwhelming and confusing. *Health information networks* may refer to a broad spectrum or continuum of systems. These include everything from an enterprise network, which serves the information management and communication requirements of a single health care system, to a global network, which provides electronic transfer of health information to international markets. (Furukawa 1997) Healthcare leaders and researchers grapple with how to define HINs particularly in the context of integrated delivery systems and the movement toward more community-based healthcare. Lee (1997) suggests that the evolution of HINs parallels the evolution of computer-based patient record (CPR) systems and integrated delivery systems. She argues that integrated delivery systems, information systems (e.g., CPR systems), and HINs are related to one other, and that each will have an impact on the successful implementation of the others.

In defining HINs, the old adage is probably true: " . . . if you have seen one HIN, you have seen one HIN." HINs are often used interchangeably with community health information networks (CHINs) or community health management information systems (CHMIS). Part of the difficulty in defining and categorizing HINs and CHINs stems from the diverse views about their roles in the healthcare marketplace. Some healthcare leaders view them as a way to gain a competitive advantage, while others view HINs as a way to provide better service to the community or to conduct population-based research. Whatever the orientation, most definitions focus on the term *community*. For example, some stress that CHINs are unique in that they provide for the electronic exchange of member information between unaffiliated organizations, while others view CHINs as building information resources throughout the community and emphasize the community link. (Dowling 1997) Regardless of the definition used, Dowling (1997, 17) suggests that there are some common points of agreement, including:

- Computer-based information systems and networks form the base technologies of CHINs.
- CHINs enable the transfer of data and information between organizations.
- The major domain of the data transferred is health and the provision of health services.
- Patient information is included in the information set.
- An objective of CHINs is to improve the efficiency and effectiveness of healthcare delivery.

Given these points of agreement, there are different levels or degrees of sophistication among HINs. The former Community Medical Network (ComNet) Society, a nonprofit membership organization established in the early 1990s to address industrywide concerns related to HINs, developed an evolutionary model representing the various levels of HINs. (Furukawa 1997) (See Figure 15.3.) This model provides a framework for understanding the evolution of HIN development and

Figure 15.3   Defining the HIN Continuum

Evolving Scope ——▶
Enterprise ⟹ Community ⟹ National ⟹ Global

Global Health Information Infrastructure (GHII)
National Health Information Infrastructure (NHII)
National Health Information Network (NHIN)
Value Added Network (VAN)/EDI Network
State Health Information Network (SHIN)
Regional Health Information Network (RHIN)
Community Health Management Information System (CHMIS)
Community Health Information Network (CHIN)
Telemedicine/Telehealth Network
Integrated Delivery Network (IDN)
Proprietary Health Information Network (PHIN)
Enterprise Network

Courtesy of TRIAD Research.

strategy across the broad boundaries of enterprise, community, national, and global networks.

An *enterprise* network is one that is established to support the information management and communication requirements of a single organization, such as a hospital/health system, managed care organization, physician group, or government agency. (Furukawa 1997) Two unique characteristics of enterprise networks include: (1) they are generally private rather than public; and (2) they are designed to serve the information needs of an *individual* integrated healthcare system. Enterprise networks are also commonly used synonymous with proprietary health information networks (PHINs) and integrated delivery networks (IDNs). These systems are the most common type of HIN in existence today and will be discussed further later in this chapter.

The next level of HIN development in this evolutionary or continuum model is the *community network* or CHIN. At this level the network's mission is to benefit quality/cost factors for delivery systems within a regional, state, or national community of care, and to capitalize on the commonalties and noncompetitive threats among providers, payors, employers, government, and others to facilitate the open, seamless sharing of clinical, administrative, financial, and educational information in a standardized electronic format. (Furukawa 1997) It is also at this level that healthcare organizations or other participants begin to focus on the health information needs of the broader community. This level of CHINs may be referred to as regional health information networks or statewide health information networks.

The two other HIN levels represented in the evolutionary model (Figure 15.3) include *national networks* and *global networks*. National networks hold great promise as state and federal governments continue to fund initiatives related to the National Information Infrastructure (NII), commonly known as the "information superhighway." Some experts predict that the NII will revolutionize healthcare delivery in the United States, and globally, by combining different information technologies into a common infrastructure that is fast, efficient, interoperable, extendible, reliable, secure, easy to use, and globally accessible. (Poggio and Caldwell 1996) Leaders in Europe, Asia, and Australia are also actively involved in developing HINs to support the health information needs of their countries. (Furukawa 1997) By transferring health information technologies to international markets, the development of a global health information infrastructure may become a reality in the next decade.

In contrast to the ComNet Society model, Dowling (1997) developed a model for illustrating the various levels of HINs with three levels: the organizational, interorganizational, and extraorganizational. In this model, patient care is at the center of all activities. (See Figure 15.4.) At the organizational level, individual healthcare organizations are building information communications and application systems that allow them to manage patient care and their institutions more efficiently and effectively. Healthcare organizations are still struggling with problems at this level including cost, systems integration, legacy systems, and vendor supply of acceptable systems. (Dowling 1997) The next level, the interorganizational level, is comparable with the enterprise network in the ComNet Society model. It is at this level that organizations or entities within an integrated delivery system build information systems to support the coordination and control of their operations. The third level of HINs is the extraorganizational level. This is the level at which agencies and community organizations come together to focus on the larger societal healthcare issues. Several examples of HINs at this level include statewide HIN efforts in Iowa and Wisconsin and the Medical College of Georgia Telemedicine Network.

Although different in the number and types of levels, these two models are similar in that they both illustrate the evolutionary nature of HINs. Different organizations are at different levels of development of HINs. Some healthcare organizations are able to share financial information electronically throughout the state, but have limited capabilities for sharing clinical information. Others are able to share both financial

History of CHINS and Barriers to Widespread Implementation

In 1993, 75 CHIN-related initiatives were known to be under way throughout the nation. By 1995, this number had grown to over 500, representing all 50 states and most metropolitan areas. (Hanlon 1996) Although a relatively new phenomenon, CHIN projects gained a great deal of attention in a short time span. Results of a national study on CHINs, entitled "CHINs-in-Progress: Evolving to the Next Level," revealed that although more than 65 percent of the healthcare organizations had established electronic connectivity with providers and payors outside their enterprises and 46 percent reported being well-positioned to become part of a community network in the near future, more than 80 percent of the 500 health information network initiatives under way had yet to collaborate fully with unaffiliated stakeholders. (Hanlon 1996) For the true benefits of CHINs to be realized, information infrastructures or "infostructures," that serve all community stakeholders (physicians, hospitals, insurers, employers, government, and consumers) must be developed. Many communities are beginning to examine the benefits of a shared infostructure. Since it is costly and inefficient to build proprietary, redundant networks that serve the same geographical regions, Hanlon (1996) suggests there may be incentive enough by enterprises to collaborate in CHIN development by simply sharing the costs and risks among multiple stakeholders.

To survive in this new integrated environment, healthcare leaders have been struggling with how to develop and implement CHINs capable of supporting the information needs of their constituents. Although more than 500 CHIN initiatives are under way throughout the United States, many are not yet fully operational. Some argue that "CHINs are the latest technology fad to grip the health care industry." (Appleby 1995, 43) Healthcare organizations have been reluctant to share proprietary information with their competitors and many have not been able to cost-justify these systems. Others have paid consultants high fees only to discover the CHIN-effort failed due to competing interests and the high price tag for establishing a community network. While these views have become increasingly prevalent, other healthcare leaders view CHINs as the building blocks of a National Health Information Infrastructure and the forerunner to a true computer-based patient record system. (Hanlon 1996) Regardless of the future of CHINs, one thing is clear: the healthcare industry is looking to information technology as a tool for increasing efficiency, reducing cost, and improving the quality of patient care. (Davenport, Backerman, and Kreitzer 1996) Healthcare organizations must be well-positioned not only technologically, but operationally and strategically, if they are to move toward a true community network. Issues related to data ownership, confidentiality, security, and data standards that have curtailed some of the earlier efforts to establish community networks must also be addressed.

Even though a number of CHIN-initiatives have not come to fruition, there are several that have been quite successful in accomplishing their goals. One example is the Wisconsin Health Information Network (WHIN). Established in 1992, the WHIN formed as a result of a joint venture between Ameritech, the Midwest's Regional Bell Operating Company, and Aurora Health Care, a Milwaukee multihospital system. The WHIN became operational in the first quarter of 1993 with two hospitals and 27 physicians. Since then, it has grown to include 16 hospitals, more than 1,300 physicians, seven payors, eight clinics, and other regional ancillary service providers. (Pemble 1997) As WHIN has grown, client/server applications have become more commonplace and the technical infrastructure of WHIN has evolved to support communication of other client/server pairs. Much of the success of the WHIN has been attributed to the fact that the information providers and users have found that the network has added value to their business. For example, by having a communitywide electronic signature application or a community repository of patient indexes, the users were more likely to use the network than to resort to the traditional means of accessing information. Those using the network found that the new systems were much more efficient and reliable than the ones they replaced. In recent years, WHIN has also provided substantial cost savings. Information providers, such as the participating hospitals, experienced an annual savings of $375,000 to $1,000,000 alone in copying costs for patient medical records. Physicians practices saved between $17,000 and $68,000 or more in electronic claims processing. (Lassila et al., forthcoming) Other studies similar to these will be needed in the future to assess the impact of CHINs on local and regional communities from an economic, patient care, and population perspective.

Figure 15.4 Three Levels of HIN

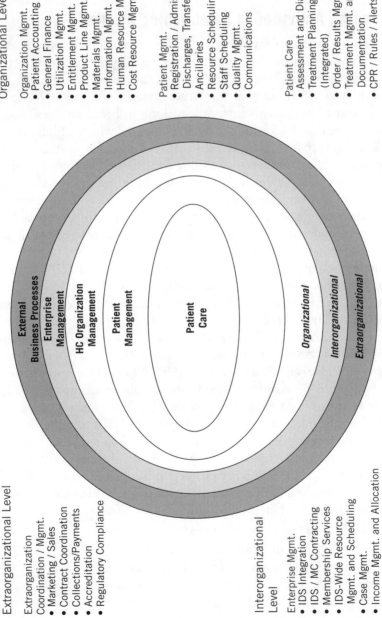

Extraorganizational Level

Extraorganization
Coordination / Mgmt.
- Marketing / Sales
- Contract Coordination
- Collections/Payments
- Accreditation
- Regulatory Compliance

Interorganizational
Level

Enterprise Mgmt.
- IDS Integration
- IDS / MC Contracting
- Membership Services
- IDS-Wide Resource
  Mgmt. and Scheduling
- Case Mgmt.
- Income Mgmt. and Allocation

Organizational Level

Organization Mgmt.
- Patient Accounting
- General Finance
- Utilization Mgmt.
- Entitlement Mgmt.
- Product Line Mgmt.
- Materials Mgmt.
- Information Mgmt.
- Human Resource Mgmt.
- Cost Resource Mgmt.

Patient Mgmt.
- Registration / Admissions,
  Discharges, Transfers
- Ancillaries
- Resource Scheduling
- Staff Scheduling
- Quality Mgmt.
- Communications

Patient Care
- Assessment and Diagnosis
- Treatment Planning
  (Integrated)
- Order / Results Mgmt.
- Treatment Mgmt. and
  Documentation
- CPR / Rules / Alerts

Source: Dowling, A. G. 1996. "Three Levels of HIN." *Information Networks for Community Health.* p. 24.

and clinical information, but only within their enterprise. Still, others are putting together the pieces needed to build a global health information infrastructure. Regardless of where organizations currently are in terms of their information systems development, it is essential to appropriately plan for the establishment of an HIN.

Planning Activities in Establishing an HIN

Developing and implementing an HIN is an enormous financial commitment. Some estimates indicate that integrated delivery systems can expect to spend between $30 to $50 million on information network technology, or as high as $250 million for the larger systems. (Bazzoli 1996) Spending on information systems integration alone in healthcare is expected to reach more than $3.5 billion in 1999, compared with $1.4 billion in 1994. The reality is that building an information network infrastructure able to provide seamless connectivity among all affiliated entities or participants is a costly endeavor. In addition, the use of information technology for integrated patient care delivery will not only involve automation, but radical change in the actual delivery process if the full potential benefits are to be realized. Therefore, it is important to properly plan for the development, implementation, and evaluation of HINs. In particular, all planning activities related to the establishment of an HIN should be a component of the healthcare enterprise's strategic information systems plan and well integrated with the overall strategic plan of the enterprise, as discussed in Chapter 7.

Healthcare leaders have used various processes and methods in planning for the development and implementation of HINs. (Hinte and Searls 1997; DeFauw and L'Heureux 1995; Wager, Heda, and Austin 1997) Although any process or method used should be tailored to the unique goals of the organization or enterprise, there are some underlying issues that must be addressed when developing an HIN, whether it is at the enterprise level or community level. Lessons learned from hundreds of pioneers in the industry can serve as road maps for new HIN initiatives, demonstrating not only where to begin, but how. Following is a list of eight fundamental activities or issues that should be addressed in *any* planning process when establishing an HIN infrastructure:

1. understand business objectives;
2. assess current information system needs;
3. identify information system requirements and user needs;
4. determine type of organization or ownership;
5. determine method of financing;
6. address legal and security issues;
7. establish infrastructure for managing network; and

8. implement process for ongoing HIN evaluation and future development.

Understand Business Objectives

Developing an HIN for an enterprise or within a community is a business decision, not a technology decision. Therefore, the decision to develop and implement an HIN should directly relate to the healthcare organization's business goals. As an example, the Greater Rochester Health System (GRHS) developed, as part of its strategic planning process, a graphical model illustrating that the consumer is central to its mission. The Health System's business goal was to provide high-quality, coordinated care in the most cost-effective manner to consumers using its services. To accomplish this goal, GRHS realized that integrated information and management systems must be available. An evaluation of the IS planning process used at GRHS revealed that physicians, administrators, and others involved in the process had tremendous enthusiasm for the project and cooperated with the various entities. They also found that because the business objectives for the organization had been established, they were able to easily map the information systems strategic initiatives to the business goals. (Hinte and Searls 1997)

Defining the business goals for an enterprise requires that healthcare leaders think in broad terms. That is, leaders must move away from a single-institution perspective to an integrated delivery system perspective. This requires a willingness on the part of administrators and executives to subordinate their individual institution's priorities to those of the broader delivery system. (Wager, Heda, and Austin 1997) This is not an easy task. Healthcare organizations have spent years competing with each other for patients, physicians, and other resources, and have often invested a considerable amount of time, resources, and energy into the systems now in use. There may be fear of losing an identity or market niche when becoming part of a larger system. Likewise, it is not uncommon for chief information officers (CIOs), information systems professionals, and health providers to want to keep the information systems that they have helped build, acquire, or implement. Consequently, it is important to actively involve key players from each of the respective institutions in defining common business goals of the enterprise. Included should be representatives from top management, clinical and ancillary areas, information systems, health information services, finance, and other major service areas. Individuals from each participating organization should also assess their organization's critical success factors and understand why participation in the HIN is important. The stated reasons should support the individual organization's business goals, or top management may likely discontinue support for the HIN in favor of initiatives that do.

Assess Current Information Systems

Besides understanding the common business goals of the entities involved in establishing an enterprise network, it is important to assess the current information systems used among the various organizations. A common approach is to begin by conducting an inventory of systems; this inventory should include the hardware, software, communication systems, and manual and automated interfaces. Typically, one of the first systems assessed is the registration systems, since a community master patient (or member) index may be needed to identify patients and organize their information, regardless of where patients have been seen and where information is captured. (Wager, Heda, and Austin 1997) Most likely, each of the institutions or facilities participating in the proposed HIN will have different methods for identifying patients and different procedures for maintaining this information. In fact, it is not uncommon to find that in one facility, different departments may be using different numbering systems or methods to identify patients. Therefore, it may be difficult for one facility to pull together all its clinical, financial, and administrative information about a single patient. (White and Messler 1997)

To link patient records contained in such disparate systems, healthcare leaders are considering various alternatives such as implementing a community master patient index system (MPI) designed to track patients across multiple facilities and through multiple episodes of care. A community MPI may provide the foundation from which to build the network infrastructure. Other current information systems, besides the registration system, should also be assessed to determine if they are well-equipped to meet the future needs of the network. Some legacy system may need to be replaced, upgraded, or surrounded with new capabilities; other information systems may be central to the success of the network. A critical evaluation of all current information systems should be conducted before future new information technologies are acquired.

Identify Information System Requirements and User Needs

Within the enterprise or integrated delivery system, there may be different types of providers and organizations that are interested in linking their information systems with the HIN. Each provider or organization will have either paper-based or computerized administrative, clinical, and/or financial information systems already in place. Therefore, it will be particularly important as part of the planning process, to identify the information systems requirements and needs of the various users. At a minimum, the information system requirements for a successful integrated delivery system should include document management; orders and results management; clinical protocols with embedded case management tools; clinical decision support; and administrative practice management functions such as enrollment management, scheduling, and utilization management. (Harris, Sockolow, and Petzko 1995) In identifying these requirements, it is important to think about IS automation from a paradigm that emphasizes an enterprisewide focus, patient-focused and managed care systems, client/server processing, object-oriented technology, and open systems. (Pawola and Klineman 1995)

The information system requirements should be fairly well-defined. For example, several system requirements for one integrated delivery system included:

- establish a single standardized numbering system to identify each patient in the network;
- capture accurate clinical and demographic information at its source as the patient care is delivered;
- develop the ability to quickly access an integrated delivery system member's medical record from anywhere in the continuum of care;
- present the necessary information elements at the right time in the care process to facilitate case management;
- share clinical information with providers inside and outside the organization and ensure the accuracy and confidentiality of the information;
- use information effectively to serve the community, conserve resources, monitor the cost and quality of care, and manage the enterprise. (Work and Pawola 1996, 29)

As part of the planning process, it is important to not only identify the IS requirements but also the infrastructure needed to support the system requirements. Some healthcare executives are designating administrators to manage processes across traditional organizational boundaries. (Drazen, Reed, and Metzger 1995) These managers are given the authority to develop and manage on a continual basis processes, such as patient registration or case management.

To build an infrastructure that is able to support the HIN requirements requires that there be a strong communication system in place. This entails, at a minimum, setting up a telecommunications network, establishing data and language standards, and planning for systems integration. Setting up the telecommunications network requires answering some key questions including:

- What is the number and geographic locations of the various sites?
- How much information and in what form (text, voice, image) must it be communicated?

- How much imaging data must be stored and sent to the various providers?
- Is telemedicine to be part of the network?
- What information will need to be available for immediate access? What information may be archived?
- Who will have access to the various types of information? How will information be secured on the network?
- How many users will need access to the system at various times during the day?
- Who will manage the network? How will it be managed?
- What plans, if any, are there to use Internet-based technology to build an Intranet enterprisewide or send information electronically via the Internet?

In addition to planning for the telecommunications network, it is also important to establish data and language standards for the HIN. Data standards ensure that information transferred among the various organizations is accurate. A universal interface engine is sometimes needed to build interfaces between individual computer applications and to ensure the smooth transfer of data. Likewise, all healthcare organizations and providers participating in the network will need to agree on language standards. It is not uncommon to find that the definition for a single test or procedure has one meaning in one hospital and another meaning in a physician office. The various participating organizations need to decide if it is best to communicate using a universal dictionary (which attempts to define the parameters for all tests and procedures the same way) or allow users to maintain their own individual standards and definitions.

Determine Type of Organization or Ownership

Healthcare organizations and providers may decide to build, buy, or partner with others when establishing an enterprise or community network. How the HIN will be organized and owned is a political issue, one that should be considered very carefully. There are about as many different strategies for organizing an HIN as there are definitions of them. However, the four most common strategies are enterprise, coalition, vendor, and virtual. (Furukawa 1997) The *enterprise* strategy uses a single stakeholder approach to link all owned or affiliated entities. Simply stated, the HIN remains internal to the organization or enterprise; the goal is to develop an information infrastructure that aids in providing care to patient populations within the enterprise of the integrated delivery system. The HIN is owned, funded, and managed by the affiliated organizations and therefore, there is a relatively high degree of control in database development and access issues. This strategy offers healthcare organizations and providers the flexibility in designing the HIN to meet unique goals and needs. It is also known as the "bottom-up" approach to HIN development, in that the HIN emerges at the institutional, or grassroots, level.

In contrast to the enterprise strategy, the *coalition strategy* generally involves a coalition of employers, providers, payors, government agencies or other stakeholders that are *not* affiliated with one another. This strategy is designed to improve quality of care and reduce costs within the community by establishing a not-for-profit organization or entity that contracts with a vendor for development and operation of the HIN. The coalition HIN is owned and funded by the coalition participants, often with some assistance from vendors. (Wakerly 1994) With this strategy, the coalition can set up its own HIN and incur the associated costs or contract with one or more vendors to build and operate the HIN. This "top-down" approach has experienced numerous setbacks related to the challenges of bringing together competitors at the same table. However, several statewide initiatives in Maine, Ohio, and West Virginia have been successful.

The third approach is the *vendor* strategy, whereby a vendor generally funds and operates the HIN as a for-profit enterprise. Funds are generated through usage, transaction, operation, and maintenance fees paid by the various participating organizations and providers. Most vendor-owned HINs are able to maintain control of the network by securing at least 51 percent ownership. The advantage to the participating organization or provider is that the vendor bears the cost of implementing the HIN hardware, software, network, and technical support staff. One disadvantage to this approach, however, is that there is generally less flexibility in system design because the vendor maintains primary control. (Wager, Heda, and Austin 1997)

The fourth major strategy is the *virtual* strategy. Rather than building a new information network, Furukawa (1997) suggests that this approach allows for the virtual sharing of health data by facilitating standards-based connectivity (including using Internet technology) between existing HINs. Healthcare organizations in Massachusetts Health Data Consortium's Affiliated Health Information Networks of New England (AHINNE) and the Foundation for Health Care Quality's Washington Health Care EDI (WHEDI) are using this approach. (Furukawa 1997) Other healthcare entities are using Internet technology and the WWW to facilitate the virtual strategy, including the Minnesota Health Data

Institute's CHMIS Initiative (MedNet) and the statewide HIN in Vermont known as VTMEDNET.

Besides these four primary forms of ownership and structure, there are also various hybrid models or variations to these strategies. For example, the HIN may be owned and managed by the state. Each strategy has its own strengths and limitations, therefore, it is important for the healthcare organization or participating provider to select a strategy or model that fits well with its business goals, IS needs, and financial status. The enterprise strategy may be a useful approach to a healthcare organization with sufficient capital to own and manage the HIN, but that also wants to control the use and development of the network. Not all healthcare organizations or providers, however, have the capital and resources to develop and maintain their own HIN, and therefore, the coalition strategy may be a more feasible approach. The coalition strategy builds on the people and resources in the community to fund the HIN. On the other hand, the vendor strategy has become more popular because much of the financial risk for the HIN initiative falls on the vendor. Finally, the virtual strategy has the potential to enable the transfer of data through the Internet without the need to establish separate, independent HINs. This strategy is likely to become more widely used because of the cost-effectiveness of the Internet and its widespread use among healthcare organizations and providers.

Determine Method of Financing

In the planning process, it is also important to determine how the HIN will be financed. Although actual expenditures will vary depending on the type of HIN and each organization's or provider's degree of involvement, it is important to budget for major categories of expenditures including the cost of staffing, feasibility studies, legal services, request for information development, vendor selection, and contract negotiations. (Wager, Heda, and Austin 1997) Revenue sources may include participant fees, private grants, government funding, and vendor-supplied capital. (Kennedy 1995)

Address Legal and Security Issues

Building HINs to support the goals of integrated delivery systems requires that healthcare organizations and providers establish mechanisms to ensure privacy, confidentiality, and security of patient information. Although there are no universal standards or guidelines that address all the legal and security issues associated with HINs, efforts are under way to change various state and federal laws to protect the privacy and confidentiality of patient information. The Fair Health Information Practices Act, reintroduced to Congress in early 1997, promises to address privacy protection for patient information at the federal level. Similarly, the Health Care Portability and Accountability Act (1996) directs the Secretary of Health and Human Services to develop and promulgate security standards for electronic health information by 1998. Many healthcare providers are expected to comply with these standards within two years. Furthermore, this legislation establishes penalties for wrongful disclosure of a patient's health information, including fines up to $250,000 and ten years' imprisonment. (McKenzie 1997) Until national standards are universally accepted, however, healthcare organizations and providers must take proactive steps to ensure that patient information is kept confidential and secure and to protect the integrity of their data.

There are a number of methods that should be employed to protect confidential information within the proposed network. Included are the use of passwords, access cards, biometric techniques (e.g., fingerprint or voice-based security), call-back devices, user security clearance levels, alert devices, audit trails, encryption, and virus-scanning programs. (White, Wager, and Lee 1996) Network administrators should also implement security devices that restrict access to the HIN to those who have a legitimate right of access. For example, *firewalls* should be in place to protect individual computers from intrusions outside the network. (McKenzie 1997) A firewall is a dedicated computer that provides network safeguards by examining and restricting incoming and outgoing communications. Healthcare organizations should also implement enterprisewide security and confidentiality policies, procedures, and practices to protect patient privacy and ensure security of patient information. Education and training should be an integral part of the integrated delivery system's plan to ensure that all users understand relevant security practices and confidentiality policies *before* being granted access to the network. Similarly, healthcare organizations should establish sanctions for violations of confidentiality and security policies that are applied uniformly and consistently to all violators. Clearly, the success of an integrated delivery system will be based on the trust it employs from patients, providers, and other users. (See Chapter 7 for further discussion of data security policies.)

Establish Infrastructure for Managing Network

In planning for an HIN, it is critical to ensure that adequate people, resources, and funding are available to provide a solid infrastructure to manage the network. In fact, the information infrastructure should be viewed as a utility rather than a capital expenditure. The success of the integrated delivery system will be largely based on healthcare providers and administrators having access to timely, accurate, and complete information in order to provide care and manage resources effectively. Establishing an infrastructure requires commitment from top administration and "buy in" from physicians, nurses, and other clinicians. Adequate staff will need to be available 24 hours a day to manage the technical support problems. Disaster recovery plans will need to be in place to ensure that adequate back-up procedures are in order. It is critical that all end-users gain trust and confidence that the HIN is accurate, reliable, and accessible.

There are many different ways in which an enterprise can establish an *information* infrastructure to support the HIN. One common approach is to build an "intranet" that can be managed and controlled at the local level, while enabling users the flexibility of using Internet-based technology. Rather than replacing legacy systems, some healthcare organizations are using intranets to access legacy data and applications through a WWW browser, a universal front-end user interface commonly used when accessing the Web over the Internet. Intranets offer many benefits including ease of use; ability to combine text, audio, and video data; little network training required; and low integration costs. Healthcare providers do not want to have to learn ten separate front-ends in order to access different systems on the network. Intranets enable providers to use one user interface to access the different applications. (See Chapter 5 for further discussion of Internet technology and Chapter 16 for further discussion of Internet applications.)

Integrated delivery systems have used intranets primarily as a means for disseminating information that was previously distributed on paper, including nursing manuals, human resource materials, clinical protocols, and provider phone books. (Siwicki 1997) These materials alone can save integrated delivery systems tens of thousands of dollars in printing costs. Some healthcare organizations are also planning to use intranets to capture clinical and financial data through their delivery systems. Examples of facilities involved in implementing intranets to support HINs include Samaritan Health System of Arizona, Marshfield Medical Center in Marshfield, Wisconsin, and Emerson Hospital in Concord, Massachusetts. (Siwicki 1997)

Implement Process for Ongoing HIN Evaluation and Future Development

In addition to building an infrastructure to support the HIN, it is also important to establish a process for evaluating the HIN on an ongoing basis. Frequently, information systems are implemented in healthcare organizations with no formal evaluation of the systems effectiveness ever performed. Reasons for not conducting system evaluation studies include cost, lack of staff and resources, and difficulty in defining system effectiveness. The system evaluations that are done generally focus on technical aspects, with little or no consideration given to the organizational and financial impact. Kaplan (1997) argues that it is critical to understand the process that contributes to the outcomes. In other words, in addition to assessing *what* differences clinical information systems make in patient care, education, medical research, and health management, evaluations should address *why* these systems make those differences or have the impact that they do. The same holds true for HINs. The process for evaluating the HIN should address issues such as:

- What are the perceived advantages and disadvantages of the HIN among end-users?
- In what ways does the HIN facilitate patient care across the continuum?
- To what degree does the HIN meet users' needs?
- What system features or components of the HIN are most critical to the success of the integrated delivery system? Which are most problematic?
- What impact has the HIN had on the enterprise from an organizational perspective (e.g., relationships between units, communication, work patterns)?
- What are the identified costs/benefits of the HIN?
- In what ways could the HIN be improved?
- How is the HIN contributing to the accomplishment of the enterprise's business goals?

Questions such as these are important to address in the ongoing evaluation and assessment of the newly established HIN. Information systems development is a cyclical process, requiring ongoing review and analysis. It is also important to include goals for future systems development in the evaluation plan.

Summary

The growth and expansion of integrated delivery systems place new demands on healthcare leaders to develop information infrastructures or HINs to support them. To accomplish the goals of integrated delivery systems (e.g., decrease healthcare costs while providing quality care across the continuum), healthcare providers and administrators need access to timely, accurate, and complete clinical and financial information.

Most integrated delivery system models today include information systems as the hub that holds or links the various entities together.

Healthcare organizations are at different stages of HIN development. Some have established enterprise systems, while others are expanding their efforts to community systems. In the future, HINs may expand to national and international levels. Regardless of where a healthcare organization is in its stage of IS development, it is essential to appropriately plan for the establishment of an information infrastructure able to support the goals of the integrated delivery system. An HIN is an enormous financial investment, and therefore, it is essential to appropriately plan for its development and implementation. The plan should indicate (1) an understanding of business objectives, (2) an assessment of current information system needs, (3) information system requirements and users needs, (4) type of organization or ownership, (5) method of financing, (6) methods by which legal and security issues will be addressed, (7) an infrastructure for managing network, and (8) a process for ongoing HIN evaluation and future development. Key issues that need to be addressed relate to data and language standards, security, confidentiality, data ownership, network management, and funding.

Discussion Questions

15.1 Distinguish between an enterprise network and a community health information network.

15.2 Discuss the history of CHINs and identify some of the barriers to full implementation of such systems.

15.3 How does the planning process for establishing an HIN within an enterprise compare with the strategic information systems planning process described in Chapter 7?

15.4 Discuss at least six critical issues that should be included in the planning process when establishing an HIN. Why is each issue important?

15.5 Why are data standards important in today's healthcare environment?

15.6 Describe the four common strategies for organizing an HIN including enterprise, coalition, vendor, and virtual.

15.7 What methods or strategies should a healthcare organization adopt to protect the integrity and security of information within an HIN?

Problems

15.1 Assume that you are the project manager for establishing an HIN within your enterprise. The enterprise consists of eight large primary care practices, a 550-bed acute care facility, a 300-bed children's hospital, two nursing centers, and an outpatient rehabilitation facility. Develop a project plan for the development and implementation of the HIN. Include in your plan a description of the key individuals involved, issues to be addressed, and methods for evaluating the success of the project.

15.2 Interview a CIO in your community whose organization is part of an integrated delivery system. Assess the degree to which their information infrastructure supports the goals of their delivery system. What are the greatest strengths and limitations of their current information infrastructure? Prepare a summary report of your interview and an assessment of the challenges they face in the future.

15.3 Identify a health services organization that has either been successful or unsuccessful in establishing an HIN at the enterprise or community level. Investigate the factors that have led to the network's success or demise. Prepare a summary report that describes the "lessons learned" throughout the HIN development process and strategies that would be useful to others about to embark on such an initiative.

References

Appleby, C. 1995. "The Trouble with CHINs." *Hospitals & Health Networks* 69 (9): 42–44.

Bazzoli, F. 1996. "Integrated Delivery Systems: The Journey Toward Enterprise Networks." *Health Data Management* 4 (3): 44–46, 48, 50.

Conrad, D. A., and S. M. Shortell. 1996. "Integrated Health Systems: Promise and Performance." *Frontiers of Health Services Management* 13 (1): 3–40.

Davenport, R. L., J. Backerman, and M. Kreitzer. 1996. "Understanding and Assessing CHIN Network Technology." *Proceedings of the 1996 Annual HIMSS Conference.* Volume 1: 36–46.

DeFauw, T. D., and D. L'Heureux.1995. "How to Strategically Align Information Resources With the Goals of an Integrated Delivery System." *Journal of the Healthcare Information and Management Systems Society* 9 (4): 3–10

Dowling, A. F. 1997. "CHINS—The Current State." In *Information Networks for Community Health*, edited by P. F. Brennan, S. J. Schneider, and E. Tornquist. New York: Springer-Verlag, Inc.

Drazen, E., B. Reed, and J. Metzger. 1995. "The CIO of the Integrated Delivery System." *Healthcare Informatics* 12 (2): 24

Furukawa, M. 1997. "Models for Evolving Community Health Information Networks." *Topics in Health Information Management.* 17 (4): 11–19.

Hanlon, P. J. 1996. "CHINS-In-Progress: Evolving to the Next Level." *Proceedings: 1996 Annual Meeting—Toward an Electronic Patient Record.*

Harris, C. M., P. S. Sockolow, D. R. Petzko. 1995. "Information Requirements for an Integrated Delivery System." *MEDINFO Proceedings.* 1553–37.

Healthcare Information and Management Systems Society and Hewlett-Packard Company (HIMSS/HP). 1997. *Annual Leadership Survey.* Chicago: The Society.

Hinte, G. M., and W. V. Searls. 1997. "The Trials and Tribulations of IDS Strategic Planning." *Proceedings of the 1997 HIMSS Conference, Volume 1*: 187–97.

Kaplan, B. 1997. "Addressing Organizational Issues in the Evaluation of Medical Systems." *Journal of the American Medical Informatics Association* 4 (2): 94–101.

Kennedy, R. 1995. "Building the CHIN Organization." *Journal of the Healthcare Information and Management Systems Society* 9: 21–28.

Lassila, K., K. Pemble, L. DuPont, and R. Cheng. Forthcoming. "Assessing the Impact of Chins: A Multi-Site Study of the Wisconsin Health Information Network." *Topics in Health Information Management.*

Lee, F. 1997. "Evolution of Computer-Based Information Systems and Networks to Support Integrated Health Care Delivery Systems." *Topics in Health Information Management* 17 (4): 1–10.

McKenzie, A. 1997. "Protecting the Confidentiality and Integrity of Patient Records." *Topics in Health Information Management* 17 (4): 62–71.

Pawola, L. M., and K. A. Klineman. 1995. "Developing Information Systems for Integrated Systems." *Healthcare Financial Management* 12 (6): 44–48

Pemble, K. R. 1997. "Information Infrastructure for Health Communities: The Wisconsin Health Information Network." In *Information Networks for Community Health*, edited by P. F. Brennan, S. J. Schneider, and E. Tornquist. New York: Springer-Verlag, Inc.

Poggio, P., and C. Caldwell 1996. "Why a Testbed is Needed". *Proceedings: Toward an Electronic Patient Record '96.* 12th International Symposium on the Creation of Electronic Health Record System and Global Conference on Patient Cards. May 11–18. 358–365.

Shortell, S. M., R. R. Gillies, and D. A. Anderson. 1994. "The New World of Managed Care: Creating Organized Delivery Systems." *Health Affairs* 13 (5): 49.

Shortell, S. M., R. R. Gillies, D. A. Anderson, J. B. Mitchell, and K. L. Morgan. 1993. "Creating Organized Delivery Systems: The Barriers and Facilitators." *Hospital & Health Services Administration* 38 (4): 447–65.

Shortell, S. M., R. R. Gillies, and K. J. Devers. 1995. "Reinventing the American Hospital." *Milbank Quarterly* 73 (2): 131–60.

Siwicki, B. 1997. "Enterprise Networks: Strategies for Integrated Delivery Systems." *Health Data Management* 5 (2): 54–63, 66.

Wager, K. A., S. Heda, and C. J. Austin. 1997. "Developing a Health Information Network Within an Integrated Delivery System: A Case Study." *Topics in Health Information Management* 17 (4): 20–31

Wakerly, R. 1994. "Models of CHIN Ownership." In *Community Health Information Networks—Creating the Health Care Data Highway*. Chicago: American Hospital Publishing, Inc.

White, A. W., and C. Messler. 1997. "Facilitating Linkage Through Universal Patient Identifiers: A Difficult Endeavor." *Topics in Health Information Management* 17 (4): 32–39.

White, A., K. Wager, and F. Lee. 1996. "The Impact of Technology on the Confidentiality of Health Information." *Topics in Health Information Management* 16 (4): 13–21.

Work, M. R., and L. Pawola. 1996. "Information Systems for Integrated Healthcare Delivery." *Healthcare Financial Management* 1: 27–30

Additional Readings

Bazzoli, F. 1994. "Health Information Networks: Where Are We Headed?" *Health Data Management* 2 (9): 38–47.

Bergman, R. 1994. "Where There's a Will . . . Computer-Based Patient Records Require Commitment, Time, and Money." *Hospitals & Health Networks* 68 (9): 36, 38, 40, 42.

Bradshaw, E., R. Leemis, P. O. Russell, R. K. Thomas, and F. Tabatabai. 1995. "An Integrated Patient Information System for a Primary Care Network." *Journal of the Healthcare Information and Management Systems Society* 9 (4): 67–71.

Brailer, D. J. 1996. "Clinical Decision Support: Managing Quality in Integrated Delivery Systems." *Quality Management in Health Care* 4 (2): 24–33.

DeLuca, J. M. 1995. "Translating the Promise of Integrated Regional Delivery Systems Into Performance." *Journal of the Healthcare Information and Management Systems Society* 9 (4): 31–37.

Fickenscher, K., and S. Buettner. 1996. "Lessons from the Trenches in Physician Integration." *Physician Executive* 22 (6): 14–18.

Griffin, J. 1996. "Modeling the Enterprisewide Information Architecture." *Healthcare Informatics* 13 (8): 50–52.

Haughorn, J. L., and L. J. Gibson. 1995. "Improving the Cost, Quality, and Access to Healthcare in Community Hospitals Through the Use of Reorganized Integrated Delivery Systems and Implementation of Sophisticated Clinical Information Systems: An Organizational Experience." *MEDINFO Proceedings*. 1558–61.

Havighurst, C. 1995. "The Power Circuit." *Health Systems Review* (21) 4: 52.

Houtz, J. H., and C. J. Okstein. 1996. "Information Systems Drive Health Care Into the 21st Century." *MGM Journal* 43 (5): 64–69.

Kralewski, J. E., A. De Vries, B. Dowd, and S. Potthoff. 1995. "The Development of Integrated Service Networks in Minnesota." *Health Care Management Review* 20 (5): 42–56.

Kuriyan, J. 1996. "Myths in the Land of Integrated Delivery Systems." *Health Management Technology* 17 (1): 54.

Moynihan, J. J., and K. Norman. 1994. "CHIN Provides Vital Healthcare Linkages." *Healthcare Financial Management*. 48 (1): 59–62, 64.

Petry, J., and P. Nimtz. 1996. "Choosing the Right HIN Ownership Model." *Proceedings: Toward an Electronic Patient Record '96*. 12th International Symposium on the Creation of Electronic Health Record System and Global Conference on Patient Cards. May 11–18, 521–28.

Simpson, R. L. 1996. "Will the Internet Supplant Community Health Networks?" *Nursing Management* 27 (2): 20, 23.

Veatch, R. 1996. "Without Question, Most of Us Wish We'd Started Earlier." *Quality Letter for Healthcare Leaders* 8 (2): 12–15.

Weaver, C. 1993. "CHINs: Infrastructure for the Future." *Trustee* 49 (6): 12–13.

16

INTERNET APPLICATIONS

Brian T. Malec

T HE FUTURE of healthcare information management will be closely allied with the Internet and the technology derived from it. This chapter introduces the history and structure of the Internet, describes healthcare applications of the Internet and Intranet, and discusses issues related to management of the technology. The chapter does not

Concepts and Applications

The recent development of the Internet has affected American commerce greatly, including healthcare organizations. Nearly 400 hospitals are using Internet technology to help deliver comprehensive care, establish links with business partners, and provide information about themselves to patients and the community.

Many healthcare organizations are implementing Intranets, which has resulted in more efficient intraorganization communication and enhanced teamwork.

After reading this chapter, readers will be able to discuss the history and the current state of the Internet. They will also be able to describe business strategies for their organizations using Internet, as well as Intranet, technology.

discuss the technical requirements for creating Internet applications but rather focuses on the management implications of Internet-derived technology for health services organizations. Since the technology is new and constantly evolving, the chapter attempts to focus on those elements of it that will survive the test of time.

Internet technology poses a challenge for healthcare organizations to harness the communication potential of this tool and make the technology work to further their organizational goals. The fact that access to information on the Internet is simple is both a blessing and a curse. On the one hand, the technology makes it easy for people to access information that an organization wishes to make available to the public. On the other hand, there is no quality control to prevent misleading or false information from being just as accessible. The effective use of this technology by healthcare organizations is a central theme of this chapter.

A related technology, the Intranet, applies Internet technology within the safer, more controlled environment of a single organization. The Intranet provides controlled access to corporate information, policies, and common databases within an organization and among a selected group of users.

History and Structure of the Internet

The Internet is a complex network of already networked computers connected together from all over the globe. It is a network of networks. As a worldwide phenomenon, the Internet can be accessed by virtually anyone with certain basic technology components. Entry into this network of computers is relatively easy because there are few rules and because by design the Internet is accessible from many locations and gateways. The information and data flowing through the Internet are constantly changing. Edwards (1995) compares it to a cloud that is constantly changing its form, size, and shape. No person, government, or organization either controls the flow of information or the actual content of the information. Individual networks, such as a university computer system or healthcare organization's system, pay for and maintain their own systems and cooperatively support the communication lines that connect them all together.

The World Wide Web (Web or WWW) is a system for finding and accessing Internet resources. Web browsers such as Netscape and Microsoft Explorer allow the user to examine vast amounts of information contained on thousands of computers. See Chapter 5 for a detailed description of Internet technology.

The Internet's early beginnings evolved from the U.S. military's need to develop a secure communication system that could not be disrupted or destroyed by an enemy attack. Beginning in 1969, the U.S. Department of Defense (DOD), through the Advanced Research Projects Agency (ARPA), funded a project that would involve the DOD, military research contractors, university research centers, and others to develop a reliable computer/communications network. (Edwards 1995, 4) ARPANET, as it was called, was designed around the concept of "dynamic message routing," which would allow the automatic rerouting of communications if one element in the system was destroyed or became dysfunctional. The system was designed so that messages sent from one source to another would not follow the same route every time. If an Internet user in Chicago sends a series of messages to Los Angeles, the actual electronic signal will probably never travel in a straight line; it will be rerouted through different "hubs" each time a new message is sent. This ensures that if a "hub" were to be destroyed or down for repairs, the users of the system would see no difference in the speed of communication.

The strength of the Internet rests on this central design. A resulting reality is that since messages and information do not go through a central location, there is no way to control the content or ensure the accuracy of the information. In the 1980s the National Science Foundation (NSF) established a network of supercomputers around the country that evolved into the physical backbone of the Internet system. NSFNET, and various commercial companies, currently provide the backbone for Internet communication in the United States. Other countries have established similar organizations that provide the core infrastructure for the Internet. (See Edwards (1995) and Health Care Cybervision (1996) for more information on the historical development of Internet technology.)

Initially, the Internet had only a few users—universities with super-computers and staff who were engaged in DOD research. But Internet use grew rapidly as the personal computer (PC) was developed, standards were set for communication among and between computers, and easy access to it was provided through commercial and other providers, like universities and businesses. As a result, the Internet has become an essential communications tool of both nonprofit and profit-making firms, including healthcare organizations.

Internet Applications for Healthcare Organizations

Many health services organizations are embracing Internet technology as an effective and inexpensive management strategy to help deliver comprehensive, integrated care. In late 1996, more than 400 hospitals and other healthcare organizations had established Web sites on the Internet. (Flower 1996)

The rapid diffusion of Internet technology, beginning in the mid-1990s, has resulted in many healthcare organizations leaping onto the Internet "with a bungee cord instead of a business strategy." (Monahan 1997, 6) This section discusses integration of Internet applications with the business strategies of the organization.

Figure 16.1 lists four major business strategies of healthcare organizations. Each of the strategies are discussed in the sections that follow, and Internet applications associated with each strategy are reviewed.

Improving Internal Business Processes and Services

Internet applications have been developed that are designed to improve internal operations and support delivery of services:

Online Customer Services. Some health services organizations are using the Internet to provide limited services to patients or health plan members. For example, systems have been developed that allow patients to renew prescriptions, complete healthcare forms, and make appointments online through the Internet. At Long Beach Community Hospital and Medical Center in California, patients can register online in order to avoid waiting at the facility. (Jaklevic 1996, 47)

Retrieval of Medical Information. Many hospitals and other healthcare organizations provide Internet service to physicians who use the system to obtain current medical information and knowledge. A growing number of medical knowledge bases are available on the Web. (See Chapter 11.)

Figure 16.1 Business Strategies and Internet Applications

1. Improving Internal Business Processes and Services
   a. Online customer services
   b. Retrieval of medical information
   c. Retrieval of business-related information
   d. Employee recruiting
2. Establishing External Linkages with Business Partners
   a. Ordering supplies and materials (electronic commerce)
   b. Obtaining insurance authorization and processing claims
3. Increasing Marketshare and Stability
   a. Advertising services
   b. Providing information on benefits and facilities
4. Providing Public Service Information to the Community
   a. Providing health promotion and wellness information
   b. Providing disease-specific information

Retrieval of Business-Related Information. The Internet can be used by managers to obtain current information that supports their activities in the organization. For example, chief information officers (CIOs) can find information about computer hardware and software on the Web. Chief financial officers (CFOs) can obtain current information on Medicare and Medicaid policies from the Health Care Financing Administration through the Internet (http://www.hcfa.gov). (See Figure 16.2.)

Employee Recruiting. Some larger organizations have established Web sites that list job announcements and position openings. For example, Columbia/HCA Healthcare Corporation (www.columbia.net) provides physician recruitment information for their many facilities and clinics. PacifiCare Health Systems, a California HMO, uses its Web site (http://www.phs.com) to provide an interactive job listing of currently available positions (see Figure 16.3). Applicants can scan the job list and submit résumés via electronic mail (e-mail) to the company's human resources department. (Zeff 1996, 20)

Establishing External Linkages with Business Partners

The Internet provides healthcare organizations with a tool for communicating with external business partners and vendors.

Ordering Supplies and Materials. Web technology has been used for online order processing between healthcare organizations and suppliers. The electronic commerce capability of the Internet provides access to vendor catalogs and permits online order placement and payment.

Obtaining Insurance Authorization and Processing Claims. The Web can be used by healthcare providers to obtain eligibility information and advanced authorization for services provided to patients. In some cases, Internet linkages are used for processing claims for insurance payment, thereby improving cash flow and reducing accounts receivable.

Increasing Marketshare and Stability

Through a Web site, health services organizations can provide present and potential customers with information about services that are available in the local marketplace.

Advertising Services. Web sites have been developed that provide detailed information about services offered by healthcare organizations. For example, the Web site of Christ Hospital and Medical Center in Oak Lawn, Illinois, provides a listing of services including cardiovascular, pediatric and childbirth services, cancer care center, psychiatry and substance abuse services, emergency services, intensive care services,

Figure 16.2 Health Care Financing Administration Web Page

| HCFA | Medicare | Medicaid | Help | Feedback | Search | FAQs |

Medicare

Medicaid

Publications & Forms

Local Info.

Stats & Data

Research & Demonstration

Laws & Regs

Public Affairs

About HCFA

Feedback

Gov't Links

Search

Help

Welcome to **HCFA**
the Medicare and Medicaid Agency
Health Care Financing Administration

Welcome to the **Health Care Financing Administration** (HCFA), the federal agency that administers the Medicare and Medicaid programs.

HCFA provides health insurance for over 74 million Americans through Medicare and Medicaid. The majority of these individuals receive their benefits through the fee-for-service delivery system, however, an increasing number are choosing managed care plans.

In addition to providing health insurance, HCFA also regulates all laboratory testing (except research) in the U.S. through the Clinical Laboratory Improvement Amendments (CLIA) program.

As part of HCFA's Initiatives, the agency has begun two projects to provide national identification systems for providers and health plans: **"PAYERID"** and the **"National Provider Identifier"**. As future initiatives arise, you will find a link to new information from the updated **"News"** column to the right. Thanks for visiting HCFA's web site. We look forward to hearing from you.

In the News Aug 05, 1997

New York Medicaid Waiver Approved Press Release; & Facts Sheets

Medicare Proposes Cuts in Excessive Home Oxygen Payments.

HCFA Restructuring Underway

Pregnancy and HIV: What you need to know

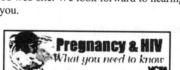

About HCFA ▼
Quick Navigate

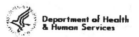
Department of Health & Human Services

Figure 16.3 PacifiCare Health Systems Web Page

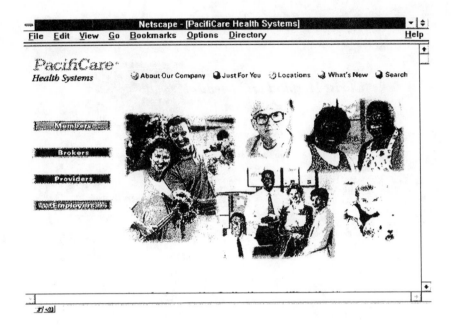

and outpatient care (http://www.advocatehealth.com/sites/christ.html).
(See Figure 16.4.)

Providing Information on Benefits and Facilities. Some health plans
and integrated delivery systems have established Web pages that offer
information on benefits available and the location of facilities offered by
the plan. For example, United Health Care of Arizona has a Web site that
enables enrollees to find a provider, locate the nearest provider on a map,
review benefits, and talk to a service representative online. (Morrissey
1997, 142)

Providing Public Service Information to the Community

Healthcare organizations have a responsibility to improve the health
within the communities they serve. Internet technology is being used
to serve this purpose.

Providing Health Promotion and Wellness Information. Web sites have
been developed that provide disease prevention information, health reminders, nutrition and healthy recipe information, information on health
education programs, poison control information, and immunization
information. For example, the Columbia/HCA Web site (http://www.
columbia.net) contains information about sports medicine services,

Figure 16.4   Christ Hospital and Medical Center Web Page

Christ Hospital and Medical

✚ *Advocate*

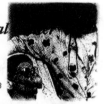

4440 West 95th Street
Oak Lawn, Illinois 60453
708-425-8000

Health Advocate Articles	Community Wellness Programs	Speakers Bureau

- 754-bed teaching center opened in 1961

- The largest private hospital in Illinois based on admissions

- Level III perinatal center -- the highest designation -- one of only 10 hospitals in Illinois to serve high-risk mothers and newborns

- Hope Children's Hospital, a new 60-bed children's hospital, treats over 5,000 pediatric inpatients annually

- Nearly 4,000 babies delivered each year

- Home of The Heart Institute for Children

- Level I trauma center

- More than 60,000 patients treated in the emergency department each year

- Over 750 physicians provide care in more than 60 specialties and subspecialties

Christ Hospital and Medical Center is a 754-bed regional health care provider serving the larger <u>southwest metropolitan Chicago communities</u>. Referrals for specialty care have helped make Christ Hospital the largest private hospital in the state, based on admissions. A teaching hospital with residency programs and medical fellowships, the hospital's exceptional medical staff includes many who also educate the country's future physicians. Along with highly trained nur sing staff and other patient care professionals, physicians provide medical care with a genuine concern for patients and their families. The hospital's mission is to restore patients' health and improve the quality of their lives.

health education classes, and wellness activities, as well as a link to a healthcare encyclopedia.

Providing Disease-Specific Information. Some HMOs and other healthcare providers use the Web to offer support services to individuals with a particular disease or medical condition. These Web sites direct patients to support groups; "chat" groups of others who have the same condition; local, state, and national organizations (e.g., American Cancer Society, American Heart Association); and other sources of medical information available on the Internet.

These examples illustrate the varied and creative ways healthcare organizations are using the Internet to further specific business strategies or respond to current market pressures to develop a Web site. The Internet can be used to help position an organization for future growth in the managed care environment. Some organizations are embarking upon Web projects because the competition is doing it, rather than for clearly defined business strategies. From a management standpoint, however, organizations need to determine first if connecting to the Internet is advancing a business strategy or is an uncontrolled and unmanaged event.

Intranet Applications for Healthcare Organizations

The term *Intranet* began to be used in mid-1995 to describe "internal Webs," or private computer networks based on Internet-derived technologies. (Benett 1996, 7) Fotsch defines the Intranet as an internal Internet network "that links an organization's communications and information in a way that makes information more accessible and navigation through all the resources and applications of the organization's computer environment more seamless." (Fotsch 1997, 26) An Intranet is more then just e-mail, although e-mail is an essential element of it.

Intranets support a wide range of organizational goals and are growing in importance in the healthcare industry. At present, Intranets usually involve communication and distribution of information across the

Figure 16.5 Categories of Intranet Applications

---

1. Improving Internal Communications
    a. Linking components of an integrated delivery system
    b. Communicating electronically clinical information
    c. Communicating electronically financial and administrative information
    d. Providing a "help desk" to respond to frequently asked questions
2. Distributing Organizational Information
    a. Posting and distributing organizational policies, procedures, and announcements
    b. Distributing internal newsletters
    c. Distributing company forms and software
3. Delivering Educational Programs
    a. Providing patient health education programs over internal networks
    b. Providing staff education programs and teleconferences

---

organization. Figure 16.5 lists three major categories of Intranet applications and gives examples of each.

Improving Internal Communications

Linking Components of an Integrated Delivery System. Intranets are being used to provide electronic communication of information among components of an integrated delivery system. (See Chapter 15.) For example, six Boston-area hospitals (Beth Israel Deaconess, New England Baptists, Mount Auburn, Deaconess Waltham, Deaconess Nashoba, and Deaconess Glover) have developed an Intranet Web site that allows medical personnel within the system to access patient data stored anywhere in the network. (HIMSS 1997, 6)

Communicating Electronically Clinical Information. Intranets are being used for electronic communication of medical information and related clinical applications. (See Chapter 11.) For example, Group Health Cooperative im Seattle has established an Intranet for use by its physicians. "It's entire Clinical Roadmaps program . . . is entirely supported by an online library of clinical guidelines and other forms of decision support powered by the organization's clinical intranet." (Hagland 1997, 22)

Communicating Electronically Financial and Administrative Information. Intranets can also be used for electronic communication of financial and other administrative information among components of an integrated delivery system or among departments of one organization. For example, an Intranet might be used to establish insurance eligibility for patients seeking care at an ambulatory clinic of a medical center.

Providing a "Help Desk" to Respond to Frequently Asked Questions. Some organizations use their Intranets to provide 24-hour access to staff at an online "help desk," which can provide answers to frequently asked questions or route users to the most appropriate source for answers.

Distributing Organizational Information

Posting and Distributing Organizational Policies, Procedures, and Announcements. Intranets are replacing voluminous organizational policy manuals and directories by making this information available online. The need for costly updating of printed manuals and directories is eliminated. The Rush Presbyterian/St. Luke's Medical Center in Chicago uses its Intranet to provide current employee information, organizational policies and procedures, a phone directory, and health and fitness information. (Skarulis 1996)

Distributing Internal Newsletters. Most healthcare organizations publish internal newsletters to provide information to physicians, employees, and other constituents. Intranets are being used to provide this information online, thus reducing publication and distribution costs.

Distributing Company Forms and Software. Intranets are being used to respond to requests for standard forms used within the organization. In addition, the system can be used to download standard software applications from a central computer software library maintained by the organization.

Delivering Educational Programs

Providing Patient Health Education Programs over Internal Networks. Intranets can provide the communications links required to deliver health education programs to patients in a hospital or other health services organization.

Providing Staff Education Programs and Teleconferences. In addition to patient education, Intranets are being used to deliver education programs and teleconferences to employees of the organization.

The applications listed are only examples of the potential use of Internet and Intranet technology. Given the rapid growth of this technology, increased utilization can be anticipated in the years ahead.

Management of Internet Technologies in Healthcare Organizations

Internet technologies have emerged so rapidly that few in-depth studies have been done to determine the benefits and costs of healthcare applications. However, in the face of this uncertainty, Internet technologies appear to provide several benefits.

1. Internet technologies are *relatively inexpensive* to purchase, compared to standard healthcare applications software and hardware. The cost of a Web browser is marginal, and stiff marketplace competition assures both competitive prices and increased access to newer and cheaper applications. Many vendors are developing "plug-in" (prepackaged) applications that cut down on application development costs. As standards are adapted, a greater number of vendors worldwide will compete for business, further reducing costs.

2. Internet technologies are *convenient to use.* Because they are becoming a part of everyday life both at work and home, an increasing number of users have access to the technology and are familiar with its basic operations. Whereas implementing a new software application in

the finance area could take months of training, it takes only days to learn how an Internet application works.

3. The World Wide Web is *international in scope,* which opens a wide range of business opportunities.

4. Of great importance, Internet technologies are *user friendly.* The Internet is not a complicated puzzle that must be mastered before people can use it. Rather it is a transparent technology that allows the user to focus on the problem, not the technology.

Internet technology also has its drawbacks, which healthcare organizations should consider when deciding whether to use the Internet to support a business strategy. These potential negatives include:

1. *Security issues.* These issues are decreasing as new developments in Internet technologies allow greater coding and encryption, which protect the transmission of sensitive corporate and patient information. Firewalls, a sophisticated software-hardware combination that stops unauthorized communications, can prevent or limit access to the Internet and even restrict the areas of the Web to which individuals can have access. (Morrissey 1996)

2. *"Lost in Cyberspace."* Some employees fall in love with the technology and spend hours a day surfing through the Web. In effect, they get lost in Cyberspace. This can impact employee productivity and, therefore, is an important issue for any organization. Some organizations permit unmonitored access to the Internet, while others keep detailed logs of utilization.. Healthcare organizations must develop policies to help manage Internet technologies. (See Chapter 7.)

3. *Slow response time.* The growth in the use of the Internet by corporations, nonprofit organizations, government agencies, and the general population has put a significant strain on the technology, which just a few years ago was used only by a few major research institutions. The traffic flow can be substantial, thus delaying a potential user's access to a Web site. A health plan member who tries unsuccessfully to get access to an organization's Web site can become frustrated, destroying goodwill. If employees are attempting to access the Web for a business-related function, such as information on a current medical protocol, Web traffic can cause a loss of productivity.

4. While Internet applications are relatively less expensive than other information systems, *the cost is not zero.* Costs include personnel, technology, maintenance, and management. One significant cost involves gathering and updating information on the Web. The startup of a Web site is often far easier and less expensive than the continual updating of the site. This relative ease of startup leads some organizations to underestimate the time needed to maintain the site.

Intranets also have potential benefits and costs that need to be reviewed before an organization invests in them. Establishment of an internal network can improve organizational communication and reduce the costs of distributing forms, documents, software, policies, and directories. In addition, intranets can unite geographically and culturally diverse units of a healthcare organization.

The potential negative aspects of intranets are similar to those of Internets. Some of these include:

1. Costs of maintaining information on the network. "The cost of creating Intranet content includes the conversion of existing documents to HTML [Hytertext Transfer Protocol], coordination of various content providers, periodic indexing of material for the benefit of search engines, and continuous updating of content." (Benett 1996, 55)
2. Privacy and security issues with associated hardware and software costs. Access must be through firewalls.
3. Cost of maintaining Intranet servers and network software.

McCormack (1996, 22) reports the following costs associated with establishment of an Intranet at Lowell General Hospital, Massachusetts:

- $20,000 in startup costs;
- $10,000 for firewalls to prevent access from outside the organization;
- $6,000 for a PC server dedicated to the Internet/Intranet application;
- $2,000 for an Integrated Services Digital Network (ISDN) router and circuit switch connections, and a $600 per month fee for the ISDN link; and
- $2,000 for monitoring software.

Internet-derived technologies can contribute to the overall success of a healthcare organization if they are implemented as a part of a carefully managed process. Consiglio suggests the following guidelines for implementing either Internet or Intranet applications:

1. get small successes early;
2. nurture pilot projects;
3. understand that Web experiments require leaps of technology, skills, and investments; and
4. focus on clearing technological, financial, political, and organizational culture hurdles. (Consiglio 1996, 96)

Nurturing small pilot Internet projects allows successes that will further encourage other projects. Pilot projects also allow Internet champions to emerge and take leadership roles in developing larger, more complex projects. Moving too quickly into a large complex project can leave an organization frustrated and confused. While the basic business concepts of the Internet's usefulness are relatively easy to understand, in reality a Web project requires large leaps in technology, technical skills, and financial resources.

Perhaps the single most important aspect of introducing Internet technology is to consider the impact this technology will have on an organization's culture. Methods of problem solving, sources of information, and power bases may shift with the effective use of Internet-derived technologies. The management of change is essential when new technologies are introduced. Benett (1996, 55) states that "Intranets work best where the corporate culture encourages teamwork and rewards information sharing."

The Health Care Cybervision project recommends the following strategies for implementing Internet/Intranet technologies.

1. Make sure that the Internet technologies complement existing information architectures within your organization.
2. Establish a corporate-wide, multidisciplinary governance group to set policies, guidelines, technologies, and usage goals for Internet technologies.
3. Evaluate the implication of these technologies on current business strategies and processes.
4. Using Internet derived-technologies, develop a network of Internet experts who can support and advise in areas of an enterprisewide information infrastructure.
5. Ensure that there is widespread access to the Internet-derived technologies, especially e-mail and WWW capabilities.

(Health Care Cybervision Project: http://www.hccybervision.com/monograph2/).

As this discussion suggests, the implementation of any new technology requires close attention to detail, compatibility of the technology with the organization's current information architecture, compatibility with the corporate culture, and measurement of the benefits and costs of the new technology. The implementation of Internet and Intranet technologies requires good management skills and careful planning.

Summary

The Internet is a complex network of already networked computers connected together from all over the globe. It is a network of networks. The Web is an enabling layer of technology that allows the end-user to browse the Internet using graphical user interfaces.

The Internet began as a project of the U.S. military, and the technology was limited at first to the military and major university research facilities. In the 1980s a new technology was developed that permitted great ease in exchanging messages across various computer platforms. Transmission Control Protocol/Internet Protocol (TCP/IP) standards made it possible for computers from different manufacturers to exchange information. In the 1980s the National Science Foundation (NSF) established a network of supercomputers around the country that evolved in 1990 into the physical backbone of the Internet system.

Web browser software was developed in the 1990s and allowed the expansion of the Internet to anyone with a PC and proper browser software. By the end of 1996, millions of individuals had access to the Internet, and more than 400 hospitals and other healthcare organizations had established Web sites.

Many organizations are embracing Internet technology as an effective and inexpensive management strategy to help deliver comprehensive, integrated care. In healthcare organizations, Intranet applications are being developed to improve internal business processes and services, establish external linkages with business partners, increase marketshare and stability, and provide public service information to the community.

The term *Intranet* describes an internal Web, or private computer network, based on Internet-derived technologies. The Intranet links an organization's communication networks with information sources to make the information more accessible and the computer environment more uniform and seamless. Healthcare organizations have developed Intranet applications in order to improve internal communications, distribute organizational information, and deliver educational programs.

Internet and Intranet technologies have positive and negative aspects in their application to healthcare organizations. The technology is relatively inexpensive, convenient to use, provides access to international markets, and is user friendly. On the negative side, Internet technology has security issues that are still being resolved. Employees can spend too much time on the network. Gaining access to the Web can result in a slow response time for potential visitors to an organization's Web site, and the cost of maintaining a site can be substantial.

An Intranet provides the ability to organize information from multiple systems across an organization and can reduce the cost of distributing organizational information including policies, procedures, announcements, and directories. Intranets are collaborative systems that can improve communications and contribute to team building.

Negative aspects of intranets include the cost of converting existing documents to the appropriate Internet format (HTML); security issues; cost of maintaining, updating, and removing information from internal home pages; development of individual skills to use the technology effectively; and the absence of a corporate culture that encourages teamwork and rewards information sharing.

The implementation of Internet-derived technologies requires careful planning. Guidelines and strategies for implementation include getting small successes early, starting with pilot projects, evaluating compatibility with present information architecture, and determining the benefits and costs of a project.

Discussion Questions

16.1. Define *Internet*. Define *Intranet*. What are the similarities and differences between the Internet and Intranets?

16.2. What are the possible business strategies that might be accomplished by using Internet technologies? Why are these strategies important in a managed care environment?

16.3. What are the principal categories of Internet applications?

16.4. What are the potential benefits of both Internet and Intranet technologies?

16.5. What are the potential problems associated with use of Internet technology?

16.6. What strategies might be useful when implementing Internet/Intranet technologies?

16.7. What impact does an Intranet have on organizational culture and why? What can be done to help improve the implementation of Intranets?

Problems

16.1. Find five Web sites for each of the following types of healthcare organizations: individual hospital, HMO or managed care organization, medical group practice or clinic, or integrated multihospital system. For each new site describe the following:

a. the content and scope of the web site;

b. the types of applications used and the business strategies that these applications support;

c. the links to other Web sites, if any, and the purpose of those links; and

d. your assessment of the quality of information found at each site.

16.2. Prepare a questionnaire and contact a CIO, or other senior staff member, of a local healthcare organization. Questions should include:

a. Does the organization have either an Internet or an Intranet?

b. How long have they used the technology and what was the initial reason for adopting the technology?

c. What has been the impact of the technology on the business objectives of the healthcare organization?

d. What challenges or new opportunities did they discover since implementing the technology?

References

Benett, G. 1996. *Introducing Intranets: A Decisionmakers Guide to Launching an Intranet.* Indianapolis, IN: Que Corporation.

Consiglio, G. 1996. "Health Care and the Internet: A Friendship in the Works." *Health Care Informatics* (July): 96.

Edwards, M. J. A. 1995. *The Internet for Nurses and Allied Health Professionals.* New York: Springer-Verlag, Inc.

Flower, J. 1996. "Log On: A Continuing Guide to the Online World for Health Care Executives, Managers, Clinicians and Patients." *Health Care Forum Journal* 39 (4): 46–51.

Fotsch, E. 1997. "Net Worth of the Internet, Intranets and Extranets." *Health Care Financial Management* 51 (3): 26, 29.

Hagland, M. 1997. "How WebCare is Changing Health Care Delivery, Hit by Hit." *Health Management Technology* 18 (4): 22–26.

Healthcare Information and Management Systems Society (HIMSS). 1997 "Web Site Triage Links Medical Records Among Boston Hospitals." *HIMSS News* 8 (6): 6

Health Care Cybervision 1996. "The Role of the Internet in Health Care." Internet Home page—http://www.hccybervision.com [accessed February 1997].

Jaklevic, M. C. 1996. "Internet Technology Moves to Patient-Care Front Lines." *Modern Healthcare* 25 (9): 47–50.

McCormack, J. 1996. "Live, on the Internet: Surgery." *Health Data Management* 4 (11): 21–22.

Monahan, T. 1997. "Who's Driving Internet Expansion?" *Healthcare Informatics* (May): 6.

Morrissey, J. 1997. "HMOs Enter Internet Age." *Modern Healthcare* 27 (14): 140–44.

———. 1996. "Securing the Internet Frontier." *Modern Healthcare* 26 (43): 56–64.

Skarulis, P. 1996. "Intranet Case Studies." Unpublished presentation at: *Healthcare CIO Symposium.* Boca Raton, Florida, November 21–22.

Zeff, P. S. 1996. "The Web as an HMO Marketing Tool." *Health Data Management* 4 (5): 20.

Additional Readings

Anthony, D. 1996. "Health Resources on the World Wide Web." *International Journal of Information Management* 16 (4): 315–19.

Bazzoli, F. 1996. "The Ins and Outs of Internet Outsourcing." *Health Data Management* 4 (2):19–20.

Brakeman, L. 1996. "It's Full Speed Ahead on the World Wide Web." *Managed Healthcare* 6 (1): 38–40.

———. 1996. "Planning is the Only Way to Prevent a Rocky Start." *Managed Healthcare* 6 (8): 54–56.

Brown, M. 1996. "Cyberspace-savvy Health Care Market Identified: Internet Not Meeting Its Needs." *Health Care Strategic Management* 14 (11): 8–9.

Claridge, A. 1996. "Harnessing Intranet Technology." *Healthcare Informatics* 13 (6): 144.

Clark, R. L. 1996. "The Intriguing Internet." *Healthcare Financial Management* 50 (8): 16.

Fotsch, E. 1996. "Intranet: Information Technology for a Limited Universe." *Healthcare Financial Management*, 50 (9): 30.

———. 1997. "Intranet Applications Can Strengthen Relationships with Physicians." *Healthcare Financial Management* 51 (1): 24.

Gonzalez, E., and S. Helen. 1995. "Internet Sources for Nursing and Allied Health." *Database* 18 (3): 46–49.

Hancock, L. 1996. *Physicians' Guide to the Internet*. Philadelphia: Lippincott-Raven.

Hoben, J. W., ed. 1996. *1997 Guide to Health Care Resources on the Internet*. New York: Faulkner & Gray, Inc.

Johnson, D. E. 1996. "Internet Will Promote Collaboration." *Health Care Strategic Management* 14 (12): 2–3.

Meyer, H. 1996. "Surfing the Net for a Health Plan." *Hospitals & Health Networks* 70 (16): 37–38.

Muscaarella, J., ed. 1996. *1997 Guide to Intranets in Health Care*. New York. Faulkner & Gray, Inc.

Negroponte, N. 1996. "Caught Browsing Again." *Healthcare Financial Management*. 50 (8): 30.

Nordhaus-Bike, A. M. 1996. "It Takes a Virtual Village." *Hospitals & Health Networks*. 70 (7): 52, 54.

Ryer, J. 1997. *HealthNet: Your Essential Resource for the Most Up-to-date Medical Information Online*. New York: John Wiley and Sons.

Siwicki, B. 1996. "Intranets in Health Care." *Health Data Management* 4 (8): 36–47.

DEVELOPING AN ELECTRONIC MEDICAL RECORD FOR AN INTEGRATED PHYSICIAN OFFICE PRACTICE

Andrea W. White and Gloria R. Wakefield

The Beaches Clinic located in Florida is a prestigious, highly specialized, 180-member integrated physician office practice offering 32 specialty services. Its mission is threefold: patient care, research, and education. Patient care is the primary mission but interdependent with the other two. The Clinic has grown impressively since its opening in 1986, and now reports having more than 33,000 patient registrations and more than 160,000 office visits per year. The Beaches Clinic was built on the premise that serving the whole patient is of paramount importance. When a patient is seen at the Clinic, the patient is assigned a primary physician who guides the patient's care and receives prompt assistance, when necessary, from the many specialists who also are employed at the Clinic. Most diagnostic and therapeutic services are performed within the Clinic. Should the patient require hospitalization, the patient is admitted to neighboring PrimaCare Hospital, with which all Beaches Clinic physicians are affiliated.

During the last three years, the Beaches Clinic has been involved in an ambitious undertaking, that of replacing its labor-intensive paper medical record system with a fully electronic patient record. The electronic patient information is now accessible to Beaches physicians from numerous terminals throughout the Clinic and from a number of terminals within PrimaCare Hospital as well. The intent of the new electronic system is to reduce administrative inefficiency, improve access to patient information to benefit patient care, and to improve access to research data. This case study will provide readers with an understanding of the process used by Beaches Clinic personnel in planning, developing, and implementing its electronic medical record.

The Paper Medical Record System— Its Benefits and Disadvantages

The original record system utilized paper medical records enclosed in a plastic pouch. The record consisted of multiple forms of heavy paper, folded width-wise in thirds, color-coded by specialty, placed back-to-back, with the forms arranged according to ease of accessibility for the individual clinicians. The records were handwritten except for the electronic information generated by the Cycare Registration System, the Cerner Laboratory System, and the SD&G Radiology System.

These records were housed in the Health Information Services Department when a patient was not undergoing treatment at the Clinic. When a patient was undergoing treatment, the record resided in the particular area of the Clinic where the patient was being treated. If a patient needed the services of several specialties, the record traveled from one area to another, and if the patient needed to be hospitalized, the record was sent to PrimaCare Hospital. This continual movement of the record created numerous opportunities for the record to be misplaced and created location difficulties for physicians wishing to access the record. The loose material generated by the patient's visits to the various areas of the clinic continually followed the record and required personnel to locate the record and file the material. It was essential that newly generated material be filed within the record before the patient's next visit so that physicians would have access to the most complete information.

As can be imagined, the number of employees required to manage the information in the record was high. About 330 Desk Attendants worked on the eight floors of the clinic and had the sole responsibility of tracking individual records, filing loose material, gathering x-ray films, and transporting the films and the record to the various locations in the clinic where the patient was being seen.

The Health Information Services Department served as the storehouse for the completed record. The department employed 17 clerical people called Completion Assistants. After a patient's treatment ended, the record returned to the Completion Assistants for final analysis and completion. The Completion Assistants made certain that the forms were signed and that all of the necessary reports were included. The Completion Assistants spent a considerable amount of time out of the department, walking on the Clinic floors trying to obtain the necessary signatures and reports. Despite their efforts, it was not unusual for the record to take up to six months to be completed and filed, and, therefore, a tremendous backlog of records waiting for processing existed. Hundreds of records could be found throughout the Clinic waiting for attention. Not surprisingly, physicians often had difficulty obtaining information when they needed it, and frequently were frustrated by the system's inefficiency.

In addition to physicians needing information, the physicians' secretaries also needed access to patient information as they frequently called and spoke to patients. Locating the record could be quite a task. It was possible that a single patient's record could have been taken to and found in numerous locations—the Completion Assistants' area, a number of different Clinic areas, a number of different physicians' offices, a number of secretaries' offices, the business office, or the legal department. A computerized chart tracking system, a part of the Cycare System, was used, which helped manage the process a great deal. Occasionally, however, some human error would occur, and the record was then not readily located. When this unfortunate situation occurred, or when needed patient information was not available in the record, a very labor-intensive "all-points bulletin" search would be initiated. If a search failed to locate the misplaced record, the physician would be forced to cancel and reschedule the patient's visit, which was most irritating and inconvenient for all concerned.

One benefit of the existing system, however, was that when everything worked, and the record was able to be accessed, physicians knew exactly where to locate the information they needed. The system called for records to have all loose material filed onto the record prior to a patient returning to the clinic. The specific services's Desk Attendants arranged the record for their physicians according to the physicians' specifications. Thus, all needed information was located in the front of the record and readily accessible to the physician providing the care. Additional information was easily accessible to the physician who knew the system and needed only to sort through a few colored forms to locate information of interest.

Planning for the Electronic Medical Record

In 1992 a group of physicians and administrators began discussing the possibility of developing an electronic medical record. The Chief Executive Officer of the Clinic, the Associate Administrator of PrimaCare

Hospital, the President of the Beaches Clinic Medical Staff, seven Clinic physicians, and the Director of the Clinic's Information Services Department formed a steering committee to look into the possibility of creating an electronic medical record for Beaches Clinic patients. This group of people recognized that the present system of record keeping was very inefficient. It required the employment of an exorbitant number of people just to manage the record.

The committee wanted a system that would allow data integration between the Clinic, the hospital, the newly developing HMO, and other primary care physician practices, which were increasingly being networked into the Beaches Medical System. They wanted all Beaches physicians to have access to patient information from a number of locations within the medical system. They wanted test results immediately accessible once the tests were completed. They also wanted pertinent patient information from the hospital available to physicians at the Clinic. Since physicians were used to having the Desk Attendants arrange the forms in the paper record specifically for each specialty, with the information that was considered important to the specialty located at the beginning of the record, they wanted the electronic record to also be maintained in a specialty-specific manner. The group wanted diagnostic and procedural billing data to be electronically transmitted to the business office. They wanted data entry to be an easy process that did not require physicians to key in anything. They also wanted the electronic statistical data to be available for research efforts. They expected that an electronic record system would reduce costs in time and labor because there would be no need to shuffle the paper record from area to area in the Clinic, and there would be no need to send the record to the hospital for an admitted patient. In essence, they wanted an electronic application that replicated the paper medical record they had, but which would be readily available in multiple locations to multiple users at the same time.

The Electronic Medical Record (EMR) Steering Committee began looking for a vendor that would be able to provide a product to meet their needs. The in-house Information Services Department at this time included only 10 people within the Clinic and 17 people within the hospital since there was minimal automation in the medical system. The Committee realized they did not have the technical expertise in-house to build the system and sent out an RFP to three vendors. The Committee members made site visits to talk to the vendors and to see their systems. The results were disappointing. What they learned was that there was no one vendor that could deliver all of what the Committee had required, and that if they wanted to continue pursuing the idea of acquiring an electronic medical record, they were going to have to choose the best of a less than ideal system.

The Committee members were unimpressed with two of the vendors, but were intrigued with the third. This vendor was owned by physicians and therefore personnel "could speak their language." The Committee was already somewhat familiar with the vendor because it also had developed the Clinic's laboratory system. This vendor explained to the EMR Steering Committee that they had developed a clinical data repository that allowed the integration of all patient data. This idea interested them, but the Committee explained that they wanted the system to serve not just as a data repository, but also to actually become their medical record. Although the vendor already had several clients, none of these clients had any intention of using the system as its medical record. The company was interested in partnering with the Beaches Clinic and working toward developing the system so that it could be used as the medical record. It offered to act as a consultant in helping the Clinic select other systems that would work well with its clinical data repository and help facilitate its functioning as a medical record. The vendor presented a very convincing proposal to the Clinic that their company could customize the system and could meet the needs of the Clinic through a developmental partnership for an alpha product would greatly enhance the support of the practice.

The Clinic EMR Steering Committee agreed to partner with the vendor, and in 1993 the vendor began planning how it would implement the system. It recommended the use of an optical imaging system and suggested an imaging vendor. The plan called for having all handwritten notes scanned into digital format from the year 1992 forward. The Health Information Services Department hired five clerical people who could scan the handwritten reports that would allow physicians to access the scanned information from the terminals. Additional systems were also brought in to support dictation and transcription.

Implementing the Pilot Program

An expanded Steering Committee, with seven physicians, one clinic administrator, one hospital associate administrator, one information systems director, and the vendor project manager decided that the best way to implement the creation of the electronic medical record (EMR) was to initiate a pilot program. The sixth floor of the Clinic, which treated internal medicine patients, was designated as the opening site. Two of the five internal medicine physicians on this floor who were selected to treat patients using the electronic medical record were serving on the Steering Committee and were eager to test the system. While learning to use the

EMR, the physicians were also to have access to and routinely use the paper medical record. In January 1994, the Pilot Program began.

When word spread that the Pilot Program was being initiated, there was some concern expressed about its feasibility. Not many Clinic physicians expected it would be successful, much less continued. With the exception of the seven physicians serving on the Committee, the Clinic physicians had only been minimally informed of the concept of changing to an EMR. There had been no formal announcement or communication informing the physicians that a plan was being considered and tested. The rumors of a change to an EMR were somewhat unsettling, but few physicians could anticipate the impact of the change. While the physicians recognized the disadvantages of the paper record system, they were at least familiar and comfortable with it. The Beaches Clinic had used paper records since its origin and still boasted of having its first medical records in hard copy. These physicians did not expect that the Clinic would break with tradition.

The Clinic Information Systems (IS) Department designated an individual to serve as a trainer for the five physicians testing the system and set up training sessions. The trainer carried a pager and was readily available to offer assistance. The IS Department also instituted a HELP line. The vendor developed training manuals and a quick reference guide, which could easily be carried in a pocket. The Pilot Program was initially planned to last three months. As the weeks progressed, the five physicians appeared pleased with the EMR. They were still able to practice with their paper medical records, but also used the EMR. Some of them used the EMR more frequently than others.

In March 1994, the Clinic administrator asked the Health Information Services Director of PrimaCare Hospital to serve in an advisory capacity on the Steering Committee and to spend some time each week consulting in the Health Information Services Department of the Clinic. This individual knew what information was required in the medical record and had expertise in the presentation of data, data integrity, and the legal aspects of confidentiality and security of patient information. She was able to act as a liaison between the IS people and the clinicians using the EMR. Eventually, this individual was appointed Director for the Health Information Services Department in the Clinic as well as in the Hospital.

The Pilot Program continued for six months, and as problems or issues developed, the Steering Committee addressed them. Although the Pilot Program had been established as a pilot program, in actuality, it functioned as the vehicle to implement the plan to move from the paper medical record to the electronic medical record, rather than as a testing and evaluation mechanism of a possible electronic medical record idea.

At the end of the six months, despite holding no formal evaluation of the system, the Steering Committee continued with the implementation, confident in its commitment to the project and in its decision that there would be no turning back. The Clinic and the vendor were moving forward in their partnership to develop the electronic medical record.

The rollout was done by specialty, with the easier specialty services rolling out first, and the more complicated services implemented later. The Primary Care practice at the hospital was also done. As the rollout progressed, physicians began expressing concern about the time it was requiring to actually use the system. They were unfamiliar with the system and required training, but this training and unfamiliarity were impacting on the physicians' productivity. Clinic physicians were employed by the Clinic and were expected to meet certain productivity standards. The new system was interfering with their ability to meet these standards. The physicians were not able to see as many of their patients and the time they spent with each patient was significantly increased as they searched for information on the EMR. Moreover, physicians found it difficult to talk to patients and maintain eye contact as they also scanned computer screens. It was hard to do both activities at the same time when they felt so unfamiliar with the system. For example, the ophthalmologists had been spending about ten minutes with each patient using the paper medical record. Now, however, they were spending about 25 minutes seeing patients as they clicked through the record trying to locate specific information they needed to evaluate the patient. Administration recognized their concerns and made arrangements for them to have decreased productivity while they learned the system.

The last departments implementing the EMR were Surgery and Hematology/Oncology. These departments were the most productive and the most complicated. They also were quite content with the present paper medical record system and the most resistant to practicing solely with the EMR. However, the Clinic Information System personnel continued the training. Formal training sessions had been established, and the IS Department practiced a "Train the Trainer" method, training personnel in the Clinic's Education and Development Department who then trained the physicians. Eventually the last departments were also comfortable with using the EMR.

Maintaining a Parallel Operation

Although it was always the Clinic's intention to develop the EMR to replace the paper medical record, it was recognized that both the electronic and the manual systems would have to be maintained for a period of time. The paper record was the official medical record of the Clinic and the only one sanctioned by state law at the time. The paper record was also necessary to serve as the backup to the electronic record during computer downtime. Initially, it was expected that implementing the Pilot Program of the EMR would have little impact on current medical record operations, and that the paper medical record system would continue to be maintained exactly as it had been during the past ten years. However, the Pilot Program immediately impacted the paper record and its operations.

The Pilot Program began on the sixth floor, which housed three specialties. The first issue to be resolved was how to simultaneously get the new paper information, which was being generated during patient visits, onto both the electronic record and the paper record, since it was needed on both records. With the exception of the sixth floor, the paper record was in use exclusively in all other areas of the Clinic. Even though patients were seen in the pilot specialty areas, they were also being seen and receiving treatment in other areas of the Clinic as well. Therefore, the newly generated information needed to be maintained in both a paper and an electronic format. This dual system created a tremendous paper chase to ensure that all results were returned to the pilot floor area where they could be scanned into the EMR. As a result, point-of-service scanners were purchased and implemented on each of the floors and also placed in the Health Information Services Department to better capture all "loose" material.

It was noted by physicians that results of tests that they knew had been performed were not present in both the EMR and the paper medical record. This became a frequent enough occurrence that a quality control process had to be implemented to check the EMR against the paper record and to be certain that all results and necessary reports were found in both the EMR and the paper record prior to a patient's scheduled appointment. As the EMR was rolled out to other floors, this quality-control process became extremely labor intensive. Approximately 30 temporary staff were hired to perform the process. In addition, ten other temporary staff were hired to maintain the filing of loose reports. The quality control process continued for two years until it was believed that the majority of scheduled appointment records had been reviewed and that the paper records and the electronic records contained the same information.

The EMR Steering Committee recognized that the Clinic needed to maintain the dual record system for at least two years. The process of rolling out the EMR to all the specialties had been planned to take place over a two-year time frame. Physicians' mixed acceptance of the EMR as well as performance and stability issues of the new system required that the process not be rushed. Also the paper medical record served as the backup during system downtime.

Three years into the conversion, the paper record continues to serve as the legal record and the downtime backup record. A legal record must have reports with authorized physician signatures and must be easily retrievable and easily hard-copied so that it can be sent to designated locations when patients authorize a release of information. The EMR system, at this time, is not able to easily satisfy these requirements. The vendor is continuing to work on enhancements and upgrades, but progress has been slow. A new product version that is under development and is scheduled to be implemented in the fourth year will soon meet all of the legal requirements and will allow the EMR to truly serve as the legal medical record. Until that time, however, both systems must be maintained.

By March 1996, everyone in the Clinic was using the EMR System. No longer were paper medical records allowed to be used by physicians along with the electronic record. Physicians were expected to practice using the EMR alone. The paper record was continuing to be maintained, however, for legal reasons. Although no survey had been conducted at the time, it was estimated that the majority of physicians had become familiar enough with the system and appeared pleased with it. User groups have now been established and are able to present their issues about the system to the EMR Steering Committee. A formal survey of physicians to solicit user input is also being conducted at the time of this writing.

Impact of the Electronic Medical Record

The new Electronic Medical Record System at the Clinic has achieved many of the goals for which it was intended. Electronic patient information is almost always available at multiple locations and by multiple users and is used to support practice. There has been minimal computer downtime, and when it has occurred, a paper medical record has been available since it is still being produced. State law has only recently been changed to allow for electronic signatures. Therefore, the electronic medical record can now serve as the official medical record once electronic signatures have been incorporated into the system. It is expected that this electronic signature implementation will be initiated sometime in the near future, eliminating the need for the dual systems.

The new system has produced dramatic changes in the number and use of clerical and technical personnel and the associated personnel costs. During the first two years of implementation, costs associated with increased personnel and equipment purchases rose dramatically. During the third year, however, costs decreased substantially and are expected to continue declining. The initial conversion required additional low-cost clerical personnel and high-cost technical staffing. Since physicians continued to dictate their reports and clinic notes rather than keying in information, the information needed to be transcribed into the new electronic system. A significant number of transcriptionists were and are needed to accomplish this task. The Director of Health Information Services had originally employed only eight transcriptionists, but she now employs 55 transcriptionists and estimates that she needs at least ten others to transcribe all of the Clinic Notes, Patient Referral Correspondence, and Outpatient Operative Reports. Some of these transcriptionists are located in the main Clinic building, but most are off-site working in a separate building several miles away. Three contract services are also being utilized to ensure a 48-hour turnaround time.

Paper test results also had to be scanned into the electronic system. The Clinic purchased optical scanners and currently employs 12 people who serve as scanning personnel, optically scanning test results into the system. These scanners are located on each of the Clinic floors and do point-of-service scanning as documents are generated on the floor. Two scanners are also used in the Health Information Services Department and scan information into newly created electronic records as previously seen patients re-enter the Clinic for evaluation and treatment.

The number of computer terminals used in the Clinic has dramatically increased. Computer terminals can now be found at each Desk Attendants' area, in each patient examining room, and on all nursing units on all of the floors. The need for in-house technology support substantially grew. Due to the continuation of system enhancements and the planned conversion of the hospital medical record, additional positions were required, increasing the in-house Clinic technical staff from the original 10 to 30 and the hospital technical staff from 17 to 35.

The importance of receiving feedback from users has been recently recognized. The Health Information Services Department during the past year employed two individuals who have been charged with talking to physicians in specific specialties to find out what information they particularly need and want to have at their fingertips. These individuals then work with the Information Systems personnel and convey those needs so that the IS Department and the vendor can design the EMR screens to be more user-friendly for the specialists. Although more work is needed in this specific customizing, the efforts are beginning to pay off. While the patient record screens are a far cry from the sophisticated, colorful, and attractive Windows computer screens so commonly in use today, the specialty screens are functional. A Windows-based graphical user interface is being developed for the next upgrade of the system.

Obviously the initial additional personnel and the technological requirements were costly to the Clinic during the first two years of implementation. By the first quarter of the third year however, a significant reduction in clerical staff associated with paper record movement was achieved. The number of Desk Attendants and Completion Assistants was substantially reduced. Paper record maintenance is currently being accomplished by the use of low-cost temporary staffing. It is expected that the need for the temporary staffing will be eliminated once the paper record functions are eliminated at the end of the fourth year of EMR implementation

Although technical staff were also increased, it is predicted that by the fourth quarter of the fifth year, the technical staff will be reduced by one third and will only be involved in performing system maintenance functions. The current Health Information Services staff, numbering 106 and presently involved in paper and electronic record functions, is expected at that time to be reduced to 25 since it will only be performing electronic record maintenance functions.

In the third conversion year, the Clinic realized a $6 million increase in revenue. This increase reduced an existing $8 million deficit to $2 million. The trend in revenue enhancement is expected to exceed the five-year revenue enhancement projections.

The benefits of the new electronic system are numerous. In 1994, approximately 50 records were listed as "unable to locate." Optical imaging of paper documents has now eliminated "lost" information. Access to medical information has been greatly improved, thus improving turnaround times for patient appointments and follow-up visits, obtaining billing information, abstracting data in registries, and conducting quality management reviews. Duplication of work in sharing information between physician offices and the hospital has been greatly reduced. No longer is information needed to be copied, faxed, or mailed to different locations. Physicians have immediate online access to patient information. Record retrieval for scheduled patient appointments has been reduced from a 24–48-hour retrieval time to retrieval at time of the appointment. Optical imaging at the point-of-service provides a complete medical record in a more timely manner than the previous practice of filing late reports in the paper record, which in some cases resulted in a record not being completed for several months.

All of these improvements have greatly enhanced the quality of patient care provided to Clinic patients and have improved the efficiency and reduced the costs of delivery. The system currently in use at Beaches Clinic is well on its way to serving as the legal and electronic medical record of the Clinic, and the members of the EMR Steering Committee are feeling confident that they have helped the Clinic make dramatic improvements in their information system and in their delivery of patient care.

Benefits of the Electronic Medical Record

- Immediate physician access to patient information from within either the hospital or the Clinic
- Improvement in creation of a timely and complete medical record, benefiting patient care
- Elimination of "lost" information in the record
- Improvement in turnaround time for scheduling patient appointments and follow-up visits
- Improvement in timeliness and access to billing information
- Improvement in capability for abstracting research data
- Improvement in access to quality management data
- Elimination of faxing, copying, and mailing of patient information between hospital and Clinic
- Reduction of clerical personnel involved in record movement and record retrieval
- Additional cost reductions projected as system performance improves

---

Discussion Questions

1. How did the organizational culture of the Clinic impact on the planning and decision-making process of this project?
2. What were the benefits and disadvantages of the process used by the Beaches Clinic in planning and implementing the EMR?
3. What might you suggest to improve upon the planning and decision-making process?
4. Why is communication essential among administrators, clinicians, information systems personnel, and the vendor?
5. Why is it essential that data integrity be ensured in a multisystem integration?

IMPLEMENTATION OF A COMPUTER-BASED PATIENT RECORD IN A FAMILY MEDICINE CLINICAL PRACTICE

Frances Wickham Lee
Steven M. Ornstein
and Ruth G. Jenkins

The Department of Family Medicine (DFM) at the Medical University of South Carolina (MUSC) has long been recognized as a leader in the development of computer applications in family medicine. They developed one of the nation's first computerized medical records in the early 1970s, and a few years ago they implemented a state-of-the-art, comprehensive computer-based patient record (CPR). The CPR is used not only to support direct patient care, but also to provide longitudinal data for evaluating preventive services, quality improvement, and other research studies. The CPR at MUSC is considered a highly successful implementation of technology to support and improve patient care.

Background

The DFM is one of several academic departments within the College of Medicine at MUSC, a large, state-supported academic medical center. The medical center includes a large tertiary care hospital, a children's hospital, a psychiatric hospital, multiple outpatient clinics (including the Family

Medicine Center), and six academic colleges—Medicine, Nursing, Pharmacy, Dentistry, Graduate Studies, and Health Professions. As is the case with most university-based healthcare departments, the MUSC DFM has three major components to its mission—clinical service, education, and research. The clinical service activities of the DFM are provided through the Family Medicine Center (FMC), located on the MUSC campus. Approximately 125 patients are seen in the clinic each day. The educational activities of the department include a residency program with 38 family practice residents, a rotation for third-year medical students, a Doctor of Pharmacy residency program, and other health profession educational activities and rotations. The education and clinical components of the department's mission are closely linked because family practice residents provide care under the direction of designated faculty physicians to the majority of patients seen at the FMC. Major research efforts of the department include ongoing projects in preventive services and computer-based patient records.

Identifying the Need for a New Medical Record System

In 1972, just two years after it was established, the DFM developed one of the first computerized medical record systems in the United States. This early system was originally developed by a medical student who believed that "there must be a better way" to document patient care than the cumbersome paper charts. The early system was maintained on a series of minicomputers, which met the department's needs for more than a decade. However, with the availability of more sophisticated, less expensive technology by the late 1980s, it became evident that a new system would be needed.

There were actually several events that occurred that moved the decision to convert to a new CPR system to the forefront. The original computerized medical record system had been developed specifically for the FMC. Although quite innovative for its time, the system software was written in an outdated computer language, required several programmers and a full-time operator to run, and ran on an aging minicomputer. On top of the multiple equipment problems, there were personnel problems as well. In 1988, the system operator quit, followed by the last programmer. In September 1989, a major hurricane hit the East Coast of the United States and caused extensive damage to the FMC. The computer system, which was already showing signs of its age, began to show further signs of deterioration. In short, the system had become expensive and difficult for the department to maintain.

Finding a Replacement CPR System

As Dr. Steven Ornstein, Director of the DFM Research Division, likes to tell it, he became "in charge" of the computerized medical record system because "he could spell computer and his research associate, Ruth Jenkins, could turn it on." Jenkins had worked closely with the system operators and programmers for about six months, and once they had resigned, she was left as the person with the most knowledge about operating the system.

Both Ornstein and Jenkins were convinced that they could find an up-to-date, affordable CPR system for the department. Not only was the existing system unable to meet the growing needs of the department, it was increasingly expensive to maintain. The cost of maintaining the minicomputer and the salaries of the programmer and operator were in excess of $100,000 per year. An additional cost to the existing system was the fact that a duplicate paper record was maintained for every patient. The medical record department at the center had four full-time equivalents (FTEs) in the fall of 1989. These medical record personnel had some involvement with the computer system, but spent the majority of their time maintaining the parallel paper record system.

While attending an Academy of Family Medicine meeting in September1989, Ornstein and Jenkins had the opportunity to see several commercial CPR products that were displayed at the meeting by various vendors. They both felt that one of these systems might be exactly what the department needed. In the absence of any department clinical information system long-range plan, after his return from the meeting to MUSC, Ornstein approached the department chairperson for input. Although the chairperson was only mildly interested in computers, he recognized that finding an up-to-date CPR system was an important project for the department. He essentially delegated the responsibility of identifying a new system to the Research Division. Consequently, in December 1989, the staff of the Research Division began to investigate commercially available CPR systems as a possible option for replacing the existing computer system at the DFM.

During the investigation, one CPR system in particular captured the attention of the Research Division. Practice Partner™ software, developed and marketed by Physicians' Micro Systems, Inc., in Seattle, Washington, included the modules the department needed for medical records, medical transcription, and appointment scheduling. The medical record module included all of the features typically found in a patient record: problem lists, progress notes, vital signs, medical history, social history, family history, medication lists, immunizations, health maintenance, laboratory results, and a section for reports of ancillary studies. The software also included sophisticated search and data export functions.

Dealing with the University Procurement Process

As a state-funded institution, MUSC is bound by detailed rules and regulations governing procurement of capital equipment. Not only was internal approval through proper channels needed before any CPR system could be purchased, but a specific bidding process was also required. Problems were encountered with both processes. First, the internal approval was delayed. The university had just entered into an agreement with another larger computer company to be a beta test site for a clinical data repository system, with hopes that it would eventually serve as the basis for a computerized medical record for the entire medical center and all of its affiliated clinics. Some of the managers within the MUSC Center for Computing and Information Technology did not feel that the DFM should be pursuing the purchase of separate CPR given the large investment that was being made for the clinical data repository system. Ornstein, however, was adamant that the clinical data repository that the university was looking at would not meet the needs of the FMC. His reasons included the fact that the system was still in development and it was being designed for a large inpatient-setting, not ambulatory care. There were many meetings scheduled throughout most of 1990 to resolve the issues between the Center for Computing and Information Technology and the department. Eventually, the department was granted approval to pursue the purchase of a separate CPR.

The state capital equipment bidding procedure requires that an RFP be sent to all potential bidders for capital projects. After a lengthy process to develop the RFP for the proposed CPR system, four potential bidders responded. Of the four, two did not have any systems that were installed and one was a minicomputer-based system. Only Practice Partner™ had an established clientele and ran on microcomputers, so it was selected and, subsequently, purchased for the DFM. It was actually installed 18 months after the department's initial investigation into a replacement system, in April 1991.

Using the Software

Once Practice Partner™ was installed, the Research Division expected a smooth transition with few delays. A departmentwide network of microcomputers had been developed for use by the clinical and administrative areas of the FMC. Computer workstations were placed in each examination room in addition to the administrative and support areas. The administrative and clinical staff had all been trained on how to use the new system. However, there were still a few delays. Some support staff were reluctant to change over to the new appointment system. Likewise, some clinicians did not like having the workstations in the exam rooms and did not give up their practice of requesting a duplicate paper record. These problems led to more meetings, discussions, and, ultimately, to the decision to stop using paper records at the FMC altogether. As a result, clinical and support staff had to adjust to the CPR, and the medical record staff was eventually reduced from four FTEs to one and a half FTEs.

Today Practice Partner™ is well integrated into the daily operations of the Family Medicine Center. Support staff, physicians, pharmacists, and others use the system to document and track the care provided to patients. All prescriptions are generated at the computer workstation. In addition to the direct patient care functions, data from Practice Partner™ is used in ongoing quality improvement projects and other research endeavors.

Some information within the CPR comes from outside the DFM. Consultation reports, letters, and other paper documents are scanned into the system. However, other information is electronically transmitted. For example, Practice Partner™ has a limited interface with the MUSC laboratory. Batched lab values for Family Medicine patients are sent over from the MUSC laboratory information system each evening and subsequently downloaded into the CPR. Plans for an interface between Practice Partner™ and the MUSC Oacis™ system have been in place for some time, but to date the interface has not been accomplished. This interface would allow lab values, radiology exam results, discharge summaries and other reports stored in Oacis™ to be electronically transmitted into the CPR at Family Medicine.

In spite of the obvious successes associated with the installation of Practice Partner™, there is some evidence that the system may not be used to its fullest capacity. For example, the Windows-based version of the software has been released and installed throughout the clinic. However, some of the clinical and support staff are reluctant to make the change from the older DOS version because they feel they have not been adequately trained on the new version. Another indicator is that only about 20 percent of the documentation into the CPR is by direct entry by the care provider, in spite of the availability of disease-specific progress note templates. The majority of the documentation comes from notes that are transcribed into the system by data-entry clerks. Finally, as a part of a course, two graduate students from the College of Health Professions conducted a systems analysis for the DFM

Research Division that suggested that the system could be used more effectively. The students identified, among other things, the need for a full-time position to be responsible for CPR training, software support, and report writing. Currently, there is no one within the center to whom these responsibilities have been assigned. The department has a network administrator who is responsible for the maintenance of the department's network, including all of the hardware and software needs of the 120 plus microcomputers. His duties, however, are primarily technical in nature; he does not have a training or clinical background. As a result, many support and clinical staff report that they do not feel adequately trained to use all the system features.

Discussion Questions

1. Summarize and evaluate the overall CPR selection process used by the Department of Family Medicine at the Medical University of South Carolina.
2. What factors contributed to the lengthy selection and procurement process for the CPR system? Could some of these have been avoided? How?
3. Do you agree that this case represents a "successful implementation of technology to support patient care"? Why or why not?
4. Evaluate the role of each of the following individuals or groups in the development of the FMC CPR system. What role do you think he/she/they should have played? Discuss other individuals or groups that you think should have been involved in the process, as well.

   Steven Ornstein, MD, Director of the Research Division
   Ruth Jenkins, Research Associate
   Department of Family Medicine Chairperson
   MUSC Center for Computing and Information Technology

5. Consider the recommendations made to the department by the College of Health Professions students. Do you agree with their assessment? Can you identify other possible problems within the department that could be contributing to the CPR being underused?
6. Do you feel that you have enough information to evaluate the use of the CPR at Family Medicine? If not, what other information would you need?

MARKET CRISIS IN METROPOLIS: OPPORTUNITY FOR STRATEGIC ADVANTAGE THROUGH INFORMATION TECHNOLOGY

Kathy S. Lassila and Karen A. Wager

Overview

"In my 25 years in the healthcare industry, I have never seen such a major disruption in the marketplace," said chief executive officer Lee Simpson during a strategic planning session of the executive management team at Sunrise Health System. "With the marketplace in disarray, we have an opportunity to expand our market share while making sure our other provider and insurer alliances remain strong. We also have the opportunity to link the various information systems within our integrated delivery system in an effort to provide a true continuum of care and contain healthcare costs. By linking these systems, I think we will be able to capture a larger market share."

The disruption in the marketplace discussed by Simpson was the severing of a five-year relationship between Borealis Health Care (one of Sunrise Health System's key competitors) and Corporeal Care (the largest insurance company in the Metropolis region, Sunrise's service area). Sunrise Health System and Borealis Health Care are two of the three dominant integrated delivery systems in the Metropolis region. The third is Promise Health Systems.

The task currently confronting the executive management team is the formulation of an information technology strategy that will support Sunrise Health Systems' movement to expand their marketshare and allow them to gain competitive advantage in the Metropolis marketplace. Some of the challenges they are confronting include: a geographically dispersed set of affiliated insurers and independently owned hospital-physician organizations; widely disparate existing hospital and clinic information systems; lack of information technology expertise within the system; and a highly unpredictable marketplace.

Following a brief description of the Metropolis region healthcare marketplace and the major players, the challenges and opportunities for Sunrise Health System resulting from the breakup of Corporeal Care and Borealis Health Care will be discussed. The implications for Sunrise Health Systems' market expansion strategy in South Metropolis on information technology strategic planning will then be presented, followed by an overview of the potential role for community health information networks.

Market and Competitive Conditions

As the three largest regional provider systems, Sunrise, Borealis, and Promise have pursued different strategies and approaches to achieving their goals, although all three networks are committed to serving the community as best they can. They share the following goals: provide high-quality health care to patients, lower healthcare costs, and improve the overall efficiency and effectiveness of their systems, so that they can continue their mission of caring for patients. However, the networks have adopted very different strategies for achieving their goals and for gaining marketshare in today's cost-conscious managed care environment.

Borealis Health Care

Borealis Health Care is a tightly organized network with most of its hospitals and clinics under its ownership. Borealis leadership believes the way to reduce the nation's healthcare tab is to make people healthier. The corresponding strategy is expansion in the primary care arena through development of Borealis' primary and community clinic arm. Their long-term strategy focusing on care management is based on the belief that doctors and hospitals, not insurance companies, must manage the care for patients.

Promise Health Systems

Promise Health Systems' overall strategy is directed from it parent system, Barley Care Company, located in another state. Promise's key strategy is an integrated "A to Z" approach to the market, focusing on offering everything related to healthcare to employers and patients. As a result, Promise Health Systems recently became an insurance company when Barley Care formed a partnership with Total Health Plans, which allows Promise to sell a point-of-service insurance plan and HMO plan. They feel the new insurance offerings open up a section in "one-stop shopping" that has not previously been available. Industry critics, however, wonder whether Promise can successfully compete as both a healthcare provider and a managed care insurer.

Rather than owning all of its clinics and hospitals, Promise forms long-term relationships with providers to secure a geographic reach and achieve the integration it wants. Promise is currently focusing on growth, particularly in the outpatient area, since a large volume of patients means it can give deeper discounts because it can spread its costs over more patients. Executive management at Promise believes they can ensure high quality and low cost by making sure they have tight integration.

Sunrise Health Systems

Both Borealis Health Care and Promise Health Systems have centralized many of their services. In contrast, Sunrise Health Systems felt each of its hospitals were strong. Sunrise prefers to let each entity in its network remain under independent ownership, although it jointly makes decisions to hold down costs and improve healthcare. Sunrise Health Systems, like Borealis Health Care, also emphasizes collecting data to show physicians which methods have the best clinical results.

Unlike Promise Health Systems, Sunrise doesn't believe it should be an insurer. Executive management instead sees the need for strategic alliances between the physician and the insurer. As a result, Sunrise has formed hospital-physician organizations and teamed up with insurers. Simpson believes that these alliances will enable them to deliver good care at a good price. Overall, Sunrise Health Systems believes this means value for employers and patients.

Challenges and Opportunities

Each of the three integrated delivery systems is geographically defined by the locations of its major hospitals. Borealis Health Care owns the three largest hospitals in Southern Metropolis, while Promise Health Systems owns three major hospitals in Northwest Metropolis. Sunrise Health Systems owns two major hospitals in Northeast Metropolis. Each of the three hospital chains is supported by a group of clinics and affiliated doctors.

In Southern Metropolis, a neighborhood doctor most likely will refer patients to a Borealis hospital, in the Northeast to a Sunrise institution, and in the rest of the region to Promise. This is what makes the decision of Borealis and Corporeal Care to sever their relationship so traumatic. It leaves the Southern Metropolis customers and doctors without access to their largest neighborhood hospitals. This geographic concentration of hospital ownership is why most area health maintenance organizations (HMOs) have maintained relationships with all three hospital groups. The HMOs market to companies whose employees live all over the area. To offer the best service, they must be involved in hospitals everywhere.

The Borealis-Corporeal Care split has rewritten this marketing arrangement. To keep its customers in South Metropolis, Corporeal will have to convince them to go beyond downtown for hospital care, or they will leave Corporeal for another HMO with broader reach. In either event, Borealis, Promise, and Sunrise come out stronger than Corporeal Care. For Corporeal Care to survive, it must come to agreements with Promise and Sunrise. Their negotiating hand is made stronger because Borealis is out of the picture. In turn, Borealis' negotiating position with other HMOs is strengthened because it has demonstrated that anyone who wants to provide convenient service to South Metropolis will have to play on its terms. Of course the risk is that all HMOs will decide Borealis' terms are unacceptable, leaving South Metropolis without convenient healthcare and Borealis in trouble. Ultimately, the consumer, and to an extent independent doctors, are caught between the three integrated delivery systems.

The area's largest healthcare provider and its largest HMO company are steering patients away from each other. Enrollments during the first quarter of next year should indicate which will be hurt more by the split. Borealis will aggressively sell its own provider pool—Borealis Health Network—directly to large, self-insured companies, cutting out the middlemen. Borealis may even form alliances with other networks. It is clear to industry leaders and consultants that no single network is able to address the entire Metropolis area, and that two of the three existing networks could cover the Metropolis region providing Borealis is one of them.

In the meantime, Corporeal Care has lost the largest hospital-and-clinic system on the city's south side, which has a loyal citywide following, just as its contracts with Metropolis' two other large hospital-based systems, Promise Health System and Sunrise Health System are about to expire. With a 33 percent share of the market, Corporeal Care needs Promise and Sunrise hospitals and clinics like never before. Executive management at Corporeal Care believes they can negotiate better discounts from Sunrise and Promise because they can deliver to them an influx of patients from area facilities.

The termination of the relationship between Borealis and Corporeal clearly poses a significant challenge. It presents systems with an opportunity to aggressively market their services to the business community and to the existing Borealis patient base at a point in time when many of them can respond quickly to either maintain the Borealis relationship or move to one of the other integrated delivery systems. How those customers respond, and which company they turn to, will be seen in the next few years.

Borealis' split with Corporeal Care, the state's largest health plan was significant and generates opportunities for Sunrise Health System. The rift throws once-predictable choices for employers and workers into the air. What will happen all depends on the price the market will bear for healthcare. The Metropolis marketplace has refused to pay large increases in insurance premiums in the past several years. Increasingly, the marketplace is determining premium levels, and the premium levels are determining the payments to healthcare providers. This means hospitals and clinics with higher fee structures will find it more difficult to get additional money, unless a reputation for excellence enables them to charge a premium or they are big enough to command more.

Implications for Information Technology Strategic Planning

Sunrise Health System's Chief Information Officer Kate Lazar listened intently, if somewhat excitedly, during Simpson's discussion of the marketplace and review of the competitive situation in the Metropolis region. With 15 years of experience in healthcare information systems, the last five of which were with Sunrise, she knew information technology would figure prominently in the support plan for Sunrise's bid for market expansion in Southern Metropolis. She hoped that this sudden push to expand into another geographical area would have a dramatic impact on Sunrise's attempts to redesign their information systems for the managed care world by providing the catalyst for major investments in information technology.

Her attempts to develop a strong computer infrastructure to equip the already geographically dispersed integrated delivery system had been a slow and painstaking struggle for the past five years, with inadequate funding for capital expenditures on information technology architecture as the primary obstacle. Most integrated delivery systems spend 1 percent to 3 percent of their total budgets on information technology, while organizations in other industries spend from 15 percent to 20 percent. She knew that Sunrise Health Systems' current capital expenditures were well below that of both Borealis and Promise, and this was an opportunity to procure funding to move her plan for Sunrise's information systems into reality.

Lazar's ultimate objective is to connect the hospitals with primary care and specialty physicians, and with referral hospitals within the state to allow the geographically dispersed provider network to capture and route data electronically. Since Sunrise is a coalition of independently owned hospitals and clinics, the various organizations possess a wide range of information systems running multiple applications on widely disparate platforms. Most hospitals currently cannot access by computer the medical records of most of the specialty clinics in the professional buildings across the street. Over the past five years, Lazar had focused on the following priorities related to electronic linkage within the provider network, which improve flexibility and accessibility to information:

- standardized format for computerized patient records;
- optical-disk storage for patient medical and business records;
- client/server computing architecture and distributed infrastructures; and
- data warehousing and clinical repositories.

Overall, the task of creating a technical infrastructure for Sunrise was formidable. All of the components of the technical infrastructure needed to integrate easily, the infrastructure needed to have the ability to expand and grow, it had to accommodate continuous technological advances, it had to handle disparate operating systems, and the price-vs.-performance benefits had to be readily demonstrable.

In addition to these priorities, Lazar and her staff were working on identifying the appropriate interface engines and software switching hubs to translate data among incompatible systems and transmit data to/from various geographical locations—the next step in creating an information network for Sunrise Health Systems. One of the options available to Sunrise Health Systems is participation in the Metropolis Health Information Network (MHIN).

Potential Role of Community Health Information Networks

MHIN is a community health information network that functions as an electronic highway that provides seamless connectivity to all components of a healthcare region. It was originally started as a joint venture between a telecommunications company and Borealis Health Care approximately five years ago and forms the backbone of Borealis' information technology infrastructure. Participation in the network is available to all providers and healthcare-related entities in the Metropolis region.

MHIN consists of information provider interfaces, a central switching system, and a user interface. The information provider interfaces, located at each information provider site, translate data into a consistent format for transmission via MHIN. Information users, primarily physician office staff, typically use a modem and personal computer to dial up to the central MHIN switching system to access information from the information providers. All users access MHIN with user interface software that provides consistent presentation and display of information, regardless of the information's source. The user interface software is relatively simple and straightforward, and users require a modest amount of initial training in order to access MHIN.

MHIN currently supports a variety of patient clinical and business transactions including patient census, patient demographics, patient searches, medical records abstracts, medication orders, claims processing and submission, medical transcriptions, laboratory results/reports, radiology images/results/reports, electronic mail, and referral processing.

Security on the MHIN network is achieved at three levels: the information provider, the information user, and the network. The information provider (source of the information) authorizes who can access the data and which transactions can be accessed. He or she also passes along security levels required by in-house systems. User access is secured by user identification names and passwords. MHIN can also disable a disk drive or printer when unauthorized printing or saving of information is detected. Finally, all data and information transmitted over the network is encrypted as it travels electronically from source to destination.

The benefits of community health information network participation have been identified as:

- reduced administrative costs related to inefficient manual processes and duplicated efforts;
- enhanced quality of services controlled by ready access to patient information;
- reduced healthcare costs through reduced administrative work, streamlined payor/claims processes, and increased clinical efficiencies;
- improved quality of care through enhanced communication and co-ordination among care providers;
- optimized capital investment in information technology; and

- improved healthcare delivery in an increasingly competitive, capitated, and information-driven environment.

Although these benefits appear significant, little solid data are available on the actual quantifiable benefits accrued by information network participants. This is due in part to the fact that health information networks are a relatively new, emerging technology.

The Future

The characteristics and functionality of MHIN make it an attractive alternative for Sunrise Health Systems. However, the biggest stumbling block in MHIN participation has been cost justification. While the initial investment in MHIN participation depends on the state of current information systems throughout the integrated delivery system and the complexity of the corresponding information provider interfaces which must be developed, the ongoing costs of participation vary based on the number of transactions handled by the network on a monthly basis. Initial estimates indicate a startup cost of approximately $375,000 per hospital to develop an information provider interface to prepare data from disparate systems for transmission via MHIN, and an ongoing monthly fee of approximately $50,000 for average monthly transaction volumes.

In addition to MHIN participation as the backbone for the network infrastructure, Lazar has explored the option of building a proprietary information network for Sunrise Health Systems. Here the cost estimates were even more dramatic. For a six-hospital integrated delivery system, quotes ranged from $700,000–$2 million for year one to $6–$27 million for year six.

Karla Waggett, chief financial officer, acknowledged the need for increasing the level of investment in information technology at Sunrise Health Information Systems as she listened to Simpson's presentation. She had fought hard and succeeded in keeping the growth of information technology investment to 10 percent annually over the past five years. But given Sunrise's focus on expanding into Southern Metropolis and the need of the integrated delivery system to facilitate electronic access to geographically dispersed providers, it was obvious that the level of information technology investment would need to rise significantly.

Waggett's primary concern was over which alternative would be the best course of action. Costs were likely to be much higher and the implementation time frame was likely to exceed two years, outside the window of opportunity for penetrating the Southern Metropolis area, if Sunrise decided to build their own proprietary network. However, she also felt there were serious issues regarding participation in MHIN. The benefits of MHIN participation were predominantly anecdotal and exceedingly difficult to quantify. Few fully-functioning health information networks were operating at the time. Also, who would bear the cost of MHIN participation? Since Sunrise Health Systems' hospitals were not owned by Sunrise, the integrated delivery system could not dictate participation in the network. How could the various hospital-physician organizations be persuaded to participate and how would the effort be financed?

During the strategic planning session, Bernard Myers, chief operating officer, listened with a frown on his face. He knew Lazar was thinking that this was a prime opportunity to make a definitive move toward investing in the information network infrastructure. He also knew that Waggett could no longer oppose a major increase in information technology investments. Myers' biggest concern came from knowing that having the right technological infrastructure was only a small piece of the battle. Unless business processes and procedures were appropriately redesigned to take advantage of the features and functionality of the system, it was unlikely that Sunrise would receive the payback it expected to get from increasing investments in information infrastructure. Process redesign was a time-consuming, costly venture for any organization, but even more so with a disparate group of hospitals and clinics. Who would lead the effort, and who would ultimately be responsible for converting the investment in information technology to the desired benefit level?

Following Simpson's presentation on the current marketplace, the executive management team listened to Lazar's options for an information infrastructure to facilitate Sunrise Health Systems' expansion into the Southern Metropolis area. It was obvious they were confronted with a major decision that could significantly impact their ability to gain marketshare and achieve their strategic business goals.

Discussion Questions

1. What are the key factors to be considered in the decision to build a proprietary information network or participate in MHIN?
2. What, if any, is the risk to Sunrise Health Systems of participating in an information network initially formed as a joint venture by Borealis?
3. Why is the decision to participate in MHIN a strategic one?
4. How concerned should Sunrise be at this point with the cost benefit of the investment in an information network?
5. How will development of a proprietary information network or participation in MHIN help Sunrise achieve its goals/strategies?

GLOSSARY OF TECHNICAL TERMS

Address. The identifier for a storage location in the computer or for an input-output unit.

Addressable sectors. Sectors of a disk, organized on the basis of concentric tracks, with addresses consisting of track and sector identifiers.

Administrative information system. An information system that is designed to assist in the performance of administrative support activities in a health services organization, such as payroll accounting, accounts receivable, accounts payable, facility management, Intranets, and human resources management.

Algorithm. A step-by-step procedure for performing a task. Computer algorithms consist of logical and mathematical operations.

Analog signal. The representation of data by physical variation of some continuous variable such as temperature, pressure, rotation, voltage, speed, or electrical resistance. *See also* Digital signal.

Applications program. A program that performs tasks for the computer user. These programs may be developed by in-house programmers or purchased from vendors as "off-the-shelf," generalized programs.

Artificial Intelligence (AI). A discipline that attempts to simulate human problem-solving techniques in a computer environment. *See* Expert System.

Asynchronous transfer mode (ATM). A networking technology that switches small fixed-length cells containing data and transmits them at high speeds, and allows for voice, data, and video to be mixed and sent over networks.

Backbone. The fastest Internet links, which carry most of the electronic traffic. Until 1993 the National Science Foundation Network was the backbone for much of the Internet in the United States. Currently, a number of commercial providers act as the backbone; i.e. Sun Microsystems.

Bandwidth. A measure of the data-carrying capacity of a transmission medium. The higher the bandwidth the larger the volume of data that can be moved across networks.

Bar-code label. Precoded marks on a printed form or plastic card, which can be read automatically by specially designed computer input devices.

Bar-code reader. An input device that allows a computer user to scan a bar code label to input data to a central computer.

Baud rate. The number of data bits (in thousands) transmitted through a media per second.

Bedside terminal. A microcomputer-based terminal that allows nurses and other clinical staff to input and receive patient data at the bedside.

Bit. A binary digit (0 or 1) that is part of a data byte. Either seven or eight bits make up one byte.

Browser. A software application that provides graphical user interface (GUI) enabling the requesting and displaying of documents and other resources from the Internet.

Bus. A set of parallel signal connection lines that link the central processing unit (CPU) with primary memory and with input/output facilities. The parallel lines of a bus permit simultaneous transmission of the bits of a single byte.

Byte. The smallest addressable piece of information in a computer's memory consisting of seven or eight bits signifying a unit of data.

Cathode-ray tube (CRT). An electronic vacuum tube with a screen on which characters and graphic patterns may be displayed by control of a beam of electrons. A terminal with a display screen is commonly called a CRT.

CD-ROM. The use of the compact disk (CD) optical technology for mass storage of computer data on a read-only basis.

Cellular Digital Packet Data (CDPD). A network architecture that permits the transmission of data similar to cellular telephones except that the user is transmitting or receiving data rather then voice message.

Central processing unit (CPU). In a computer, the controlling and processing center that processes data, performs the actual calculations, and supervises and coordinates the various functional units of the system.

Client/Server Architecture. The front-end, or "client," part of the system consists of applications for the end-user such as word and data processing, and other interfaces. The back-end, or "server," part of the system contains the database management, printing, communication, and application programs.

Clinical Data Repository. A database that consists of information from various sources of care and from various departments and/or facilities. The database may represent a longitudinal description of an individual's care.

Clinical (or medical) information system. An information system that provides for the organized processing, storage, and retrieval of information to support patient care activities.

Closed system. A completely self-contained system that is not influenced by external events. *See also* Cybernetic system; Open system; System.

Coaxial Cable. A type of copper cable capable of transmitting high-speed digital signals and wide-bandwidth analog signals. It is fast, cost-effective, and easy to install, but subject to rust and corrosion.

Compiler. A computer program that translates instructions and subroutines written in a high-level programming language into language understood by the computer (machine language).

Computer programming. The process of coding a set of instructions or steps in a given data processing language that directs the computer and coordinates the operation of all hardware components.

Computer virus. A computer program that intentionally tries to alter applications programs, operating systems, and data files on a computer hard drive or floppy disk. Viruses may be intentionally or unintentionally transmitted from one computer to another by floppy disks, communication links, or downloading from the Internet.

CPU. *See* Central processing unit.

Critical path network. A tool used to define the interrelationships on a time scale for all events and activities that must be accomplished in order to complete a predetermined objective.

CRT. *See* Cathode-ray tube.

Cybernetic system. A self-regulating system that contains the following automatic control components: sensor, monitor, standards, and control unit. *See also* Closed system; Open system; System.

Cyberspace. A term used to describe the whole range of information resources available through computer networks. It is also used to describe a world in which computer and people coexist.

Data. Facts secured from empirical observations or research. Data in and of themselves often have little value and take on meaning only after sorting, tabulation, and processing into a more usable format.

Database. A series of records stored together, with each record consisting of a set of data fields.

Database Management System (DBMS). A collection of data carefully organized so as to be of value to the user. The software that is used to manipulate the database is commonly known as a database management system or DBMS.

Data Definition Language (DDL). A software language used to define and describe the data in a database.

Data dictionary. A file that contains the name, definition, and structure of all the data fields and elements in a database file.

Data field. One piece of information stored in a data record as part of a database.

Data Manipulation Language (DML). A software language used to access, edit, and extract information from the data contained in a database.

Data record. A series of individual fields stored together in a database. Each record in the file has the same number and type of fields.

Data Redundancy. A situation in which the same data item appears in several files, perhaps from multiple departments, of a healthcare organization's computer system.

Data Warehouse. A data warehouse enables the collection and organization of disparate data sources into an integrated subject-oriented view of the data to facilitate decision making.

Debugging. The process by which computer programs are tested and programming errors are identified and corrected.

Decision-support system (DSS). A system that supports an organization's ability to aid in management decision through data retrieval, modeling, and reporting of results to management.

Deterministic system. A system in which the component parts function according to completely predictable or definable relationships. Most mechanical systems are examples of this type of system.

Digital data. Data stored in binary digital (rather than analog) form using a representation of 1s and 0s.

Digital signal. The representation of data as a numerical series of discrete units. Digital signals in a computer system are represented in a binary coding system by the on or off (1 or 0) condition of the electronic switch. *See also* Analog signal.

Direct-access computer storage. Data files stored so that any data item can be accessed without the need for sequential searching. Also called *random access storage.*

Disk directory. A disk file used to list all the program files or data files stored currently on the disk.

Disk drive. A peripheral data storage device using a magnetically coated disk. The disk drive consists of a mechanism to provide rotation of the disk (spindle), a read-write head to establish and detect magnetic patterns on each disk surface being accessed, and a mechanism to position the head appropriately for access.

Distributed processing. A data processing system in which the workload is spread out through a network of computers that can be located in different organizational units.

Documentation. Written information about a computer program or system.

DOS. Disk operating system for IBM-compatible microcomputers. *See also* Operating system.

Dot matrix printer. A slow, low-quality, inexpensive computer printer that uses an impact process for printing.

DSS. *See* Decision-support system.

Dumb terminal. A device that can provide input to and display output from a central computer but that cannot perform any independent processing.

Electronic Mail (e-mail). The communication between one or more people, over computer networks, using text and file attachments.

Encryption. The scrambling of electronic transmission using mathematical formulas or algorithms in order to protect the confidentiality and security of communications.

Ethernet. A widely used local-area network (LAN) technology that permits the transmission of data at high speeds across computer networks.

Executive information system (EIS). A generalized data storage and retrieval system that is designed to provide management information to the top executives of an organization.

Expert System. A decision-support system that can reproduce the reasoning process that a human decision maker would go through in reaching a decision, diagnosing a problem, or suggesting a course of action. Components of expert systems include knowledge base; database; inference engine; a user interface, and workspace.

Fiber distributed data interchange (FDDI). A network consisting of two identical fiber optic rings connected to local-area networks and other computers.

Fiber-optic cable. A bundle of hundreds or thousands of tiny glass cables in which data may be transmitted as light pulses. Fiber optic cables can transmit light even when bent and are now taking the place of much larger copper cables.

Fiber-Optic Medium. Communication transmission media that use light pulses sent through a glass cable at high transmission rates with no electromagnetic interference.

File Transfer Protocol (FTP). Refers to a communication standard under which files are moved from one computer to another. Prior to Web browser technology,

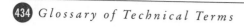

FTP was the only protocol available to receive/download or send/upload files from one Internet resource to another.

Firewall. Hardware and/or software that restricts traffic to and from a private network from the general public Internet network.

Floppy disk. A minidisk or thin, circular piece of round coated plastic used as one type of direct or random access computer memory. The original floppy disks were flexible. Today's disks are enclosed in hard shell cartridges.

Flowchart. The steps to be programmed and the sequence in which they are to be performed, displayed as a graph consisting of symbolic shapes, legends, and connecting flow lines,

Front-end processor. A small power processor, typically a minicomputer or microcomputer CPU, that can perform certain processing tasks to lighten the load of a mainframe or powerful minicomputer.

Gateways. Gateways represent the interface between two networks that use dissimilar protocols to communicate.

Gigabyte. One billion bytes. *See* Byte.

Hard disk. An external, random access storage device for a computer system.

Hardware. The physical components of a computer system.

Health Level-7 (HL7). An industry-based organization that establishes standards for the exchange of data among disparate systems within and across software vendors.

Hierarchical database. A database in which data is stored in nodes in a tree structure with the root node as the top node. Each node has one "parent" node and may have multiple "child" nodes.

High-level language. A computer programming language that is independent of the limitations of a specific computer and uses statements that resemble the problem being solved. *See also* Compiler; Interpreter.

Home Page. *See* Web Page.

Host. A computer to which other, smaller computers (nodes) in a network are connected and can communicate.

HTML (HyperText Markup Language). The software language that defines a format (fonts, graphics, hypertext links and other format details of Web pages) for creating documents for the World Wide Web.

HTTP (HyperText Transfer Protocol). The protocols used to deliver documents to a Web browser (Netscape or Microsoft Explorer) from a Web server.

Hub. A hardware device with multiple user ports to which computers and input/output devices can be attached.

HyperText. A method of presenting information on a Web site in which there are links to other documents. The HyperText "link" is the Universal Resource Locator (URL) for another Web page or other resources.

Indexed file. A file containing records accessible in sorted order according to one or more index fields. A separate sorted file or index contains records consisting only of the index field value(s) from the indexed file and one or more pointers to the location(s) of record(s) containing the value(s) in the indexed file.

Information. A meaningful aggregation of data or knowledge that can be evaluated for a specific use or set of uses.

Information Superhighway. An all-encompassing phrase that implies a communication infrastructure that will include the Internet, cable television networks, and telecommunication wireless networks.

Inkjet printer. A medium-speed, medium-quality computer printer that operates by spraying characters onto the page.

Input. Data fed into a computer system, either manually (such as through a keyboard or bar-code device) or automatically (such as in a bedside patient monitoring system).

Integrated system. A set of information systems or networks that can share common data files and can communicate among themselves.

Intelligent terminal. A terminal that has the capability of a microcomputer to process data independently of the main system.

Interactive system. A system that can provide nearly instantaneous responses to inquiries from a terminal because it has immediate access to all necessary data.

Internet. An open network of computer networks that permit people and computers to communicate and share applications through standard open protocols.

Internet Protocol (IP). An addressing scheme that identifies each machine on the Internet and is made up of four sets of numbers separated by "dots."

Interpreter. An interactive high-level language that analyzes source codes on a statement-by-statement basis.

Intranet. A private computer network contained within an organization that uses Internet software and transmission standards (TCP/IP).

ISDN (integrated services digital network). A network that uses a local telephone company branch exchange (PBX) to allow separate microcomputer workstations, terminals, and other network nodes to communicate with a central computer and with each other.

Java. An object-oriented software language, developed by Sun Microsystems, for writing Web applications. An individual application is call an "applet" and can be embedded within an HTML document.

Key. One or more fields of a record used in identification of that record.

Kilobytes (K or KB). Technically, storage medium capacity of 2 to the 10th power or 1,024 bytes. Informally, 1,000 bytes.

Knowledge Engineering. An analysis and design process by which the information components and decision-making processes of an individual are specified and modeled.

LAN. *See* Local-area network.

Laptop Computer. Powerful microcomputer that is characterized by its small size, light weight, portability, and range of capabilities.

Laser printer. A high-speed, high-quality computer printer that can function with several graphic formats and type-font options.

LCD Screen. An LCD, or liquid crystal display, is a thin lightweight computer screen generally associated with laptop computers and making use of flat panel technology.

Life cycle. The life cycle of software is the sequence of specification, design, implementation, and maintenance of computer programs. For models of computer hardware, the life cycle is the sequence in market status of development, announcement, availability, and obsolescence.

Light pen. An electronic, penlike device by which the user of a video computer terminal points to data displayed on a cathode-ray tube and retrieves that information or executes a command.

Local-area network (LAN). A computer network providing communication between computers and peripherals within an organization or group of organizations over a limited area. The network consists of the computers, peripherals, communication links, and interfacing hardware.

Magnetic disk storage. On-line or off-line data storage in which each data character is stored as a 0 or 1 in magnetic form. Magnetic storage includes hard and floppy disks, multiple disk packs, and reel-to-reel and cassette tapes.

Mainframe. This term is used to characterize relatively large computer systems, which normally have very large main memories, specialized support for high-speed processing, many ports for online terminals and communication links, and extensive auxiliary memory storage.

Master Patient Index (MPI). A relational database containing all of the identification numbers that have been assigned to a patient anywhere within a healthcare system. The MPI assigns a global identification number as an umbrella for all patient numbers, thus permitting queries that can find all appropriate data for a particular patient regardless of where that person is within the system.

Megabyte (M or MB). Technically, storage medium capacity of 2 to the 20th power or 1,048,576 bytes. Informally, 1 million bytes.

Menu. A list of options, displayed on a CRT screen, to allow the user to select the function to be performed or another, more specific menu. Programs operated through the use of menus are called *menu-driven*.

Microcomputer. A relatively small computer system, with the CPU, main memory, disk drives, CD-ROM, and interface cards and connectors installed in a small case or box.

Microprocessor. A microprocessor is the CPU chip, or semiconductor, component of a microcomputer.

Minicomputer. A computer possessing capabilities at a level somewhere between those of a microcomputer and those of a mainframe computer. Typically, they can support dozens or more than 200 terminal devices and may be linked together to share processing tasks.

MIPs. Millions of internal computer operations per second.

Modem. A term derived from MOdulator/DEModulator unit used to describe a data communication device that modulates and demodulates data between input/output devices and a data transmission link.

Multiplexing. The process of combining two or more signals into a single signal, transmitting it, and then sorting out the original signals. The devices that combine or sort out signals are called *multiplexers*.

Multipurpose Internet Mail Extension (MIME). Used in conjunction with SMTP (see below) to allow users to attach different file types to their e-mail messages (e.g., graphics, audio, and video).

Network. An interconnected collection of autonomous computer and peripheral devices. *See also* Local-area network; Wide-area network.

Network Computing (NC). The interface between computer devices (PCs and workstation) and networking devices which allow for the transparent access to: information; shared applications; and other computing devices by way of the network. In effect the network becomes the computer.

Network controller. An electronic device that automatically routes and controls the exchange of data among the nodes of a computer network.

Network interface card (NIC). A plug-in board used in microcomputers and workstations to allow them to communicate with a host computer and other nodes in a local-area network.

Object-Oriented Database. An information retrieval system that manages complex objects containing data and procedures for manipulating these data. Object-oriented databases are effective at storing complex objects such as documents and World Wide Web pages.

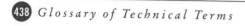

OCR. *See* Optical character reader scanner.

Open system. A system that exchanges energy, information, or material with its environment, thus, an open system has the capability of adjusting to the environment over time.

Operating system. A set of integrated subroutines and programs that control the operation of a computer and manage its resources.

Optical character reader (OCR) scanner. A hand-held or stationary full-page scanning device that can recognize different text character fonts and convert them into a word processing format.

Optical disk. A disk in which data is stored and/or retrieved nonmagnetically as 0s and 1s in pit areas (pits) and nonpit areas (lands) on a disk. A laser light beam distinguishes between pits and lands. Optical disk types include CD-ROM, Laser Video, and WORM. *See also* CD-ROM; WORM.

Optical scanner. A device that uses the scanning of light patterns to generate analog or digital signals in order to report marking patterns on a document such as a card, sheet, or label.

Output. Any data or information that a computer sends to a peripheral device or other network.

Packaged systems. Generalized computer systems, marketed by a number of commercial firms, that are designed to fulfill the information needs of any healthcare provider or organization.

Parallel processing. The use of multiple central processing units (CPUs) linked together generally for the purpose of more efficiently completing complex tasks.

PC. *See* Personal computer.

Peripheral. A device attached to a computer, such as a printer, CRT display, keyboard, disk drive, or tape drive, that transfers information to and from the computer.

Personal computer (PC). Name commonly used to refer to a microcomputer.

Point-to-Point Protocol (PPP). A TCP/IP protocol used with serial lines such as dial-up telephones. Similar to SLIP, but slightly faster and contains error checks.

Pointer. A field in a record containing the address of data or of another record.

Program. A set of instructions to the computer. Applications programs are ordinarily written in a high-level language and then translated into machine language instruction usable by the computer. Programs are also referred to as source codes.

Programming language. A software system used for writing computer programs. Used to translate functional requirements into computer commands. Examples include FORTRAN, C++, and SQL

Protocols. Rules and conventions for communication between computers.

Query language. A computer language that allows computer users to retrieve easily specific records from one or more database files.

RAM. *See* Random access memory.

Random access memory (RAM). Storage that permits access to the data stored at a particular address. It is affected by loss of power and is therefore also called *volatile memory*.

Read-only memory (ROM). Permanent instructions or files that cannot be altered by ordinary programming. It is not affected by loss of power and is therefore also called *nonvolatile memory*.

Real time. Performance of information processing within the constraints of interaction with physical processes, immediate human use, or another computer system. The results of a given transaction must be delivered in time to control a physical device, to capture data temporarily available, or to provide a response for a user waiting at a terminal.

Relational Database Model. This type of database stores data in individual files or tables with data items arranged in rows and columns. At least one data item (the key) is common in each table and is used to link two or more tables for ad hoc queries.

ROM. *See* Read-only memory.

Search Engine. Internet software applications that help to locate resources on the Internet, such as Yahoo, Achoo, and others.

Serial Line Internet Protocol (SLIP). A TCP/IP protocol for use over dial-up telephone lines. Allows a personal computer to connect to the Internet.

Simple Mail Transfer Protocol (SMTP). A TCP/IP protocol that defines how e-mail is exchanged between computers.

Software. The programs that control the operation of a computer, including applications programs, operating systems, programming languages, and productivity tools.

Source code. The form in which programs are entered for processing by a high-level language. *See* Program.

SQL. *See* Structured query language.

Structured query language (SQL). A standard, widely used database interface and query system based on the relational data base model. The intent was to permit users to specify queries with an English-like command structure involving a minimum of attention to the way in which the database was to be manipulated internally.

System. A network of parts or elements joined together to accomplish a specific

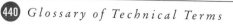

purpose or objective. Every system must include input, a conversion process, and output. *See also* Closed system; Cybernetic system; Open system.

Systems analysis. The process of collecting, organizing, and evaluating facts about information system requirements and about the environment in which the system will operate.

Tape drive. A tape recorder specially designed to work in a computer system for the recording, storage, and retrieval of data. Data stored on tape are accessible in sequential (not direct) fashion.

Telecommunications. Hardware and software that allow computers to communicate with other computers over data or phone lines or in local- or wide-area networks. Telecommunications hardware includes modems, multiplexers, and network interface cards. *See also* Modem; Multiplexing; Network interface card.

Telnet. A TCP/IP terminal emulation protocol that enables a user to logon to a remote computer and use its applications as if the user were directly connected to it.

TeraBytes. Used in computing to equal one trillion bytes or one million megabytes of stored information.

Terminal. A device consisting of a CRT unit that allows a computer user to perform processing on a host computer directly. Dumb terminals have no processing hardware of their own. Intelligent terminals have some hardware allowing some types of independent processing, such as data error checking and editing, graphics processing, and forms processing. *See also* Dumb terminal; Intelligent terminal.

Throughput time. The total time span from collection of the first data element to the preparation of the final report in a given system.

Transaction Processing Systems (TPS). Foundation or legacy systems that form the bulk of the day-to-day activities of an organization, such as financial, clinical, admissions, and business office systems.

Transmission Control Protocol/Internet Protocol (TCP/IP). A collection of data communication protocols used to connect a computer to the Internet. TCP/IP is the standard for all Internet communication.

Turnkey system. A computer system in which all the hardware and software are supplied by the same vendor and are ready to be used for a certain application without much in-house alteration.

UNIX. A multiuser operating system particularly useful for software development and known for the use of the shell utility as the primary interface for communication between the user and the system. The UNIX shell manages user/system dialogue.

Unshielded Twisted Pair (UTP). Similar to telephone cable, but with higher standards for protection against electromagnetic interference.

URL (Uniform Resources Locator). A standardized set of characters that identifies the location of an Internet document. For example: http://www.csun.edu/hs.html.

VDT. *See* Video display terminal.

Video display terminal (VDT). A computer input/output terminal that combines a keyboard and a cathode-ray tube. Video display terminals provide direct online access to computer files.

Virtual memory. A storage technique that permits the operating system to address more storage locations than are available in main memory. Disk storage is used to provide the additional memory and thus serves as an extension of main memory.

Voice recognition system. Digital systems that can store templates of utterances and later use this information to determine whether a particular person is speaking or to identify a word or phrase. Such technology can be used for data entry or for security purposes.

Web Page. A document, on either the Internet or an Intranet, written in HTML or Java that employs graphically oriented user interfaces and support hypertext links. A "home page" would be the first Web page of a particular site.

Wide-area network (WAN). A network in which long-distance lines allow computers and local-area networks to communicate.

Windows 95 and Windows NT. Operating systems that allow data from two or more programs to be displayed on a video display terminal at the same time. The use of graphical user interfaces supports a user-friendly environment and allows for multitasking of software applications.

Workstation. A microprocessor-based computer connected to a larger host computer in which some independent processing is performed. Workstations may or may not contain a hard drive (if not, they are called *diskless*) and typically have much better graphics capabilities than intelligent terminals.

World Wide Web (WWW). The "Web" is the software-enabling layer of the Internet that permits users to find and access resources on the Internet. The "Web" uses browser software technology, such as Netscape and Microsoft Explorer, to "surf" the net using HTML-based, hypertext-linked, Web pages.

WORM. An optical disk in which data may be written once but read as many times as needed (Write Once Read Many). *See also* Optical disk.

INDEX

Accrediting organizations, 12, 33, 98, 298, 323, 344

Address, in memory, 48, 51

Addressable sectors, 429

Administrative systems, 291–307
   applications, listed, *293*
   defined, 5, 18–19, 429
   for managed care, 348–52, *350–51*, 354
   and networks, 8, 386, 393

Agency for Health Care Policy and Research, 11

ALGOL language, *83*

Algorithms, 429
   and decision-support systems, *317*
   and information retrieval, 140, 155
   probabilistic, 278

Allina Health System (MN), 180

Ambulatory care systems, 13, 15, 19, 266, 273–74, 284
   See also Outpatient services

American Health Information Management Association (AHIMA), 189, 220

Analog signal, 115, 429

Appalachian Regional Healthcare (KY), 283

Appendix A, 233–39
   Patient Support Systems, Medical Univ. (SC), 233–39

Appendix B, 240–43
   Roper Care Alliance (SC), 240–43

Application software, 429
   general purpose, 94–99
   increase in, 7–8
   and operating systems, 91
   ownership of, 228

Application-specific software, 99–101, 109
   criteria for, 185, 220–22, *221*, 230
   evaluation of, 219–22
   and file dependence, 140–*41*
   for managed care organizations, 352–55, *353*
   for physicians practice management, 240–42
   and system development, 194, 196, 209–11
   turnkey products, 222, 224, 270, 292, 325, 440

Arithmetic/logic unit (ALU), 47, 48

Artificial intelligence (AI), 279, 316, *317*, 330, 429
ASCII files, 235–36
Assembly language, *81*, 89
Asynchronous transfer mode (ATM), 120, 122–23, 429
Audio, 154, 155
Aurora Health Care (WI), 365
Austin Regional Clinic, 125

Back-end functions. *See* Servers
Backup systems, 153–54, 182
  disk, 55
  emergency, 250, 376
  manual/paper, 409
  tape, *52*, 53
  utility programs for, 93
Bandwidth, 430
Bar code technology, 61, *62*, 270, 430
BASIC language, *83*, 84, *85*, 90, *243*
Batch mode, 110, 235
Baylor University Medical Center, 95
Beaches Clinic (FL), 401–12
Benchmarking, 322
Beth Israel Health Care System (NY), 273
Binary large objects (BLOBS), 154
Binary number system, 49, 80–82, 88, 115
Bit [binary digit], 49, 115, 430
Boston-area hospitals: and intranet, 392
Brigham and Women's Hospital (MA), 112
Browsers, 129, 376, 394, 397, 430
Bus network topology, *120*–21
Byte, defined, 49, 430
Byte magazine, 82

Cabrini Medical Center, 267
Capitation:
  and information systems, 188, 295, 299, 309
  and managed care, 340, 341–42, *345*, 346, *348*

and reimbursement, 9, 10–11, 19
Carpal tunnel syndrome, 59
Carrier Sense Multiple Access with Collision Detection (CSMA/CD), 120, 121
Cathode-ray tube (CRT), 430
CD-ROM drive, 54, *55*
Cellular Digital Packet Data (CDPD), 125–26, 430
Center for Health Services and Policy Research, 360
Central computers, *110*–11
  See also Mainframe computers
Central processing unit (CPU), 430
  and shared processing, 70
  and smart cards, 57
  subcomponents of, 44–48, *45*, *47*
  and time-slicing, 91–92
Character data, 49
Charleston Area Medical Center, 275
Chief information officer (CIO), 245, 251–*53*, 256, 257, 369, 387
Children's Hospital (PA), 123
Christ Hospital and Medical Center (IL), 387
City of Hope Medical Center (CA), 122, 267
Cleveland Health Quality Choice Coalition, 12
Client/server architecture, 111–14, 157, 172, 178, *243*, 254, 430
Clinical data repositories, 158–61, 431
  in case studies, 233–39, 405, 416
  and decision-support systems, *314*
  flowcharts for, *238*, *239*
Clinical pathways, 349
Clinical systems, 6, 284–85
  case study for, 413–18
  decision support (CDSS), 5–6, 277–80, 285
  defined, 5, 18, 431
  and physician order entry, 267–68
  and quality of care, 264

research and education in, 5–6,
283–84
and resource consumption, 160–61
See also Patient care systems
Closed system, defined, 29, 431
Coaxial cable, 115, 120, 431
COBOL language, *83*, 140
Coding, 15, 84, 188, 206, 266
Columbia/HCA Healthcare
Corporation, 129, 387, 391
Commercial Building Telecommu-
nications Cabling Standard,
115
Community environment, 5, 16, *32*,
35
See also Demographics
Community health information
networks (CHINs), *366*
development of, 16, 365
and integrated delivery systems,
16, 126, 361–64
Community Medical Network
Society (ComNet), 363, 364,
366
Compact disk (CD-ROM), 54–55,
56, 430
Competition, market, 419–27
and information systems, 5–6, 35,
188, 292, 319–*20*, *321*, 348
and strategic objectives, 16
Compilers, 89, 431
Complex instruction-set computing
(CISC), 49
Computer-aided systems/software
engineering (CASE), 89, 207,
210
Computer-assisted instruction
(CAI), 155–56, 283
Computer-based Patient Record
Institute (CPRI), 14
Computer files, 138–42, 235–36
Computer models:
and model manager, 313–*14*
for treatment costs, 16–17
"What-If," 314, 316, *317*, 326, 328

Computer networks. *See* Networks
Computers:
classes of, 68–73, 129
See also Hardware
Computer-supported cooperative
work (CSCW), 304
Computer virus, 153, 182, 431
Confidentiality, patient:
and computer-based records, *14*,
15, 152–53
legislation regarding, 375
and radio transmission, 117
See also Security, data
Consultants, 38, 173–74, 220, 228–29
Contractual services:
and decision-support systems,
311–*12*
and information resource
management, 179, 250
negotiations for, 226–27
selection of, 222–30, 254–56
for software development, 194,
196–97, 209–10
for transcription, 410
See also Request for Proposals
(RFP)
Control unit, computer, 47–48, 51
C or C++ language, *83*, 84–85, 87,
243
COSTAR record system, 84
Costs, healthcare, 10
administrative, *14*
component identification for, 36
containment of, 11–12, 14, 19, 264,
276, 355
and decision-support systems, 329
and healthcare reforms, 8, 9–10
and human resources, 297
and managed care, 344
Critical path network, 431
Customer satisfaction, 12, 15, 234,
320
Cybernetic systems:
components of, 30–*31*, *32*, *34*, *39*
defined, 23, 431

Cyberspace, 394, 431

Data, vs. information, *35*, 316
Data analysis, *200*, 202, 206–07, 210,
 318
Database management systems
 (DBMS), 137–62, 432
 and decision support systems, *314*,
  315, *317*, 331–33
Databases, 431
 analysis of, 206
 benefits of, 142–43
 clinical, 275, 279, 283
 design of, 218, 332
 distributed, 156–57, 178
 external, 318–*19*
 hierarchical model for, *144*–48, 434
 hypermedia databases, 155–56
 management, 155, 309, 313–*14*,
  315–18, 324–26
 and outcomes measurement,
  147–48, 160–61
 and spreadsheet software, 96
 and system implementation, 247
 See also Data warehouse; Relational
  database model
Data definition language (DDL),
 148–49, 150, 432
Data dictionary, 148, 151, 184, 432
Data entry, 58–65, *60*, 74, 110, 206
Data fields, 138–*39*, 432
Data manipulation language (DML),
 148, 149–51, 432
Data Processing Departments, 69,
 108–09, 311
Data redundancy, 140–42, 151, 170,
 432
Data warehouses, 14, 172, 178, 325,
 335, 432
Decentralized Hospital Computer
 Program (DHCP), 147–48
Decision-support systems (DSS), 31
 clinical, 5–6, 277–80, 371
 and databases, 155, 309, 313–*14*,
  315–18, 324–26

description of, 310–15, *313*, *314*,
 317, 334, 432
 strategic, 5–*6*, 309–35
Demographics:
 changes in, 13, 249, *320–21*
 and environmental information,
  5–6, 35, 318
 and managed care, 343, 345, *347*,
  351
 and profitability models, 311
Department of Veterans Affairs
 (VA), 147
Desktop publishing, 95–96
Diagnosis, computer-aided, 5, 47, 176
 See also Decision-support systems
  (DSS)
Digital signal, 115, 117, 432
Direct access storage devices
 (DASDs), 53, 432
Disk drive, 53, *54*, 432–33
Disk operating system (DOS),
 92–93, 433
Distributed processing, 112–*14*,
 156–57, 292, 433
Documentation, 151, 228, 247–49,
 248, 406, 433
DXplain decision-support system, 84

Education, computer-assisted, 285
 clinical, 5–*6*, 283–84
 hypermedia systems for, 155–56
 and intranet, 393
Egleston Children's Hospital (GA),
 14
Electronic data interchange (EDI),
 13–14, 123
Electronic mail. *See* E-mail
Electronic medical records
 (EMR). *See* Patient records,
  computerized
Electronic Numerical Integrator and
 Calculator (ENIAC), 46
E-mail, 433
 and integrated delivery systems, 16
 intranet, 392

and office automation, 304
organization policies for, 187
résumés sent by, 387
as unstructured text, 123
Emerson Hospital (MA), 376
Emory University System of Health
Care (GA), 126
Employers:
and CHINs, 16
information needs of, 355
and managed care, 9–10, 344,
345–46, *351*, 352
and outcomes information, 12–13
Encryption, 183, 187, 375, 394, 433
Ethernet, 118, 120, 123, 433
Exclusive provider arrangements
(EPAs), 9–10, 16, 345, 348
Executive information systems
(EIS), 5, 176, *317*, 331–33, 335,
433
Expert systems, 278, 316, *317*,
329–31, 335, 433

Facilities management systems, 5–6,
274, 298–300, 306
Fair Health Information Practices
Act, 375
Family Practice Clinics (SC), 274
Fiber-distributed data interchange
(FDDI), 120, 122, 123, 433
Fiber-optic technology, 116, 120,
121, 172, 267, 433
File/server architecture, 112, *113*, 178
Financial information systems,
293–96, 305
and clinical data repositories,
160–61
components of, 294–*95*, 393
and decision support, 13, 326–27
and integrated delivery systems,
188
and managed care, 346–*47*, 349
and Medicare, 292
Firewalls, 129, 153, 187, 375, 394,
395, 434

Flat-panel technology, 65–66
Floppy disk, 53–*54*, *55*, 434
Flow analysis, 207
Flowcharts, process, 434
for clinical data repository, *238*
information retrieval, *239*
and system development, 203–*04*,
218
Forté Version 1.1, 88
FORTRAN language, 82, *83*, *86*
Front-end processors, 70, 242, 434

General systems theory, 23–31
Geographic information systems
(GIS), 327, 343, *347*, 348, 351
Gigabytes, 53, 55, 434
Gigahertz, 125
Greater Rochester Health System
(GRHS), 369
Group Health Cooperative (WA),
392
Group Health Cooperative of Puget
Sound, 282
Groupware, 304

Handwriting recognition devices,
63–*64*
Hard disk, 53–*54*, *55*, 434
Hardware, 45–46, 434
acquisition of, 246
components of, 46–68, *47*, 73–74
and operating system, 91
testing, 247–*48*
Harvard Business Review, 175
Harvard Community Health Plan,
208
Health Care Cybervision project,
396–97
Healthcare environment:
changes in, 8–17, 19, 188, 249,
342–43, 353–54
factors in, *26*, 30, *34*, 294
feedback from, *26*, *29*
and system adaptability, 27, 29–30

Health Care Financing Administration (HCFA), 281–82, 387
Healthcare Informatics, 292
Healthcare Information and Management Systems Society (HIMSS), 18, 264, 342
Health Care Portability and Accountability Act, 375
Health Evaluation through Logical Processing (HELP) system, 279
Health information networks (HINs), 359–78
Health Level-7 (HL7) standard, 100, 159, 184–85, 233, 434
Health maintenance organizations (HMOs), 9
  financial forecasting for, 16
  information systems for, 17, *353*, 387
  and outcomes information, 12–13, 344–45
Health Plan Employer Data and Information Set (HEDIS), 13, 344–45, *351*, 352
Health services organizations:
  business goals of, 5, 37, 177, 369–70, *386*
  input/output patterns for, *28–29*
  management control in, 31–37, *32*, *34*
  and reorganizations, 15, 107–08, 188–89, 249, 273
  as system, 25–31, *26*, *28*, *32*
Henry Ford Health System (MI), 257
High-level languages, 82–86, 89–90, 436
Holy Cross Health System, 189
Home health systems, 282–83, 285, 328
Home page. *See* Web Page
Human resource information systems (HRIS), 5–6, 296–98, *297*, 305

Hypertext, 128, 155, 435
Hypertext markup language (HTML), 395, 434
Hypertext transfer protocol (HTTP), 434

Image processing, 47, 55, 85, 266, 271–73
Incentives, *32*, 33, 342, 343
Information, attributes of, *35–36*, 40, 316–17
Information resource management:
  outsourcing/contracting for, 179
  principles of, 36–37, 40
  and system implementation, 5, 194–95, 245–49
  See also Chief Information Officer
Information Services Department (IS):
  in case study, 404, 406–07
  functions of, 70, 119, 153–54
  staffing for, 179, 252–54, *253*, 258
Information systems:
  categories of, 5–6, 18–19
  centralized, *110*–11, 143, 177, 188
  decentralized, 8, 177, 178, 188, 269
  manual, 24–25, 247, 402–03, 407–08
  objectives for, *35–36*, 216, *217*, 234, *247–48*, 251
  operation and maintenance of, 195, 218, 228, 249–50, 254, 258
  trends in, 17, 170, 254
Information systems, costs of, 368
  analysis of, 36, 39, 207, 210, 218, 248
  and vendor products, 221–22, 226
Information systems, *See also* Master plan; Systems analysis
Infrastructure, technology, 171–72
  and system planning, 177–78, 368
  and telecommunications, 371–72
Inova (VA), 180
Inpatient services, 13, 15, 19, 299

Input devices, computer, *47*, 58–65,
  60, *62*, *64*
Institute of Medicine (IOM), 13–*14*,
  265–66, 284
Integrated delivery systems (IDS),
  361
  and clinical laboratory, 33–*34*, 270
  and continuum of care, 14, 265,
    275
  development of, 9, 10, 13, 14, 19,
    363
  and information systems, 180,
    187–89, 359–78
  and insurance products, 13, 16–17,
    19
  and interfaces, 172
Integrated information systems,
  359–78, 435
  for clinical/financial data, 160–61
  configurations for, 177–78, 190
  enterprisewide, 15–16, 126, 159–60
  vs. interfaced systems, 100–01, 177
  for minicomputers, 71
  See also Standardization, data
Integrated Services Digital Network
    (ISDN), 115, 127, 396, 435
Intellectual property, 186, 187
Interfaces, 113
  bridge, 117
  browsers, 129, 376, 394, 397, 430
  creation of, 196, 372
  gateway, 118, 233, 235–36, 434
  and system design, 177, 219, *243*
  translator, 160
Interfaces, user:
  command-based, 92–93
  and decision-support systems, *313*,
    314, 326, *330*
  friendly, *313*
  graphical (GUI), 92–93, 411
  interactive, 92
Intermountain Health Care System
    (UT), 17
Internet, 397, 435
  access to, 127–28

  and clinical databases, 283
  and data security, 186–87, 394
  and gateways, 118
  history of, 126, 384–85, 397
  organization policy for, 186
  and virus introduction, 153
Internet applications, 383–98
  benefits of, 394
  consumer information, 346, *351*,
    352
  implementation of, 396–97
  integrated delivery systems, 16,
    372
  negative aspects of, 394–95
  virtual data sharing, 373–74
  See also World Wide Web (WWW)
Interpreters, 89, 90, 435
Interviews, 199–200, *201*, 210
Intranets, 129, 384, 435
  applications of, 304–05, 391–93,
    392, 397–98
  benefits of, 376, 398
  negative aspects of, 186, 395–96

Job control language (JCL), 92
Joint Commission on Accreditation
    of Healthcare Organizations
    (JCAHO), 33, 98, 323
Jukebox, 56–*57*

Kilobytes (kb), defined, 49, 436

Laboratory systems, 33–*34*, 269–70
L. A. Care (CA), and Medi-Cal,
    354–55
Laptop computers, 73, 124–25, 283,
    436
Laser Cards, 57
Legal issues:
  and decision-support systems, 279
  electronic signatures, 409
  and integrated delivery systems,
    374–75
  mandated standards, 33
  paperless record systems, 266

and telemedicine, 281–82
vendor contracts, 227, 230, 256
Light pen, 61, 436
Linear programming, 322
Links. *See* Pointers
Liquid crystal display (LCD), 65–66, 436
Local-area networks (LANs), 109, 436
  and digital signals, 115
  and ethernet, 118, 120
  and fiber-optic transmission, 116, 120
  and file/server architecture, 112
  and network interface, 117
  and spread spectrum technology, 125
Long Beach Community Hospital and Medical Center, 386
Long-term care systems, 282–83, 285
Lowell General Hospital (MA), 395
Lutheran General Health Systems (IL), 257

Machine cycle, 48, 49
Machine language, 80–*81*, 88, 89
Magnetic cores, 49
Magnetic disk storage, 53, 436
Magnetic tape storage, 52, 69
Mainframe computers, 436
  and centralized processing, *110*–11, 118
  future of, 70–71
  history of, 6, *7*, 69–70, 91, 108–09
  operating systems for, 70, 92, 110
  utility programs for, 94
Managed care, 311, 341–42
  and capitation, 10–11, 342, 343–44, *347*, 348, *350*
  and cost accounting, 295, 346–*47*, *350*
  expansion of, 8–10, 17, 19, 98, 113
  and outpatient services, 15, 17, 342, *350*

Managed care information systems, 341–55
  administrative, 348–52, *350–51*, 354
  application software for, 352–55
  information needs of, 124, 148, 265, 311, 342–46
Managed care organizations (MCOs), 343, 348–52, *350–51*, 354–55
Managed Care Workstation (VA), 147–48
Management, executive:
  and decision-support systems, 309–35, *313*
  and system development, 172–74, *173*, 199, 255–56
Management control process, 31–36, *32*, *34*, 208
Management service organizations (MSOs), *347*, *353*
Manuals, instruction. *See* Documentation
Marketing strategies, 5–*6*, 320–*21*, 327, 387–91
Marshfield Medical Center (WI), 376
Massey, Calvin, 354
Master patient index (MPI), 158–59, 176, 178, 189, 266, 370, 436
Master plan, system, 169, 172–76, *175*, 189, 255–56
Materials management systems, 5–*6*, 36, 300–02, 306
Mayo Clinic (FL), 129, 329
Medicaid, 281–82, 345, *350*, 354
Medical University of South Carolina (MUSC), 233–39, 413–18
Medicare, *350*
  and HMOs, 354
  and patient care, 275, 281
  and preadmission information, 299
  and prospective payment systems, 292, 312
MEDLINE clinical database, 275, 283

Megabyte (mb), defined, 49, 436–37
Memory, computer, 48–51, *50*, 54, 55, 80
Methodist Hospital (IN), 125
Meyers, Kim Charles, 267
Microcomputers, 72–73, 437
 backup systems for, 153
 and desktop publishing, 95
 as network controllers, 118
 operating systems for, 92
 and shared processing, 70
Minicomputers, 437
 in health services organizations, 109, 414–15
 in networks, 112, *114*, 118
 operating systems for, 92
 and shared processing, 70, 71
Minneapolis Veterans Administration Medical Center, 270
Mnemonics, 81–82
Modems, 117, 127, 235, 437
Modern Healthcare, 17, 264–65
Mouse, 59, 93
Multimedia, 155, 266
Multiplexers, 117, *118*, 437
Multipurpose Internet mail extension (MIME), 437
Multisourcing, 254
Multitasking, 65, 91, 343
MUMPS [M] language, *83*, 84, *243*

National Academy of Science, Institute of Medicine, 13–*14*, 265–66, 284
National Committee on Quality Assurance (NCQA), 13, 344
National Information Infrastructure (NII), 364
Natural languages, *81*, 88, 149–50
Nelson, Stan, 257
Network architecture configurations, 190
 in case studies, 241, 354
 central mainframe architecture, *110*–11, *114*, 118

client/server architecture, 111–14, 157, 172, 178, 430
distributed processing architecture, 112–*14*, 156–57, 433
file/server architecture, 112, *113*
Network computers (NC), 129, 437
Network controllers, *110*, 118, 437
Network database model, 144–46, *145*
Network interface cards (NICs), 117, 437
Networks, 107–31
 benefits of, 107
 components of, 114–19, 130
 defined, 109, 437
 and electronic data exchange, 6, 8, 188, 266, 360
 and groupware, 304
 internal decentralized, 8, 177, 178, 188, 269
 national, 6, 13–14, 284, 285, 364
 processing function for, 109–10
 topologies for, 119–23, *120*, 177
 and wireless communications, 124–26
 See also Health information networks; Intranets
Niche strategies, *320*, 369
Nursing:
 management level, 327, 329
 and patient care, 124, 275–77, 284–85
 and staffing schedules, 298

Oacis Healthcare Network, 267
Object code, 89–91
Objectives, organizational:
 and market competition, 16
 and system planning, 174–76, *175*, 368
Object-oriented technology, 89, 154–55, 326, 371, 437
Office automation systems, 5–6, 94–95, 303–05, 306

Open systems, 29, 186, 371, 438
Operating systems, 91–93, 101, 438
  for networks, 118–19, 185
Optical jukebox storage system,
  56–57
Optical technologies:
  cards, 57–58
  disks, 54, 56–57, 172, 438
  imaging systems, 405, 411
  mark readers, 61
  scanners, 62–63, 410, 438
Optimization models, 316, *317*, 322
Organizations, professional, 17–18,
  189
"Oryx," 323
Outcomes measurement:
  and cost containment, 11–12, 14,
    19
  and databases, 147–48, 160–61
  and decision-support systems, 5–6,
    13, 16, 279
  information needs for, 322–23, *324*
  and managed care, 12–13, 344–45,
    351
  and patient care systems, 15,
    147–48, 268, 284
  and patient satisfaction, 12, 15,
    234, 320
  and quality improvement, 11–13,
    19
Outpatient services, 15, 17, 299–300,
  342, *350*
  See also Ambulatory care systems
Output devices, *47*, 65–68, 74
Outsourcing, 254–55, 258
  See also Contractual services

PacifiCare Health Systems (CA), 387
Packaged systems. *See* Application
  software
Parallel system testing, 249, 409–11
Park Nicollet Medical Center (MN),
  15
Pascal language, *83, 86*
Patient care continuum, 14, 265, 275

Patient care systems, *28*
  ambulatory care, 13, 15, 19, 266,
    273–74, 284
  and automated instrumentation,
    5–6, 72, *280–81*, 285
  and bedside terminals, 276, 430
  and "care maps," 275, 349
  and nursing information, 124,
    275–77, 284–85
  and outcomes information, 11–12,
    15, 147–48, 268, 284
  and physician order entry, 268, 284
  and preventative care, 15, 274–75,
    342, 391
  and telemedicine, 273, 281, 285
Patient records, computerized
  (CPRs), 5, *6*
  access to, 152–53, 234
  case studies for, 267, 401–18
  development of, 13–15, 19, 265–66,
    284, 363, 401–12
  functions of, *14*, 265
  and hypermedia databases, 155
  See also Master Patient Index
Patient Support Systems (SC), 233*n*
Pen-based computers, 63–*64*
Performance:
  analysis of, *350*
  employee, 296, 297
  monitoring for, 188, 250
  planned controls for, 33–*34*, 36
  standards for, 32, 208, 323
  See also Productivity
Personal computers (PC), 8, 39, 91,
  109, 112–*14*, 438
Personnel:
  changes in, *32, 34*
  and fear of change, 37–38
  for Information Services (IS), 179,
    252–54, *253*
  recruitment of, 298, 387
  as resource, 31–*32*, 33–*34*
  as system users, 181, 251, 266
  technical, 195, 196, 216, *253*
  See also Training

Pharmacy systems, 124, 270–71, 278–79

Physician-hospital organizations (PHOs), 10

Physician office systems, *272*
  See also Practice management systems

Picture archiving and communication system (PACS), 55–56, 272–73, 284

Pixels, 63, 65

PL/1 language, *83–84*

Pointers, 144, 145, 155, 440

Pointing devices, 59

Point-of-care systems, 276–77

Portable computers, 73, 124–25

Practice management systems, 240–43, 266, *272*, 273–74

Preferred provider organizations (PPOs), 9, 17, 345, 346, 348, *353*

Preventive care, 15, 274–75, 342, 391

PrimaCare Hospital (FL), 401–12

Primary storage, 47–51

Printers, 66–68

Probabilistic systems, 27

Productivity, 13–*14*, *32*, 295, 322, 407
  See also Performance

Profitability, 17, 311, 351–52

Program-generating software, *81*, 89–90

Programming, computer, 6, 431
  in-house, 194, 209, 210, 216, 218, 246, *253–54*

Programming languages, 438–39
  and data extraction, 140, 324
  evolution of, 80–89, *81*, 101

Programs. *See* Software

ProMedica Health System (OH), 123

Protocols, clinical, *32*, *34*, 264, 275, 371

Protocols, communication, 118, 119, 120, *243*, 439

Providers:
  and expert systems, 330–31

information needs of, 346–48, *347*, 355, 386

and integrated delivery system, 6, 13, 16, 274

Quality improvement:
  and information systems, *14*, 195, 265, 273
  and Total Quality Management (TQM), 250–51

Quality of care, 8
  and clinical systems, 264
  and managed care, 344–45, 355
  and nursing systems, 276–77
  and outcomes measurement, 11–13
  planned controls for, *32–33*

Query-by-example, *150*

Query language, 149–51, 155, 439

Questionnaires, *200–02*, 210, 318

Radiology systems, 72, 271–73

Radio transmission, 116

Random access memory (RAM), 51, 439

Read-only memory (ROM), 50–51, 80, 439

Real-time processing, 110, 125

Receivers, *115*, 117–18

Records, 138–40, *139*, 432

Reduced instruction-set computing (RISC), 49, *243*

Reengineering, process, 177, 207–08, 322

Reimbursement, 9, 10–12, 281–82, 292

Relational database model:
  and decision-support systems, 315, 324, 329
  description of, 145–48, *146*, 439
  and groupware, 304
  and system development, 172, *243*

Remote job entry (RJE), 110

Report cards, 12–13, 19, 344, 345

Report preparation:
  and managed care, 349

and report writers, 315, *317*, 327, 334

Request for Information (RFI), 216, 219, 223, 226

Request for Proposals (RFP), 223–26
in case studies, 354, 404, 416
and system design process, 209, 216, 219, 230

Research:
and clinical information systems, 5–6, 283–84, 285
and computerized patient records, 13–*14*, 152–53, 157, 158
and intellectual property, 186, 187

Resource allocation systems, 6, 155, 321–22, 328

Ring network topology, *120*, 121

Rollerball, 59–*60*

Roper Care Alliance (SC), 240*n*–43

Rush Presbyterian/St. Luke's Medical Center (IL), 393

Samaritan Health System (AZ), 376

Satellite transmission, 116, 270

Scanning devices, 61–63, 408, 410

Scheduling systems, 298–300, 305–06

Secondary storage, 51–58, 80, 138, 148, 153–54

Security, data, 161–62
executive role in, 256
and human resource system, 297
and Internet, 186–87, 394
mechanisms for, 143, 149, *182*–83
and system development, 177, 181–83, 218
and virus protection, 153, 182
See also Confidentiality; Firewalls

Semiconductors, 49

Sequential access computer storage, 51, 52–53, 138–39

Serial line Internet protocol (SLIP), 439

Servers, *111*–12, *113*, 118, 129, 235–36, 267

Sharp Healthcare (CA), 180

Shielded twisted pair (STP) cable, 115, 120

Silicon chips, 49, *50*

Simple mail transfer protocol (SMTP), 439

Simulation programs, 72, 283–84, 285

Smart cards, 57–58

Software, 80, 101, 439
antivirus, 153, 182, 375
code generation, *81*, 89–90
decision support, 16, 319
language translation, 89–91
network control, 118–19
oversight of, 185–86
and programming languages, 80–89, *81*, 101, 140
system management, 91–94
testing of, 247–*48*
See also Application software

Software development, 254
and contractual services, 194, 196–97, 209–10
for decision support systems, 323–24
object oriented, 89
resources for, 178–81, 219–20

Source code, 89–90, 228, 439

Spreadsheets, 65, 88, 95–96, 311, 326

Spread spectrum technology, 125

Standardization, data:
and data definition, 15, 181, 188, 372
and data dictionary, 151
and system centralization, 143
and system integration, 158, 159–60, 184–85, 371

Star network topology, *120*, 121–22

Statistical analysis, 47, 71, 96–98, 202, 314

Statistical packages, 97–98, *317*

Steering committees, 189–90
in case study, 404–09
and system design, 181–82, 185
and system planning, 169, 172–74, 176–77

St. John's Regional Medical Center, 298

St. Joseph Hospital (CO), 125

Strategic decision-support systems, 309–35
  and decision process, 311–*12*
  defined, 5–*6*, 19
  development of, 19, 323, *325*, 333
  and executive systems, 5, 176, *317*, 331–33, 335, 433
  and financial modeling, *6*, 13, 326–27
  and outcomes measurement, 5–6, 13, 16, 322–23
  and performance, 5–*6*, 322
  for planning and marketing, 5–6, 319–*20*, *321*, 327
  and resource allocation, *6*, 155, 321–22, 328
  and risk analysis, 13, 16, 188
  See also Decision-support systems

Structured query language (SQL), 88, 150–51, 326, 439–40

Stuyvesant Polyclinic (NY), 267

Supercomputers, 69, 385, 397

Support services, *28*, 242

Syntax, 80, 90

Systematized Nomenclature of Human and Veterinary Medicine (SNOMED), 160

System design, 229–30
  alternative approaches to, 209–10, 211, 216
  and application software, 194, 241
  case study for, 233–39
  executive role in, 256, 333
  outsourcing/contracting for, 194, 196–97, 222–29
  specifications for, *217*, 234–36, 257

System evaluation, 195, 250–51, 257, 377

System implementation, 5, 194–95
  and data exceptions/errors, 248, 249, 251
  steps in, 245–49, *246*, 257–58

System planning, 37
  consultants and, 173–74
  and end-user computing, 180–81, 190, 266
  for integrated delivery systems, 170, 180, 187–89, 368
  operating budget for, 172, 179–80
  organization of, 172–76, *173*
  purposes of, 170–72, *171*
  resource allocation in, 172, 176–77
  and technology infrastructure, 177–78, 368
  See also Master plan

Systems, 23–25, 39, 440

Systems analysis, 193–211
  benefits of, 208–09
  data collection for, 199–207, 210
  and decision support systems, 333
  defined, 24, 194, 198, 211, 440
  and process reengineering, 207–08
  and project organization, 195, *196*
  steps in, *198*–99, 208
  and systems development life cycle, 193–95, *194*, 210–11, 245
  tools for, 199–207, *200*

System testing, 247–49, *248*, 257–58

Tape drive, 51, *52*–53, 138–39, 440

Teamwork:
  computer-supported, 304
  and information systems projects, 5, 196–97, 211, 256

Technical systems specialists, 5, 249–50, *253*–54

Telecommunications, 107–31, 440
  cabling standards for, 115–16
  and networks, 268, 371–72
  technical staff for, 253
  and teleconferencing, 304, 393

Telemedicine, 273, 281, 285, *366*, 372

Terminals, 65, 440, 441
  bedside, 276, 430
  dumb, 70, *110*–11, 129, 433
  intelligent, 435

in networks, *110*, 118
Throughput time, 125, 440
Token ring protocol, 121
Total Quality Management (TQM), 250–51
Touch screen, 60
Training, personnel:
  in case study, 406–07
  as corrective action, *32, 34*
  and human resource systems, 296
  in implementation process, 194, 246–47, 257, 268
  vendor role in, 218, 225, 228, 247
Transaction audits, 154, 183
Transaction processing systems (TPS), 294, 317–18, 325, 346, 440
Transmission control protocol/Internet protocol (TCP/IP), 127, 129, *243*, 397, 440
Transmission media, *115*–18, 120
Treatment planning, computer-aided, 5, 16–17, 264, 278
Tree structures, *144*
Turnkey products, 222, 224, 270, 292, 325, 440

Ummel, Stephen L., 257
Uniform resources locator (URL), 128, 441
United Health Care (AZ), 391
University of Rochester Medical Center (NY), 274
University of Wisconsin Hospitals and Clinics, 296
UNIX operating system, 85, *243*, 440–41
Unshielded twisted pair (UTP) cable, 115, 120, 441
Utility programs, 93–94
Utilization, facility, 298–99
Utilization, service:
  analysis of, 148, 311, *347*, 349, *350*
  and demand fluctuation, 27
  and population-based data, 15, 35

Vendors:
  in case study, 240
  CSC Healthcare Systems, 354
  and decision-support packages, 324–25
  and Internet technologies, 387, 394
  MEDSTAT Group, 319
  network management by, 373
  Physicians' Micro Systems: Inc., 415
  resource guides for, 267, 292, *293*
  Sachs Group, 319
  selection of, 352–53
  as software source, 179–80, 181, 219–21, *220*
Video, 154, 155, 266
Video conferencing, 304
Video display terminal (VDT), 65, 441
Visual displays, 65–66
Voice recognition systems, 64–65, 88, 150, 441
Voice synthesis, 68

Web pages, 128, 155, 186, 385, 395, 441
Wide-area networks (WANs), 109, 119, 125–26, 430, 441
Windows 95, 92, 93, 441
Windows NT, 93, 119, *243*, 441
Word length, CPU, 48–49
Word processors, 94–95
Workstations, 71–72, *111, 113*, 124, 153, 172, 441
World Wide Web (WWW), 384, 441
  access to, 127–28
  and software vendors, *220*
  See also Browsers; Internet; Web pages
WORM memory, 54, 55, 441
WYSIWYG display, 96

Zip files, 235

ABOUT THE AUTHORS

Charles J. Austin, Ph.D., is Professor in the Department of Health Administration and Policy in the College of Health Professions at the Medical University of South Carolina. He previously served as Professor and Chair of the Department of Health Services Administration at the University of Alabama at Birmingham. He has served in numerous academic leadership positions, including President of East Texas State University, Vice President for Academic Affairs at Georgia Southern University, and Dean of Graduate Studies at Trinity University in San Antonio, Texas.

Dr. Austin has served on the health administration faculties of the University of Colorado, Xavier University, Trinity University, the University of Alabama at Birmingham, and the Medical University of South Carolina. His nonuniversity experience includes service as Chief of the Information Systems Division of the National Library of Medicine and systems analyst for the Procter and Gamble Company.

He has served as Chairman of the Board of the Association of University Programs in Health Administration, Chairman of the Accrediting Commission on Education for Health Services Administration, Chairman of the Editorial Board of the *Journal of Health Administration Education*, and Chairman of the Higher Education Committee of the American College of Healthcare Executives. He is the author or coauthor of five books and numerous articles published in professional and scholarly journals.

Dr. Austin holds a B.S. degree (summa cum laude) from Xavier University, an M.S. in health administration from the University of Colorado, and a Ph.D. from the University of Cincinnati.

Stuart B. Boxerman, D.Sc., is Associate Professor and Deputy Director of the Health Administration Program at Washington University School of Medicine, St. Louis, Missouri. He teaches courses in statistics, quantitative methods, and health information systems. He also holds an appointment in the University's Masters Program in Information Management and has held an academic appointment in computer science at a graduate engineering center of a state university.

In addition to his academic experience, Dr. Boxerman has gained industrial experience in computing and information system technology with a defense contractor, an electric utility, and an architectural firm. This experience has included analyses to determine system needs, systems design, programming, and presentation of "in-house" seminars on computer fundamentals and specific programming languages. Current research activities include the quantification of the value of information, specific benefits derived from using decision-support systems in health-care settings, and the application of electronic medical record systems in ambulatory care facilities.

Dr. Boxerman has been active in task forces and faculty forums sponsored by the Association of University Programs in Health Administration, including the Quantitative Methods Task Force, the Information Management Faculty Forum, and the Curriculum Development Task Force for Information Management. He currently serves as the editor of the *Journal of Health Administration Education* and has written numerous articles published in professional and scholarly journals. He is a Diplomate of the American College of Healthcare Executives and a member of the Healthcare Information and Management Systems Society, the Institute for Operations Research and the Management Sciences, and the Association for Health Services Research.

Dr. Boxerman holds B.S. and M.S. degrees in electrical engineering and a D.Sc. in applied mathematics and computer science, all from Washington University, St. Louis.

Brian T. Malec, Ph.D., is Professor of Health Administration in the Department of Health Sciences at California State University, Northridge. He also served as Chair of the Department of Health Sciences. Dr. Malec was a professor of health administration at Governor's State University for sixteen years and served in several academic positions there.

Dr. Malec has published in the area of health administration education and is a frequent presenter at national and international conferences. He was coeditor, along with Charles Austin, of a special issue of the *Journal of Health Administration Education*.

Dr. Malec is Chair of the Faculty Forum on Information Management for the Association of University Programs in Health Administration. He has been active in the American College of Healthcare Executives as a Faculty Fellow and as a member of the Regents Council for the Los Angeles Chapter of ACHE. He is a member of the Healthcare Information Management and Systems Society and the American Economics Association.

Dr. Malec holds a B.S. in education and a M.A. in economics, both from Northern Illinois University, and a Ph.D. in economics from Syracuse University.

Karen A. Wager is Assistant Professor and Director of the Master in Health Sciences–Health Information Administration Program (MHS–HIA) at the Medical University of South Carolina. She has over 15 years of experience in the health information administration field. As program director of the MHS–HIA, Ms. Wager also teaches graduate courses in health information systems and systems analysis and design. Her research interests include computer-based patient records in primary care, building health information networks to support integrated delivery systems, and the use of the Internet in healthcare.

Ms. Wager holds a B.S. in health record administration from the University of Pittsburgh and an M.H.S. degree in health information administration from the Medical University of South Carolina. She is currently a candidate for the Doctor of Business Administration degree in Information Systems from the University of Sarasota.